Disorders of Feeding and Swallowing in Infants and Children

PATHOPHYSIOLOGY, DIAGNOSIS, AND TREATMENT

Disorders of Feeding and Swallowing in Infants and Children

PATHOPHYSIOLOGY, DIAGNOSIS, AND TREATMENT

Edited by

David N. Tuchman, M.D.
Rhonda S. Walter, M.D.

SINGULAR PUBLISHING GROUP, INC.
SAN DIEGO, CALIFORNIA

Published by Singular Publishing Group, Inc.
4284 41st Street
San Diego, California 92105-1197

Typeset in 10½/12 Palatino by CFW Graphics
Printed in the United States of America by McNaughton & Gunn

Library of Congress Cataloging-in-Publication Data

Disorders of feeding and swallowing in infants and children :
  pathophysiology, diagnosis, and treatment / edited by David N.
Tuchman and Rhonda S. Walter.
      p.   cm.
  Includes bibliographical references and index.
  ISBN 1-56593-092-4
  1. Deglutition disorders in children.   2. Ingestion disorders in
children.   I. Tuchman, David N.   Walter, Rhonda S.
  [DNLM: 1. Deglutition Disorders—in infancy & childhood.
2. Feeding behavior—in infancy & childhood.   WI 250 D61106 1993]
RJ463.I54D58   1993
618.92′31—dc20
DNLM/DLC
for Library of Congress   93-19636
                                                                      CIP

Contents

Contributors

Roberta L. Babbitt, Ph.D.
Director Pediatric Feeding Disorders
  Program
Director, Outpatient Behavioral
  Disorders Clinic
Kennedy Krieger Institute
Assistant Professor
Department of Psychiatry and
  Behavioral Sciences
The Johns Hopkins University School
  of Medicine

Jane Benson, M.D.
Assistant Professor of Radiology
Johns Hopkins University
Department of Radiology
Johns Hopkins Hospital
Baltimore, Maryland

John L. Carroll, M.D.
Assistant Professor of Pediatrics
Eudowood Division of Pediatric
  Respiratory Sciences
The Johns Hopkins University School
  of Medicine
Baltimore, Maryland

David A. Coe, M.A.
Research Specialist
The Kennedy Krieger Institute
Baltimore, Maryland

Theodore A. Hoch, Ed.D.
Assistant Director, Pediatric Feeding
  Disorders Program
Kennedy Krieger Institute
Instructor, Department of Psychiatry
  and Behavioral Sciences
The Johns Hopkins University School
  of Medicine

Rebecca N. Ichord, M.D.
Clinical Instructor
Department of Pediatric Neurology
Johns Hopkins Hospital
Baltimore, Maryland

Maureen A. Lefton-Greif, Ph.D., CCC-Sp
Department of Otolaryngology Head
  and Neck Surgery
Division of Audiology and Speech
  Language Pathology
Johns Hopkins Medical Institutions
Baltimore, Maryland

Susanna A. McColley, M.D.
Assistant Professor of Pediatrics
Eudowood Division of Pediatric
  Respiratory Sciences
The Johns Hopkins University School
  of Medicine
Staff Pulmonologist
Mount Washington Pediatric Hospital
Baltimore, Maryland

Linda Miller Schuberth, M.A. OTR/L
Senior Occupational Therapist
Pediatric Feeding and Swallowing
  Disorders Clinic
The Kennedy Krieger Institute
Baltimore, Maryland

David N. Tuchman, M.D.
Assistant Professor of Pediatrics
Johns Hopkins University
Baltimore, Maryland
Division of Pediatric Gastroenterology
  and Nutrition
Department of Pediatrics
Sinai Hospital of Baltimore
Baltimore, Maryland

David Eric Tunkel, M.D.
Department of Otolaryngology/Head &
  Neck Surgery
Division of Pediatric Otolaryngology
Johns Hopkins University School
  of Medicine
Baltimore, Maryland

Rhonda S. Walter, M.D.
Developmental Pediatrician
Alfred I. Dupont Institute
Wilmington, Delaware

Preface

Intact feeding and swallowing mechanisms are essential to the overall well-being of infants and children. Although virtually every child experiences painful swallowing at some point in development, the impairment is usually transient (e.g., the "sore throat" experienced during an upper respiratory infection). However, a significant number of children are chronically afflicted with oral motor dysfunction. If severe, disordered deglutition may result in dehydration, malnutrition, aspiration, and/or potentially life-threatening sequelae. The field of pediatric feeding and swallowing disorders encompasses a diverse spectrum of entities, reflecting multiple etiologies. Assessment and treatment is best rendered by a multidisciplinary team comprised of physicians, nurses, occupational therapists, speech-language pathologists, behavioral therapists, and nutritionists. *Disorders of Feeding and Swallowing in Infants and Children: Pathophysiology, Diagnosis, and Treatment* is a reference text for clinicians working with swallowing impaired pediatric patients, written by a group of specialists who share their expertise regarding management of these disorders.

Although impaired swallowing function occurs both in children and adults, the pediatric population offers some unique problems. All children experience growth and maturation that continually changes their "baseline" swallowing function. Clinicians must evaluate each child from the perspective of his or her developmental stages — cognitive, motor, social, and behavioral — as well as from chronologic age. This perspective requires training distinct from the approach utilized in adult medicine. In addition, young children often are unable to articulate pertinent medical symptoms. Parental reports, although crucial to the investigative process, are often incomplete (a priori second-hand information). The inability of neurologically impaired or cognitively limited children to fully provide information may further hamper attempts to localize pathology.

This book represents an attempt to add to the growing body of knowledge about pediatric feeding and swallowing disorders. It provides a working knowledge of pertinent pediatric anatomy, as well as the pathophysiologic underpinnings of impaired swallowing. Considerable discussion is devoted to the structure and function of the swallowing apparatus, as well as the "differential diagnosis" of impaired swallowing in the child. This text is by no means exhaustive. It should, however, aid clinicians in identifying probable areas of swallowing dysfunction and potential complications; and choosing among the diagnostic modalities available and potential management and treatment options.

There is a need for trained clinicians who work consistently with pediatric patients with feeding and swallowing problems. Utilizing a team approach, "feeding and swallowing specialists" can ensure that each patient receives optimal evaluation and care, as well as provide a multidisciplinary forum for enhancing clinical expertise.

Acknowledgments

The editors wish to express their gratitude to Pamela Greenburg for her administrative and secretarial assistance.

To our families

Physiology of the Swallowing Apparatus

CHAPTER

David N. Tuchman, M.D.

Swallowing, or deglutition, involves a complex series of events which occur in the proximal portion of the gastrointestinal tract and functions to deliver substances from the oral cavity to the stomach. The act of deglutition is highly integrated, involves the central and peripheral nervous systems, and requires the coordination of more than 20 muscles acting in concert over a period of about 2 seconds. Since there is close approximation of the airway and the foodway, the swallowing apparatus must be capable of delivering its contents without allowing entry of substances into the airway, a condition known as "safe-swallowing."

In addition to transporting fluids and nutrients, the swallowing mechanism also delivers salivary secretions into the esophagus and stomach. Saliva lubricates the oral cavity, pharynx, and esophagus; aids in the digestion of starches and fats; helps maintain a non-acid milieu in the esophageal lumen; and may also play a role in maintaining the mucosal integrity of the esophagus and stomach by delivering proteins, such as epidermal growth factor, to the luminal surface (Sarosiek et al., 1988).

In adults, swallowing frequency is approximately 600 times per day. An indi-vidual swallows approximately 200 times during eating, 300 times while awake, and 50 times during sleep (Dent, Dodds, Friedman, Sekiguichi, Hogan, & Arndorfer, 1980; Dodds, 1989; Lear, Flanagan, & Moses, 1965; Lichter & Muir, 1975). Swallowing clears the oral cavity of saliva which flows at a rate of about 0.5 mL/minute (Dodds, Hogan, Reid, Stewart, & Arndorfer, 1973, Helm, Dodds, Hogan, Soergel, Egide, & Wood, 1982). During sleep, salivation decreases markedly (Lichter & Muir, 1975).

In the adult, the volume of water per swallow equals 17 mls. In children, ages 1.25 to 3.5 years, this value is 4.6 mls per swallow. Interestingly, when data are expressed on a weight basis, children swallow 0.33 mls/kg/swallow versus adults who swallow 0.24 mls/kg/swallow (Herbst, 1981; Jones & Work, 1961).

Embryologic Development of the Swallowing Apparatus

For a more detailed discussion of the embryologic development of the structures of the swallowing apparatus and proximal gastrointestinal tract, the reader is referred to general texts of embryology and gastroenterology (Bosma, 1985; Boyle, 1982; Herbst, 1981; Moore, 1973; Walker et al., 1991; Williams & Warwick, 1984).

Development of the Oral Cavity and Pharynx

In the human fetus, the primitive foregut is a straight tube which is lined by endoderm. At its cephalic end, this tube is separated from ectoderm by the oropharyngeal membrane which is located on the floor of the primitive oral cavity or stomodeum (Figure 1–1). The oral cavity, lined by ectoderm, develops between the fourth and eighth week of fetal life as a depression on the ventral surface of the embryo located cephalad to the first pharyngeal or branchial arch. The oro-pharyngeal membrane ruptures at the fifth week of gestation, allowing communication between the stomodeum (oral cavity) and pharynx, thereby bringing the digestive tract into communication with the amniotic fluid cavity (Arey, 1965; Moore, 1973).

The endoderm of the foregut is separated laterally from the surface ectoderm by a layer of mesenchyme which splits into vertical bars known as the pharyngeal or branchial arches. Each arch forms a swelling on the surface of the embryo and on the wall of the foregut. The grooves on the surface are known as pharyngeal clefts (between the arches), and the grooves which form on the lateral wall of the foregut are known as pharyngeal pouches.

The branchial arches give rise to the development and formation of the face and neck. The pharynx develops from multiple structures including the cephalic end of the foregut, the branchial arches, and pharyngeal pouches. The first and second branchial arches develop into the mouth, tongue, and muscles of mastication. The neck appears between the mouth and the heart, anterior to the hindbrain vesicle. The mesoderm of the third arch develops

into the superior constrictors of the pharynx while the endoderm provides the epithelial lining of the tongue, pharynx, a portion of the epiglottis and the pyriform sinuses. The mesoderm of the fourth arch gives rise to the inferior constrictors of the pharynx, and its endoderm provides the remaining epithelium of the hypopharynx.

The mouth is formed from the stomodeum and partly from the floor of the cephalic portion of the foregut. The epithelium of the lips, gums, and the enamel of the teeth originate from ectoderm. The tongue begins to form from the tuberculum impar, a triangular elevation which appears in the endodermal floor of the pharynx at the fourth week (Figure 1–2). Two lateral lingual swellings, derived from the first branchial arch, develop on each side of the tuberculum impar and increase in size so that they eventually merge, overgrow the tuberculum impar and form the anterior two-thirds of the tongue. The copula, another medial swelling located behind the tuberculum impar, extends forward, becomes v-shaped and is eventually engulfed by growth into this area of the anterior end of the third branchial arch (hypobranchial eminence). The hypobranchial eminence extends into the copula, fuses in the midline, and forms the posterior third, or root, of the tongue. The epiglottis is formed when the posterior third of the copula is split off from the tongue by a transverse groove.

Development of the Esophagus

The esophagus begins to develop from the embryonic foregut by the end of the first month. It arises from an anterior narrowing of the pharynx, at the level of the fourth branchial arch where the tracheal bud arises, and extends off the cephalic border of the vitelline (yolk) sac (Figure 1–3). The esophagus is initially a short tube, but extends in length as the heart and diaphragm descend. During the third week of fetal life a midline cleft, the laryngo-trache-

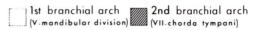

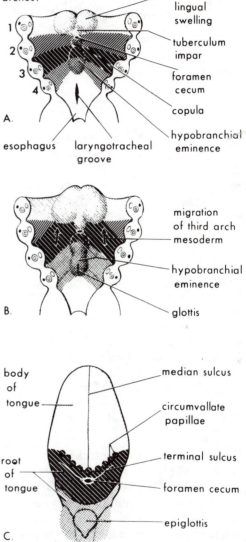

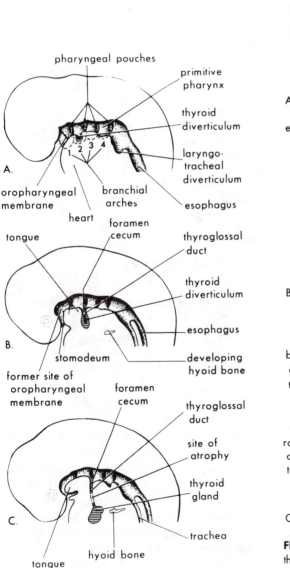

FIGURE 1-1. Schematic sagittal sections of the head and neck region of embryos at **A.** 4, **B.** 5, and **C.** 6 weeks. (From Moore, K. L. [1973]. The developing human. *Clinically oriented embryology.* Philadelphia: W. B. Saunders, p. 145, reprinted with permission).

FIGURE 1-2. A. and **B.** Schematic horizontal sections through the pharynx showing successive stages in the development of the tongue during the fourth and fifth weeks. **C.** Adult tongue showing the branchial arch derivation of the nerve supply of the mucosa. (From Moore, K. L. [1973]. The developing human. *Clinically oriented embryology.* Philadelphia: W. B. Saunders, p. 146, reprinted with permission).

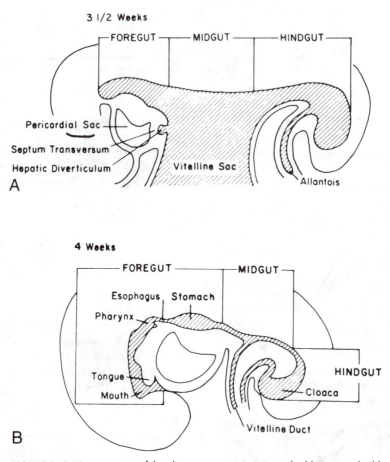

FIGURE 1–3. Segmentation of the alimentary tract. **A.** 3½-week-old. **B.** 4-week-old fetus. (From Boyle, J. T. [1982]. Congenital disorders of the esophagus. In S. Cohen & R. D. Soloway [Eds.], *Diseases of the esophagus.* New York: Churchill Livingstone, p. 98, reprinted with permission.)

al groove forms the ventral floor of the pharynx (Figure 1–4). The groove elongates and the lung buds appear from the caudal aspect. The combined laryngo-tracheal-esophageal tube is separated completely by folding and fusion of the lateral walls of the foregut in a caudal-cephalad progression. By 33 days, the tubes of the airway and foodway are completely separated except at the level of the larynx.

The esophagus initially is lined by stratified epithelium which is two to three cells deep. This proliferates between the fifth and sixth week so that the esophagus is almost a solid core. As the esophagus length-

ens, vacuoles appear during the sixth week, are most marked during the eighth week, and subsequently coalesce by the tenth week so that the esophageal lumen becomes re-canalized. During this process, the esophageal lumen is never completely occluded. Beginning in the tenth week, ciliated cells are noted in the mid-portion of the esophagus which, by the twelfth week, line its entire length. Columnar epithelium is replaced by squamous epithelium beginning in the mid-esophageal body at about 16 weeks. By the seventh month of gestation, squamous mucosa extends throughout the esophagus. At birth, the

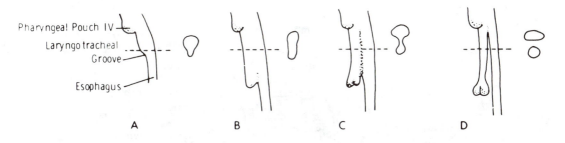

Pharyngeal Pouch IV

Laryngotracheal Groove

Esophagus

A   B   C   D

FIGURE 1–4. A–D. Separation of esophagus and tracheobronchial tree. Broken line depicts area in anatomical cross section shown to right of each longitudinal drawing. (From Boyle, J. T. [1982]. Congenital disorders of the esophagus. In S. Cohen & R. D. Soloway [Eds.]. *Diseases of the esophagus.* New York: Churchill Livingstone, p. 98, reprinted with permission.)

length of the esophagus, measured from the upper to lower esophageal sphincters, is from 7 to 14 centimeters with a diameter of 5 to 6 millimeters. In the adult, the esophagus is approximately 25 centimeters in length (Weaver, 1991).

Development of Lips, Palate, and Mandible

The facial structures of the embryo develop from 5 to 8 weeks of fetal life. The upper lip is formed by medial growth of the bilateral maxillary processes of the first pharyngeal arch. These processes eventually meet in the midline and fuse with each other and with the medial nasal process. The medial nasal process is the main contributor to the philtrum. The lower lip is formed from the bilateral mandibular processes of the first pharyngeal arch which grow medially and fuse in the midline.

The mesenchyme which forms the first pharyngeal arch divides into two processes, a short maxillary process and a long mandibular process. The mandibular processes merge with each other in the fourth week, eventually giving rise to the lower jaw, the lower lip, and the lower portion of the face. The mesenchymal core of the first pharyngeal arch is transformed into a cartilaginous bar named Meckels' cartilage. The body of the mandible develops dur-

ing the sixth week as intramembranous bone develops around and lateral to Meckels' cartilage.

Initially, in early fetal life, the nasal and oral cavities communicate directly. The primary palate, which carries the four incisors, is formed by the median palatine process and develops by the end of the fifth week (Figure 1–5). Posterior to the primary palate, two horizontal plates known as the lateral palatine processes originate from the maxillary process and grow medially. These plates fuse to form the secondary palate and also unite with the primary palate and nasal septum. Fusion of these structures occurs in an anterior to posterior direction. The primary and secondary palates form the hard palate. The soft palate forms as the two folds grow posteriorly from the posterior edge of the palatal process. The uvula is the last structure to form. Union of the soft palate occurs by the eighth week and fusion of the uvula by the 11th week.

Anatomy of the Oral Cavity, Pharynx, and Esophagus in the Adult

The major peripheral elements involved in the act of deglutition include components of the face, oral cavity, pharynx, and esoph-

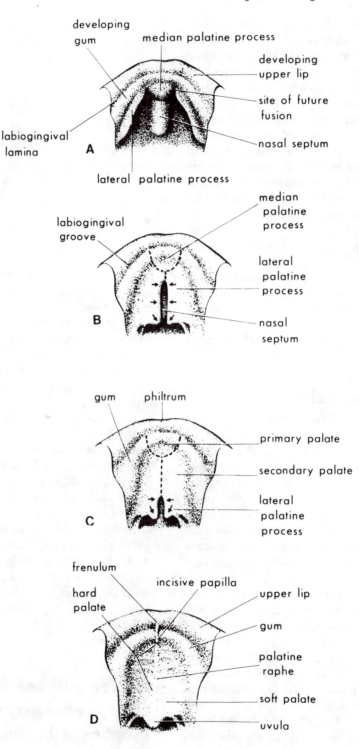

FIGURE 1-5. Development of the palate from the sixth to twelfth weeks of fetal life. Broken lines indicate sites of fusion of the palatine processes. Arrows indicate medial and posterior growth of the lateral palatine processes. (From Moore, K. L. [1973]. The developing human. *Clinically oriented embryology.* Philadelphia: W. B. Saunders, p. 154, reprinted with permission.)

agus. Portions of the pharynx that participate in swallowing include the pharyngeal (muscular or soft) palate, the pharyngeal portion of the tongue, the oropharynx, and the hypopharynx (Bosma, Donner, Tanaka, & Robinson, 1986). These regions of the pharynx are illustrated in Figure 1–6. In contrast to the naso- and oropharynx, the mandible, hyoid bone, and thyroid cartilage form the mobile skeleton of the hypopharynx (Bosma et al., 1986). Figures 1–7 and 1–8 illustrate the anatomy of the oral cavity and pharynx in the adult.

The esophagus is a tubular structure linking the pharyngeal and gastric cavities. The striated muscle portion of the esophageal body is located in its proximal third and begins at the inferior border of the esopha-

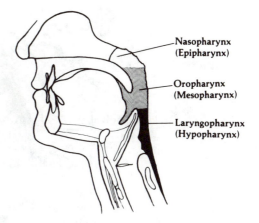

FIGURE 1–6. Regions of the pharynx. (From Bosma, J. F., Donner, M. W., Tanaka, E., & Robertson, D. [1986]. Anatomy of the pharynx, pertinent to swallowing. *Dysphagia, 1,* 22–33, p. 24, reprinted with permission.)

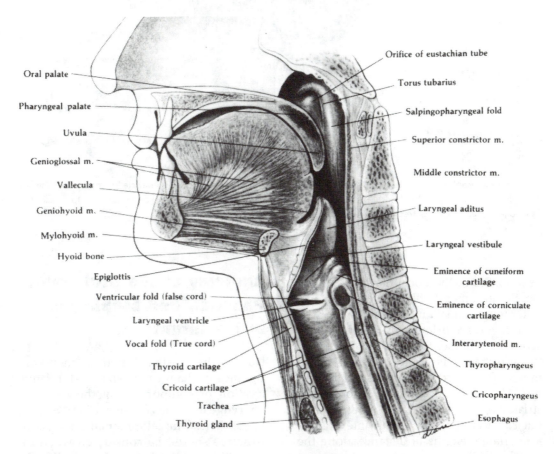

FIGURE 1–7. Anatomy of the oral cavity and pharynx of the adult. Sagittal view. (From Bosma, J. F., Donner, M. W., Tanaka, E., & Robertson, D. [1986]. Anatomy of the pharynx, pertinent to swallowing. *Dysphagia, 1,* 22–33, p. 24, reprinted with permission.)

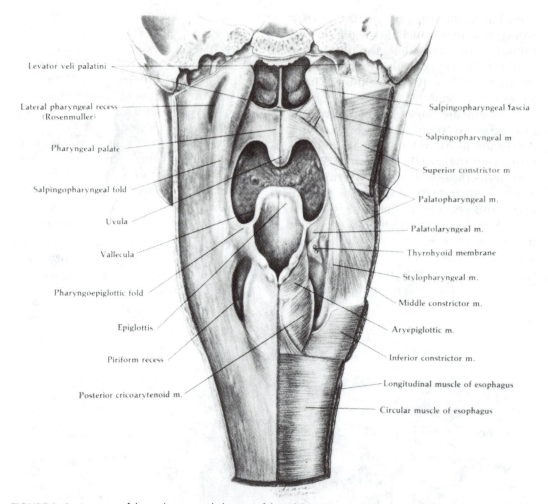

FIGURE 1-8. Anatomy of the oral cavity and pharynx of the adult. Posterior view, with muscle layer absent on the left. (From Bosma, J. F., Donner, M. W., Tanaka, E., & Robertson, D. [1986]. Anatomy of the pharynx, pertinent to swallowing. *Dysphagia, 1,* 22–33, p. 27, reprinted with permission.)

geal border of the cricopharyngeus muscle. Striated muscle fibers, which have an outer longitudinal and a thicker inner circular layer, are oriented in an oblique or screw-like course. The distal two-thirds of the esophagus is composed of smooth muscle fibers arranged in a similar manner. The junction between smooth and striated muscle is not sharply demarcated but consists of fibers which interdigitate for variable lengths of distance along the mid-esophagus.

Anatomy of the Oral Cavity, Pharynx, and Esophagus in the Infant

During the postnatal period, there are significant changes in size and relative location of components of the oral and pharyngeal cavities (Bosma, 1985; Kramer, 1985). These developmental changes in structure should be considered when interpreting pediatric imaging studies. In general, the central mobile elements of the oropharynx in the infant are large in comparison to their containing chambers (Figure 1–9). For example, the tongue is large compared to the oral cavity, and the arytenoid mass is nearly mature in size compared to the small-sized vestibule and ventricle of the larynx.

In the infant, the tongue lies entirely within the oral cavity and the larynx is positioned high in the neck resulting in a small oropharynx (Laitman & Crelin, 1976) (Figure 1–10). Between 2 and 4 years of age, the tongue begins to descend so that by approximately 9 years of age its

posterior third is located in the neck (Laitman & Crelin, 1976). The larynx also moves in a caudal direction. Based on autopsy studies, the larynx descends from the level of the third to the fourth cervical body during the prenatal period, an arrangement that persists during infancy (Noback, 1923). During childhood the larynx descends to a level opposite the sixth cervical vertebra and finally, in adulthood, moves to the level of the seventh cervical vertebra. As maturation progresses, the face vertically elongates and the chambers of the oral cavity and oropharynx enlarge (Bosma, 1985).

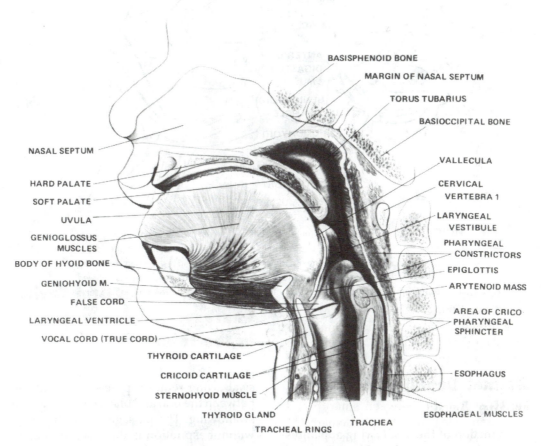

FIGURE 1–9. Midsagittal anatomic schematic from the oral cavity and pharynx of an infant. (From Kramer, S. S. [1985]. Special swallowing problems in children. *Gastrointestinal Radiology, 10,* p. 242, reprinted with permission.)

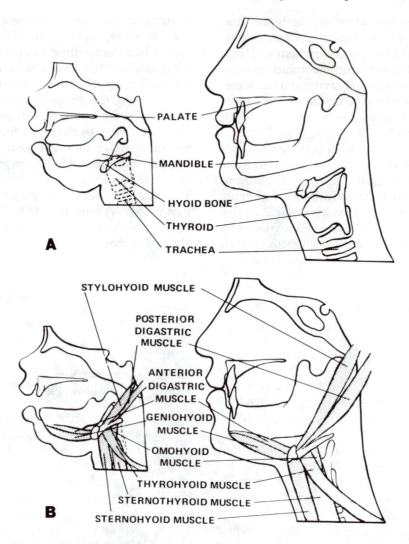

FIGURE 1-10. A. Drawing of infant and adult anatomy shows alteration in shape and orientation of the pharynx that accompanies growth and the descent of the larynx. Laryngeal cartilages and hyoid bone are shown in their relationship to the mandible. Airway is depicted (*hatched area*). **B.** Drawing illustrates change in orientaton of muscles (*stippled*) that suspend the larynx in the infant and the adult. (From Kramer, S. S. [1985]. Special swallowing problems in children. *Gastrointestinal Radiology, 10,* 241–250, p. 243, reprinted with permission.)

Normal Deglutition in the Adult

The function of the swallowing apparatus is to transport materials from the oral cavity to the stomach without allowing entry of substances into the airway. Safe swallowing requires precise coordination between the oral and pharyngeal phases of swallowing. The passage of an oral bolus without aspiration is the result of a complex interaction of the cranial nerves and muscles of the oral cavity, pharynx, and proximal esophagus (Miller, 1982; Morrell,

1984). Deglutition is generally divided into three phases based on functional as well as anatomic characteristics. These divisions are the oral (which includes the preparatory stage), pharyngeal, and esophageal phases of swallowing (Miller, 1982; Morrell, 1984).

Oral Phase

The oral phase of swallowing is voluntary and involves a preparatory stage. In the unimpaired individual, the oral cavity functions as a sensory and motor organ, effecting changes in the physical properties of the food bolus to make it swallow-safe. During the preparatory stage, the oral bolus is modified by chewing and mixing with saliva. Control of the bolus in the oral cavity is aided by placement of the tip of the tongue against the maxillary alveolar ridge or superior incisors. The anterior portion of the tongue forms a cup-shape to hold boluses of large volume (Dodds, 1989; Logemann, 1986). The tongue functions to manipulate oral contents, positioning the food bolus laterally over the molars for effective mastication. Biplane (posterior and lateral) videofluoroscopy synchronized with intraluminal manometry has been used to demonstrate deglutitive tongue functions such as bolus containment, volume accommodation, and bolus propulsion (Kahrilas, Lin, Logemann, & Ergun, 1993). Physical properties of the food bolus altered by oral activity include bolus size, shape, volume, pH, temperature, and consistency (Coster & Schwarz, 1987).

Once the preparatory phase is complete, the oral phase continues and the bolus moves into the region of the pharynx. This is accomplished by a rolling, or peristaltic, motion of the tongue against the palate in a caudal direction. As the bolus enters the pharynx, the soft palate contracts and elevates and comes into contact with the posterior pharyngeal wall. This forms a seal between the chambers of the naso- and oro-pharynx and effectively prevents pharyngonasal reflux. Palatal motion is accomplished by contraction of the levator veli palatini, tensor veli palatine, and palatopharyngeus muscles (see Figure 1–8). A strong seal at this level helps maintain the propulsive forces necessary to transport the bolus through the hypopharynx, upper esophageal sphincter, and into the esophagus.

Pharyngeal Phase

There are multiple sensory fields within the oro-pharyngeal region which may trigger the pharyngeal phase of deglutition. Touch, liquids, and soft pressure are capable of evoking a swallow when applied to the soft palate, uvula, dorsum of the tongue, the pharyngeal surface of the epiglottis, the faucial pillars, glossoepiglottidinal sinus, the posterior pharyngeal wall, and the pharyngo-esophageal junction (Miller, 1986).

During the pharyngeal phase, the swallow is reflexive and involves a complex sequence of coordinated motions. This phase, which lasts approximately 1 second, generally consists of two basic movements: elevation of the whole pharyngeal tube including the larynx, followed by a descending peristaltic wave. During the initial segment, the posterior portion of the tongue sequentially descends (moves caudad) while maintaining contact with the posterior pharyngeal wall. Pharyngeal constrictors contract sequentially in a descending sequence giving rise to a peristaltic "pharyngeal stripping wave." The bolus propagates through the pharynx at a rate of about 9 to 25 centimeters per second, an action which, in the adult, takes about 100 milliseconds (Dodds, 1989; Miller, 1982).

During the pharyngeal phase, the larynx elevates, moving in a superior and anterior direction. This is accomplished by contraction of the suprahyoid muscles (such as the myelohyoid, geniohyoid, and diagastric), and the thyrohyoid muscles (see Figures 1–7 and 1–10B) (Kahrilas, Dodds, Dent, Logemann, & Shaker, 1988). Movement of the larynx in this fashion serves to engulf the bolus on entry into the pharynx and aids in opening the upper esophageal sphincter via the forces of traction. During deglutition, the laryngeal orifice closes at the level of the epiglottis and at the level of the true vocal folds by contraction of the thyroarytenoid, aryepiglottic, and oblique arytenoid muscles. In addition, obliteration of the laryngeal vestibule occurs as the larynx is positioned "beneath" the base of tongue. A liquid bolus is generally diverted into two streams as it flows around the epiglottis and into the pyriform fossae.

Pharyngeal constrictors and elevators "inject" food from the pharynx into the esophagus with a large force at velocities as high as 100 cm per second (Buthpitiya, Stroud, & Russell, 1987; Fisher, Hendrix, Hunt, & Murrills, 1978). Pharyngeal propulsion of food into the esophagus has been compared to forcefully pressing the plunger on a syringe (Fisher et al., 1978). Approximately 600 to 900 milliseconds after the onset of the pharyngeal phase, food passes through the upper esophageal sphincter and enters the esophagus. The cricopharyngeus muscle, the main component of the upper esophageal sphincter, relaxes for approximately 500 milliseconds during the swallow to allow passage of the bolus (Shipp, Deatsch, & Robertson, 1970). Normal adults complete the pharyngeal swallow in approximately 1,500 milliseconds (Curtis & Hudson, 1983). Timing data for children are not well established.

Esophageal Phase

Upper Esophageal Sphincter

The upper esophageal sphincter (UES), also known as the pharyngoesophageal segment, is a manometrically defined high pressure zone located in the region distal to the hypopharynx (see Chapter 11 for a discussion of manometry). The sphincter is tonically closed at rest and opens during swallowing, vomiting, and belching (Palmer, 1976). The length of the high pressure zone in adults is from 2.5 to 4.5 centimeters, averaging about 3 centimeters (Palmer, 1976). Although the cricopharyngeus muscle is the major component of the upper sphincter, its length is about 1 centimeter and therefore additional muscles such as the inferior pharyngeal constrictor muscle and the muscle fibers of the proximal esophagus most likely contribute to the high pressure zone (Asoh & Goyal, 1978; Ellis, 1971; Goyal, 1984; Palmer, 1976; Welch, Luckmann, Ricks, Drake, & Gates, 1979). The pressure profile of the UES is asymmetric with higher pressures noted in the anterior and posterior directions (Winans, 1972). Orientation of a recording device must take this asymmetry into account when measurements are obtained in this region. Pressures measured in the region of the UES have a dual origin, originating from an active component secondary to contraction of the cricopharyngeal muscle and passive forces attributable to tissue elasticity (Kahrilas, Dodds, Dent, Haeberle, Hogan, & Arndorfer, 1987). Table 1–1 reports normal values for the pharyngoesophageal region of control in infants obtained by using a low-compliance, water-perfused manometry system where directional orientation of the catheter is maintained (Sondheimer, 1983).

The cricopharyngeus muscle inserts bilaterally at the inferior-lateral margins of the cricoid lamina, and as a result, cartilage and sphincter move in unison. The UES, which is closed at rest, relaxes during swallowing as the larynx elevates. Relaxation of the sphincter precedes opening by approximately one-tenth of a second (Kahrilas et al., 1988). The sphincter opens by forces of traction on its anterior wall exerted by contraction of the suprahyoid and infrahyoid muscles. The duration and diameter of

TABLE 1-1. Pharyngeal manometric measurements in control infants.

Measurement	M ± SD	Range
Resting UES pressure (cm H₂O)	28.9 ± 10	18.0–44.0
Pharyngeal peristaltic wave		
amplitude (cm H₂O)	74.7 ± 19.9	37.0–102.0
velocity (cm/s)	8.5 ± 3.6	3.2–15.0
duration (s)	0.59 ± 0.18	0.4–0.86

Source: From Sondheimer, J. M. (1983). Upper esophageal sphincter and pharyngeal motor function in infants with and without gastroesophageal reflux. *Gastroenterology, 85,* 301–305 (p. 303, reprinted with permission).

sphincter opening is influenced by bolus size and viscosity which implies that sphincter response is not stereotypic but is responsive to sensory feedback (Jacob et al., 1989; Kahrilas et al., 1988).

Proposed functions of the UES include prevention of esophageal distention during normal breathing (Palmer, 1976) and protection of the airway against aspiration following an episode of gastroesophageal reflux (Hunt, Connell, & Smiley, 1970; Gerhardt, Shuck, Bordeaux, & Winship, 1978). The latter remains controversial. Early studies demonstrated that upper esophageal sphincter pressure increased in response to intra-esophageal acidification in infants (Sondheimer, 1983) and adults (Gerhardt et al., 1978) suggesting that the UES functions as a dynamic barrier against esophagopharyngeal reflux which may occur consequent to gastroesophageal reflux. However, recent studies using more sophisticated methodology have not confirmed these findings (Kahrilas, Dodds, & Vanagunas, 1987; Vakil, Kahrilas, Dodds, & Vanagunas, 1989). Other modifiers of UES pressure include sleep, which is associated with decreased sphincter pressure, and factors associated with increased pressure including respiration, esophageal distention, and stress (Cook, Dent, Shannon, & Collins, 1987; Kahrilas et al., 1987). Palmer (1976) has reviewed neurologic control of the upper esophageal sphincter.

Esophageal Body

Esophageal function has been reviewed in detail by others (Diamant, 1989; Nurko, 1991). Following pharyngeal transit, food enters the esophagus and via primary peristalsis is transported to the stomach. Primary peristalsis is a coordinated, progressive contraction throughout the esophageal body which is elicited by a swallow (see Figure 1–11). This differs from secondary peristalsis which is initiated by an esophageal stimulus such as intra-luminal distention. In this instance, onset of the peristaltic wave occurs at the point of stimulation and propagates distally. Tertiary peristalsis, which is pathophysiologic, refers to simultaneous contraction throughout the esophageal body which does not progress (nonperistaltic).

The velocity of contraction of a primary peristaltic wave in older children and adults is from 2 to 4 centimeters per second. Peristaltic amplitude is 53.4 ± 9.0 mm Hg in the upper esophagus, 35.0 + 6.4 mm Hg in the midesophagus, and 69.5 + 12.1 mm Hg in the lower esophagus (Nurko, 1991). In the region of the mid-esophagus, at the junction of smooth and striated muscle, peristaltic pressure is lower and velocity of propagation slows. Duration of contraction is 2 to 4 seconds in the proximal esophagus and increases as the wave moves distally (Nurko, 1991).

Neurologic control of peristalsis in the esophagus is related to both central

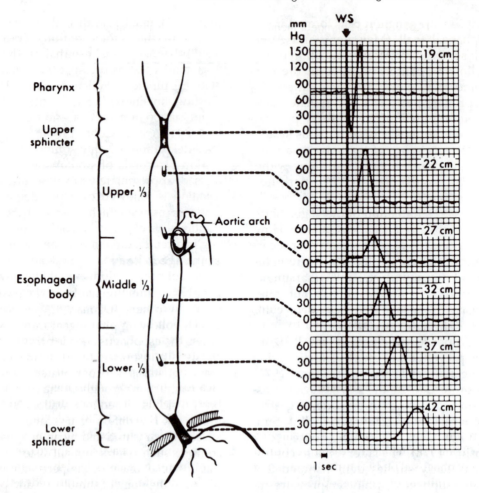

FIGURE 1–11. Manometric pressure changes with a swallow of a liquid bolus (WS = wet swallow). Proximal and distal tracings are from the upper (UES) and lower (LES) esophageal sphincters, respectively. Following a swallow, UES pressure falls transiently. Following this, LES pressure decreases and remains low until the peristaltic wave progresses in an aboral direction through the esophageal body. (From Margulis, A. R., & Burhenne, H. J. [Eds.]. [1983]. *Alimentary tract radiology* [3rd ed.]. St. Louis, MO: C. V. Mosby, p. 533, reprinted with permission.)

and peripheral mechanisms. In the striated portion of the esophagus, peristalsis is under control of the central nervous system. This portion of the esophagus receives only somatic excitatory innervation originating from lower motor neurons of the nucleus ambiguus located in the brainstem with preganglionic fibers traveling in the vagus nerve. Postganglionic vagal fibers directly innervate striated muscle fibers. Peristalsis is activated when the swallowing center stimulates the

nucleus ambiguus to sequentially fire neurons in a cranial-caudal sequence (for additional discussion, see Chapter 3). Primary peristalsis in the striated esophagus is abolished by bilateral vagotomy (Kahrilas, 1989; Nurko, 1991).

In the smooth muscle portion of the esophageal body, also innervated by the vagus nerve, neurons originate from the dorsal motor nucleus. In contrast to striated muscle, vagal fibers in the smooth muscle portion synapse with ganglion cells located in the esophageal wall (Meissner's and Auerbach's plexuses). After stimulation by the swallowing center, neurons in the dorsal motor nucleus fire simultaneously, and primary peristalsis occurs. Therefore, although initiation of a primary peristaltic wave requires central nervous system input, sequencing of the wave is a function of intrinsic neural pathways within the esophageal muscle (i.e., peripheral coordination).

Direct stimulation of the vagus nerve will result in a peristaltic sequence. However, the vagus is not necessary for secondary peristalsis because this is preserved following vagotomy (Kravitz, Snape, & Cohen, 1966; Roman, 1966). Peristalsis may occur independently of the central nervous system and is mediated by intramural neurons of the esophageal body.

Lower Esophageal Sphincter

The lower esophageal sphincter (LES) is represented by a physiologic high pressure zone located in the distal portion of the esophagus. The LES functions as a major determinate of gastroesophageal competence and provides a barrier against reflux of gastric contents into the esophagus (Fisher, Malmud, Roberts, & Lobis, 1977). There are, however, other factors which aid in the prevention of reflux (for a more detailed discussion see Chapter 13). The LES, which is closed at rest, relaxes during deglutition to allow passage of esophageal contents into the stomach.

The LES is anatomically indistinct from the more proximal region of the esophagus, but differs from the esophageal body in length-tension characteristics and response to neural and hormonal stimuli (Christensen, 1970; Lipschutz & Cohen, 1971). In adults, LES pressure ranges from 15 to 30 mm Hg using intra-gastric pressure as baseline or zero pressure reference point. Cross-sectional representation of the pressure profile of the LES demon-

strates asymmetry, with higher pressures noted in the lateral regions (Winans, 1972). In the normal esophagus, the LES maintains a resting pressure that fluctuates with respiration (Welch & Gray, 1982). Resting tone in the LES is maintained by a combination of myogenic and neurogenic factors (Goyal & Cobb, 1981).

Relaxation of the sphincter occurs within 2 seconds of swallowing and persists for approximately 8 to 10 seconds. Relaxation is followed by a postdeglutition rise in pressure which most likely reflects continuation of peristaltic contractions moving in a caudal direction in the esophageal body. LES relaxation is mediated by activation of preganglionic vagal fibers which stimulate intramural postganglionic neurons to release a noncholinergic, nonadrenergic inhibitory neurotransmitter (Goyal & Rattan, 1978). LES relaxation also occurs during vomiting, rumination, and belching. LES pressure is subject to modification by many substances, including neuropeptides, hormones, drugs, and foods (Goyal & Rattan, 1978) (see Table 1–2).

The LES increases in length during development measuring approximately 1 centimeter in infants less than 3 months, 1.6 centimeters in children older than 1 year, and 2 to 4 centimeters in adults (Goyal & Cobb, 1981; Moroz, Espinoza, Cumming, & Diamant, 1976). Early work in animals and humans suggested that sphincter pressure was initially low during infancy and increased with advancing age. However, these studies were performed with nonperfused catheters and may have provided inaccurate results. More recently, measurements utilizing water-perfused, low-compliance systems have demonstrated the LES pressures in normal full-term newborns and children are comparable to adult levels (Moroz et al., 1976; Moroz & Beiko, 1981; Vanderhoof, Rappaport, & Paxon, 1978). In preterm infants, LES pressure is lower, correlates with gestational age, and eventually reaches normal levels at full-term (Newell, Sakar, Durbin, Booth, & McNeish, 1988).

TABLE 1–2. Effect of pharmacologic and other agents on LES pressure.

Increases LES	Decreases LES
Alpha-adrenergic agonists	Beta-adrenergic agonists
Cholinergic agonists	Alpha-adrenergic antagonists
Beta-adrenergic antagonists	Anticholinergics
Metoclopramide	Dopamine
Domperidone	Calcium-channel blockers
Cisapride	Caffeine
Protein meals	Theophylline
Gastrin	Cholecystokinin
Substance P	Vasoactive intestinal peptide
Motilin	Gastric inhibitory peptide
Raised intra-abdominal pressure	Smoking
	Pregnancy
	Fat
	Chocolate
	Ethanol
	Peppermint

Source: From Nurko, S. (1991). Esophageal motility. In W. A. Walker, P. R. Dunia, J. R. Hamilton, J. B. Walker-Smith, & J. B. Watkins (Eds.), *Pediatric gastrointestinal disease* (p. 232). Philadelphia: B. C. Decker, reprinted with permission.

Normal Deglutition in Infants and Children

Deglutition In-Utero

Deglutition occurs at approximately 16 to 17 weeks of gestation, although a pharyngeal swallow has been described in a delivered fetus at a gestational age of 12.5 weeks (Humphrey, 1967). The volume of swallowed amniotic fluid increases with increasing gestational age. Initially, the fetus swallows 2 to 7 milliliters (mls) per day, increasing to 13 to 16 mls at 20 weeks gestation until, at term, the normal fetus swallows approximately 450 mls of amniotic fluid per day out of a total amniotic fluid volume of 850 mls (Milla, 1991; Pritchard, 1966).

In-utero, deglutition plays a number of important roles. These include maintenance of normal amniotic fluid volume (Grand, Watkins, & Torti, 1976; Pritchard, 1966) and promotion of normal growth and development of the gut by the delivery of trophic factors to the immature gastrointestinal tract (Mulvihill, Stone, Fonkalsrud, & Debas, 1986). In addition, a direct relationship between fetal swallowing and amniotic fluid volume has been demonstrated in an animal model (Minei & Suzuki, 1976). Abnormalities in amniotic fluid volume have been associated with altered fetal swallowing (Barkin et al., 1987).

Brace (1989) examined factors that affect regulation of fluid balance in the fetal lamb, including measurements of swallowing function. Amniotic fluid volume was calculated using an indicator dilution technique which measured the rate of disappearance of radio-labeled red blood cells. Following long-term infusion of saline into the fetal circulation, small increases were noted in fetal blood volume, whereas amniotic fluid volume, the daily amount of amniotic fluid swallowed, and fetal urine flow increased greatly. Other modifiers of fetal swallowing include changes in plasma osmolality and drug-induced systemic hypotension (Ross, Sherman, Ervin, Day, & Humme, 1989, 1990).

Developmental Changes in Feeding Behavior

The development of normal feeding behavior in the infant and child has been reviewed in detail elsewhere in this text and by others (Bosma, 1985, 1992; Kramer, 1985). Briefly, in the normal infant the oral phase of swallowing is characterized by a pattern known as suckle feeding. Suckle feeding is followed by the development of transitional feeding (ages 6 to 36 months), and, eventually, mature feeding which is characterized by biting and chewing. Maturation of feeding behavior, characterized by more complex feeding movements, occurs mainly as a result of central nervous system maturation and not as a consequence of changes in the physical characteristics of end-organs (e.g., development of teeth) (Bosma, 1986). Feeding behavior matures as motor activity is directed by higher centers such as the thalamus and the cerebral cortex, a process termed "encephalization" of feeding (Bosma, 1985).

Sucking/Suckle Feeding: Developmental Aspects

Sucking, a vital participant in the act of feeding for the infant, may be characterized as nonnutritive or nutritive. Nonnutritive sucking is defined as rhythmic movements on a nonfeeding nipple. Nutritive sucking involves delivery of a liquid bolus from a nipple with the oral phase of swallowing known as suckle feeding. Suckle feeding entails reflex feeding activity which is organized at the subcortical level, either at the pons or medulla (Kramer, 1985). Suckling is a rhythmic movement which involves good lip seal and compression of

a nipple (Figure 1–12). The lower jaw and tongue compress against the upper jaw and palate to create negative intra-oral pressures of 60–160 mm Hg (Colley & Creamer, 1958). The posterior portion of the oropharynx is closed off by apposition of the tongue and soft palate, allowing the region of the posterior oral cavity to act as a reservoir (Kramer, 1985). During suckling, the soft palate may move towards the tongue, a motion that does not normally occur in the adult swallow (Kramer, 1985). The tongue functions to move the bolus out of the oral cavity and into the pharynx. During the pharyngeal phase, the larynx elevates, although its motion is less than in the adult due to its high in the neck position (Shapiro & Healy, 1988). A prominent pharyngeal wave is seen during this phase, a finding generally not noted in the adult swallow (Kramer, 1985). Radiographic images of normal, term infants exhibiting suckle feeding from the breast and bottle have been recorded by a number of investigators (Ardran, Kemp, & Lind, 1958a, 1958b; Kramer, 1985; Logan & Bosma, 1967).

Gryboski (1969) defined developmental stages of sucking and swallowing behavior using manometric recording devices placed in the proximal gastrointestinal tract. In preterm infants, an initial phase is characterized by mouthing movements which are not associated with effective sucking (see Figure 1–13). This is followed by the development of an "immature suck-swallow pattern" described as short sucking bursts preceded or followed by swallows. Sucking rate during this phase was measured at approximately 1 to 1.5 sucks per second. A "mature suck-swallow pattern" was seen after a few days in larger infants and up to 3 months later in the most premature infants (Figure 1–14). This pattern was characterized by prolonged bursts of sucking (10–30) at a rate of 2 sucks per second. Multiple swallows occurred during these bursts at a frequency of approximately one to four times during each burst. In infants weighing less than 1,800 grams, simultanous esophageal contrac-

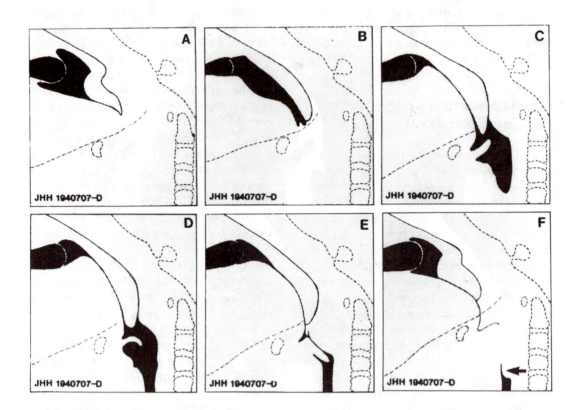

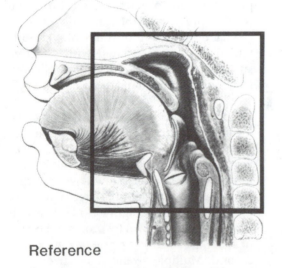

Reference

FIGURE 1–12. Drawing of normal infantile suckle feeding (lateral projection)). During oral suckling, barium (*black*) expressed from nipple collects posteriorly in the mouth, but is confined by the apposition of the soft palate and the tongue (**A**). With vigorous suckling, the soft palate configuration changes and, at times, may bow forward as the soft palate-tongue relationship is maintained. As the tongue moves the collected liquid into the pharynx (**B, C**), the pharyngeal sequence is initiated. The soft palate elevates, apposes the posterior pharyngeal wall, and closes off the nasopharynx. Pharyngeal constriction begins as a posterior pharyngeal wave in the superior pharyngeal constrictor. The larynx is elevating, the epiglottis is beginning to tilt, and the laryngeal vestibule is closed (**C**). Pharyngeal contraction seen as a prominent posterior pharyngeal wave transports the barium through the pharynx and the open cricopharyngeal sphincter into the esophagus (**D**). No barium enters the closed, elevated esophagus. At the end of the pharyngeal constriction, the pharynx is completely empty (**E**). After barium has passed into the esophagus and the cricopharyngeal sphincter has closed, the airway (*white*) immediately reopens (**F**). Note barium outlining the lower margin of the cricopharyngeal sphincter (*arrow*). (From Kramer, S. S. [1985]. Special swallowing problems in children. *Gastrointestingal Radiology, 10*, 241–250, p. 244, reprinted with permission.)

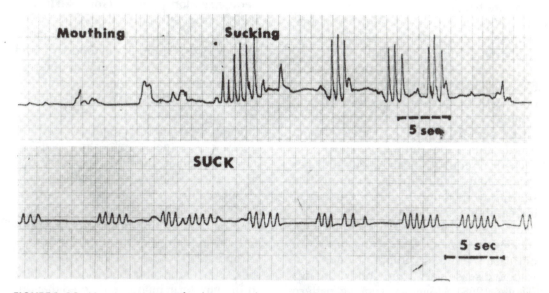

FIGURE 1-13. Manometric tracing of suck pattern in the preterm infant. Tracings were obtained with water-filled catheters. **Top:** Mouthing predominates with only short sucking bursts. **Bottom:** Short sucking bursts of 1 per second, no mouthing. (From Gryboski, J. D. [1969]. Suck and swallow in the premature infant. *Pediatrics, 43,* 96–102, p. 98, reprinted with permission.)

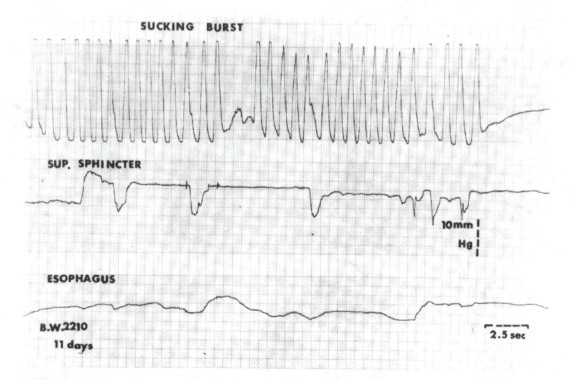

FIGURE 1-14. Manometric tracing illustrating the "mature suck-swallow pattern." Note long sucking periods in top lead. Swallowing is represented by multiple relaxations of the superior (or upper) esophageal sphincter. (From Gryboski, J. D. [1969]. Suck and swallow in the premature infant. *Pediatrics, 43,* 93–102, p. 98, reprinted with permission.)

tions (tertiary) were noted during sucking. With increasing weight and age,
esophageal contractions became progressively more coordinated and propulsive.

Wolfe (1968) characterized nonnutritive sucking as segmentally divided into
periods of sucking bursts with a sucking
frequency of two sucks per second followed by periods of rest. Nutritive sucking
was described as a continuous sequence of
sucks at a frequency of about one suck per
second. Rates of nutritive and nonnutritive
sucking were found to differ, tending to
increase with developmental age (Wolfe,
1968) (see Table 1–3). The nonnutritive
sucking pattern of infants with a history of
perinatal stress and without obvious neurologic disease vary from control infants
(Wolfe, 1968). However, sucking pattern
may be normal in infants with major central nervous system abnormalities.

Christensen, Dubignon, and Campbell (1976) examined the influence of intra-oral stimulation on nutritive sucking in
full-term infants and found that sucking
rate was dependent on nipple size (sucking rate was less when using a larger nipple). These data are similar to the response
seen during nonnutritive sucking (Dubignon & Campbell, 1968). Other factors that
influence nutritive sucking include maternal sedation (Casaer, Daniels, Devlieger,
DeCock, & Eggermont, 1982), length of

feeding session (Crump, Gore, & Horton,
1958), visual stimuli (Milewski & Sigue-
land, 1975), and taste of the fluid (Maller &
Turner, 1973). Kron, Stein, Goddard, and
Phoenix (1967) noted significant differences in sucking when comparing milk formula to corn syrup. Sucking rate and volumes ingested increased with increasing
concentrations of carbohydrate and increasing sweetness, suggesting that the
human infant is capable of sensory discrimination (Dubignon & Campbell, 1969;
Maller & Turner, 1973).

In infants, oral intake appears to be regulated by modification in sucking rate rather than a change in intraoral pressures
(Kron et al., 1967). However, Daniels, Casaer, Devlieger, and Eggermont (1986)
studied preterm infants and noted that differences in feeding efficiency could not be
explained by differences in sucking rate.

Nonnutritive Sucking

Nonnutritive sucking may improve weight
gain during gavage feeding in preterm infants. Bernbaum, Pereira, Watkins, and
Peckham (1983) studied the nutritional effects of nonnutritive sucking in a group of
low-birth-weight infants receiving formula
by enteral tube and found that, compared
to control infants, the group receiving non-

TABLE 1–3. Comparison of nonnutritive and nutritive sucking rates

| | | Sucking Rates (Mean Frequency per Second) | | | |
| | | Nonnutritive | | Nutritive | |
Age	Number of Infants	Mean	Range	Mean	Range
37–38 weeks (preterm)	3	1.7	1.7–1.8	0.92	0.86–0.96
4–6 days	10	2.1	1.9–2.3	1.0	0.8–1.2
14–60 days	10	2.2	2.0–2.6	1.3	1.3–1.6
7–9 months	5	2.7	2.4–2.7	1.5	1.3–1.6

Source: From Wolfe, P. H. (1968). The serial organization of sucking in the young infant. *Pediatrics, 42,* 945, reprinted with permission.

nutritive sucking gained significantly more weight. The mechanism accounting for this finding is not clear, although it is theorized that nonnutritive sucking may result in more efficient nutrient absorption or may decrease energy requirements secondary to lessening of infant activity or restlessness (Field et al., 1982; Neeley, 1979).

Nonnutritive sucking may have effects on pulmonary function as well. In preterm infants, nonnutritive sucking is associated with an increase in transcutaneous oxygen tension and respiratory frequency (Paludetto, Robertson, Hack, Shivpuri, & Martin, 1984; Paludetto, Robertson, & Martin, 1986). This is in contrast to findings during nutritive sucking which demonstrate lowered oxygen tension during feeding (Paludetto et al., 1986). The mechanisms accounting for the different effects of nutritive versus nonnutritive sucking on pulmonary function remain unknown.

Other investigators have shown that nonnutritive sucking may favorably affect the rate of feeding time and gastric emptying in infants receiving nutrition via enteral tube (Widstrom et al., 1988). Nonnutritive sucking during tube feeding may increase vagal activity and influence secretion of gastrointestinal hormones such as gastrin and somatostatin.

Mature Feeding

Development of Biting and Chewing

From shortly after birth until 5 months of age, biting is a reflexive action which occurs in response to pressure on the upper and lower gums. These early movements include a vertical bite and release mechanism (Milla, 1991). After 5 months of age, the infant begins to integrate these motions into biting and chewing (Milla, 1991; Morris, 1978). Rotary chewing begins at about 1 year of age as the infant gains the skills necessary to maintain the intra-oral bolus over the molars for grinding by control of lip closure and cheek action (Milla,

1991). Mature biting and chewing develops fully by 24 months of age and is characterized by a rotary chewing motion with an ability to lateralize intra-oral contents using the tongue.

Masticatory performance has been gauged by measuring a number of parameters including pulverization of a standard food (peanuts, carrots), the number of chews needed to prepare a bolus for swallowing ("the swallowing threshold"), and biting force (Herbst, 1981; Shiere & Manly, 1952). Efficiency of chewing reaches adult levels by 16 years of age.

References

Ardran, G. M., Kemp, F. H., & Lind, J. A. (1958a). A cineradiographic study of bottle feeding. *British Journal of Radiology, 31,* 11–22.

Ardran, G. M., Kemp, F. H., & Lind, J. A. (1958b). A cineradiographic study of breast feeding. *British Journal of Radiology, 31,* 156–162.

Arey, L. B. (1965). *Developmental anatomy.* Philadelphia, PA: W. B. Saunders.

Asoh, R., & Goyal, R. K. (1978). Manometry and electromyography of the upper esophageal sphincter in the opossum. *Gastroenterology, 74,* 514–520.

Barkin, S. Z., Pretorius, D. H., Beckett, M. K., Manchester, D. K., Nelson, T. R., & Manco-Johnson, M. L. (1987). Severe polyhdramnios: Incidence of anomalies. *American Journal of Radiology, 148,* 155–159.

Bernbaum, J. C., Pereira, G. R., Watkins, J. B., & Peckham, G. J. (1983). Nonnutritive sucking during gavage feeding enhances growth and maturation in premature infants. *Pediatrics, 71,* 41–45.

Bosma, J. F. (1985). Postnatal ontogeny of performances of the pharynx, larynx, and mouth. *American Review of Respiratory Disease, 131*(Suppl.), S10–S15.

Bosma, J. F. (1986). Development of feeding. *Clinical Nutrition, 5,* 210–218.

Bosma, J. F. (1992). Development and impairments of feeding in infancy and childhood. In M. E. Groher (Ed.), *Dysphagia — Diagnosis and management* (pp. 107–141). Boston: Butterworth Heinemann.

Bosma, J. F., & Donner, M. W. (1980). Physiology of the pharynx. In M. A. Paparella & D. A. Shumrick (Eds.), *Otolaryngology* (pp. 332–345). Philadelphia, PA: W. B. Saunders.

Bosma, J. F., Donner, M. W., Tanaka, E., & Robertson, D. (1986). Anatomy of the pharynx, pertinent to swallowing. *Dysphagia, 1,* 23–33.

Boyle, J. T. (1982). Congenital disorders of the esophagus. In S. Cohen & R. D. Soloway (Eds.), *Diseases of the esophagus* (pp. 97–120). New York: Churchill Livingstone.

Boyle, J. R., & Cohen, S. (1984). Does intrinsic LES tone increase as an adaptive response to increased intra-abdominal pressure? *Digestive Diseases and Sciences, 29,* 760–764.

Boyle, J. T., Tuchman, D. N., Altschuler, S. M., Nixon, T. E., Pack, A. I., & Cohen, S. (1985). Mechanisms for the association of gastroesophageal reflux and bronchospasm. *American Review of Respiratory Diseases, 131*(Suppl.), 516–520.

Brace, R. A. (1989). Fetal blood volume, urine flow, swallowing, and amniotic fluid volume responses to long-term intravascular infusions of saline. *American Journal of Obstetrics and Gynecology, 161,* 1049–1054.

Buthpitiya, A. G., Stroud, D., & Russell, C. O. H. (1987). Pharyngeal pump and esophageal transit. *Digestive Diseases and Sciences, 32,* 1244–1248.

Casaer, P., Daniels, H., Devlieger, H., DeCock, P., & Eggermont, E. (1982). Feeding behaviour in preterm neonates. *Early Human Development, 7,* 331–346.

Christensen, J. (1970). Pharmacologic identification of the lower esophageal sphincter. *Journal of Clinical Investigation, 49,* 681–691.

Christensen, S., Dubignon, J., & Campbell, D. (1976). Variations in intra-oral stimulation and nutritive sucking. *Child Development, 47,* 539–542.

Colley, J. R. T., & Creamer, B. (1958). Sucking and swallowing in infants. *British Medical Journal, 2,* 422–423.

Cook, I. J., Dent, J., Shannon, S., & Collins, S. M. (1987). Measurement of upper esophageal sphincter pressure, effect of acute emotional stress. *Gastroenterology, 93,* 526–532.

Coster, S. T., & Schwarz, W. H. (1987). Rheology and the swallow-safe bolus. *Dysphagia, 1,* 113–118.

Curtis, D. J., & Hudson, T. (1983). Laryngotracheal aspiration. Analysis of specific neuromuscular factors. *Radiology, 149,* 517.

Crump, E. P., Gore, P. M., & Horton, C. (1958). The sucking behavior in premature infants. *Human Biology, 30,* 128–141.

Daniels, H., Casaer, P., Devlieger, H., & Eggermont, E. (1986). Mechanisms of feeding efficiency in preterm infants. *Journal of Pediatric Gastroenterology and Nutrition, 5,* 593–596.

Dent, J., Dodds, W. J., Friedman, R. H., Sekiguichi, T., Hogan, W. J., & Arndorfer, R. C. (1980). Mechanisms of lower gastroesophageal reflux in recumbent asymptomatic human subjects. *Journal of Clinical Investigation, 65,* 256–267.

Diamant, N. E. (1989). Physiology of the esophagus. In M. H. Sleisenger, & J. S. Fordtran (Eds.), *Gastrointestinal disease* (pp. 548–559). Philadelphia, PA: W. B. Saunders.

Dodds, W. J. (1989). The physiology of swallowing. *Dysphagia, 3,* 171–178.

Dodds, W. J., Hogan, W. J., & Helm, J. F. (1981). Pathogenesis of reflux esophagitis. *Gastroenterology, 81,* 376–394.

Dodds, W. J., Hogan, W. J., Reid, D. P., Stewart, E. T., & Arndorfer, R. C. (1973). A comparison between primary esophageal peristalsis following wet and dry swallows. *Journal of Applied Physiology, 35,* 851–857.

Dubignon, J., & Campbell, D. (1968). Intra-oral stimulation and sucking in the newborn. *Journal of Experimental Child Psychology, 6,* 154–166.

Dubignon, J., & Campbell, D. (1969). Sucking in the newborn in three conditions: Nonnutritive, nutritive, and a feed. *Journal of Experimental Child Psychology, 6,* 335–350.

Ellis, F. H., Jr. (1971). Upper esophageal sphincter in health and disease. *Surgical Clinics of North America, 51,* 553–565.

Field, T., Ignatoff, E., Stringer, S., Brennan, J., Greenberg, R., Widmayer, S., & Anderson, G. C. (1982). Nonnutritive sucking during tube feedings: Effects on preterm neonates in an intensive care unit. *Pediatrics, 70,* 381–384.

Fisher, M. A., Hendrix, T. R., Hunt, J. N., & Murrills, A. J. (1978). Relation between volume swallowed and velocity of the bolus ejected from the pharynx into the esophagus. *Gastroenterology, 74,* 1238–1240.

Fisher, R. A., Malmud, L. S., Roberts, G. S., & Lobis, I. F. (1977). The lower esophageal sphincter as a barrier to gastroesophageal reflux. *Gastroenterology, 72,* 19–22.

Gerhardt, D. C., Shuck, T. M., Bordeaux, R. A.,

& Winship, D. H. (1978). Human upper esophageal sphincter: response to volume, osmotic and acid stimuli. *Gastroenterology, 75,* 268–274.

Goyal, R. K. (1984). Disorders of the cricopharyngeus muscle. *Otolaryngologic Clinics of North America, 17,* 115–130.

Goyal, R. K., & Cobb, B. W. (1981). Motility of the pharynx, esophagus and the esophageal sphincters. In L. R. Johnson (Ed.), *Physiology of the gastrointestinal tract* (p. 359). New York: Raven Press.

Goyal, R. K., & Rattan, S. (1978). Neurohumoral, hormonal, and drug receptors for the lower esophageal sphincter. *Gastroenterology, 4,* 598–619.

Grand, R. J., Watkins, J. B., & Torti, F. M. (1976). Development of the human gastrointestinal tract: A review. *Gastroenterology, 70,* 796–810.

Gryboski, J. D. (1965). The swallowing mechanism of the neonate. I. Esophageal and gastric motility. *Pediatrics, 35,* 445–452.

Gryboski, J. D. (1969). Suck and swallow in the premature infant. *Pediatrics, 43,* 96–102.

Helm, J. F., Dodds, W. J., Hogan, W. J., Soergel, K. H., Egide, M. S., & Wood, C. M. (1982). Acid neutralizing capacity of human saliva. *Gastroenterology, 83,* 69–74.

Herbst, J. J. (1981). Development of sucking and swallowing. In E. Lebenthal (Ed.), *Textbook of gastroenterology and nutrition in infancy* (pp. 97–107). New York: Raven Press.

Humphrey, T. (1967). Reflex activity in the oral and facial area of the human fetus. In J. F. Bosma (Ed.), *Second symposium on oral sensation and perception* (pp. 195–233). Springfield, IL: Charles C. Thomas.

Hunt, P. S., Connell, A. M., & Smiley, T. B. (1970). The cricopharyngeal sphincter in gastric reflux. *Gut, 11,* 303–306.

Jacob, P., Kahrilas, P. J., Logemann, J. A., Shah, V., & Ha, T. (1989). Upper esophageal sphincter opening and modulation during swallowing. *Gastroenterology, 97,* 1469–1478.

Jones, D. V., & Work, C. E. (1961). Volume of a swallow. *American Journal of Diseases of Childhood, 102,* 427.

Kahrilas, P. J. (1989). The anatomy and physiology of dysphagia. In D. W. Gelfand & J. E. Richter (Eds.), *Dysphagia — Diagnosis and treatment* (pp. 11–28). New York: Igaku-Shoin.

Kahrilas, P. J., Dodds, W. J., Dent, J., Haeberle, B., Hogan, W. J., & Arndorfer, R. C. (1987). The effect of sleep, spontaneous gastroesophageal reflux and a meal on UES pressure in humans. *Gastroenterology, 92,* 466–471.

Kahrilas, P. J., Dodds, W. J., Dent, J., Logemann, J. A., & Shaker, R. (1988). Upper esophageal sphincter function during deglutition. *Gastroenterology, 95,* 52–62.

Kahrilas, P. J., Lin, S., Logemann, J. A., Ergun, G. A., & Facchini, F. (1993). Deglutitive tongue action: Volume accommodation and bolus propulsion. *Gastroenterology, 104,* 152–162.

Kramer, S. S. (1985). Special swallowing problems in children. *Gastrointestinal Radiology, 10,* 241–250.

Kravitz, J. J., Snape, W. J., & Cohen, S. (1966). Effect of thoracic agotomy and vagal stimulation on esophageal function. *American Journal of Physiology, 238,* 233–238.

Kron, R. E., Stein, M., Goddard, K. E., & Phoenix, M. D. (1967). Effect of nutrient upon the sucking behavior of newborn infants. *Psychosomatic Medicine, 29,* 24–32.

Laitman, J. T., & Crelin, E. S. (1976). Postnatal development of the basicranium and vocal tract region in man. In J. F. Bosma (Ed.), *Symposium on development of the basicranium* (pp. 206–219). Washington, DC: Government Printing Office.

Lear, C. S., Flanagan, J. B., Jr., & Moores, C. F. (1965). The frequency of deglutition in man. *Archives of Oral Biology, 10,* 83–99.

Lichter, I., & Muir, R. C. (1975). The pattern of swallowing during sleep. *Elecytroencephalography and Clinical Neurophysiology, 38,* 427–432.

Lipshutz, W. H., & Cohen, S. (1971). Physiologic determinates of lower esophageal sphincter function. *Gastroenterology, 61,* 16–24.

Logan, W. J., & Bosma, J. F. (1967). Oral and pharyngeal dysphagia in infancy. *Pediatric Clinics of North America, 14,* 47–61.

Logemann, J. A. (1986). *Manual for the videofluorographic study of swallowing.* San Diego, CA: College-Hill Press.

Maller, O., & Turner, R. E. (1973). Taste and acceptance of sugars in human infants. *Journal of Comparative and Physiologic Psychology, 84,* 496–501.

Margulis, A. R., & Burhenne, H. J. (Eds.). (1983). *Alimentary tract radiology* (3rd ed., p. 533). St. Louis, MO: C. V. Mosby.

Menon, A. P., Schefft, G. L., & Thach, B. T. (1984). Frequency and significance of swallowing during prolonged apnea in infants. *American Review of Respiratory Diseases, 130,* 969–973.

Milewski, A. E., & Siqueland, E. R. (1975). Discrimination of color and pattern novelty in one-month human infants. *Journal of Experimental Child Psychology, 19,* 122–136.

Milla, P. J. (1991). Feeding, tasting, and sucking. In W. A. Walker, P. R. Durie, J. R. Hamilton, J. A. Walker-Smith, & J. B. Watkins (Eds.), *Pediatric gastrointestinal disease* (pp. 217–223). Philadelphia: B. C. Decker.

Miller, A. J. (1982). Deglutition. *Physiologic Review, 62,* 129–184.

Miller, A. J. (1986). Neurophysiologic basis of swallowing. *Dysphagia, 1,* 91–100.

Minei, L. J., & Suzuki, K. (1976). Role of fetal deglutition and micturition in the production and turnover of amniotic fluid in the monkey. *Obstetrics and Gynecology, 48,* 177–181.

Moore, K. L. (1973). The developing human. *Clinically oriented embryology* (pp. 136–166). Philadelphia: W. B. Saunders.

Moroz, S., Espinoza, J., Cumming, W., & Diamant, N. (1976). Lower esophageal sphincter function in children with and without gastroesophageal reflux. *Gastroenterology, 71,* 236–241.

Moroz, S. P., & Beiko, P. (1981). Relationship between lower esophageal sphincter pressure and serum gastric concentration in the newborn infant. *Journal of Pediatrics, 99,* 725–728.

Morrell, R. M. (1984). The neurology of swallowing. In M. E. Groher (Ed.), *Dysphagia and management* (pp. 3–35). Boston: Butterworths.

Morris, S. E. (1978). Assessment of children with oral motor dysfunction. In J. M. Wilson (Ed.), *Oral motor function and dysfunction in children.* Chapel Hill: University of North Carolina Press.

Mulvihill S. J., Stone, M. M., Fonkalsrud, E. W., & Debas, H. T. (1986). Trophic effect of amniotic fluid on fetal gastrointestinal development. *Journal of Surgical Research, 40,* 291–296.

Neeley, C. A. (1979). Effects of nonnutritive sucking upon the behavioral arousal of the newborn. *Birth Defects, 15,* 173–200.

Newell, S. J., Sarkar, P. K., Durbin, G. M., Booth, J. W., & McNeish, A. S. (1988). Maturation of the lower oesophageal sphincter in the preterm baby. *Gut, 29,* 167–172.

Noback, G. J. (1923). The developmental topography of the larynx, trachea and lungs in the fetus, new-born, infant and child. *American Journal of the Diseases of Childhood, 26,* 515–533.

Nurko, S. (1991). Esophageal motility. In W. A. Walker, P. R. Durie, J. R. Hamilton, J. A. Walker-Smith, & J. B. Watkins (Eds.), *Pediatric gastrointestinal disease* (pp. 224–235). Philadelphia: B. C. Decker.

Palmer, E. D. (1976). Disorders of the cricopharyngeus muscle: A review. *Gastroenterology, 71,* 510–519.

Paludetto, R., Robertson, S. S., Hack, M., Shivpuri, C. R., & Martin, R. J. (1984). Transcutaneous oxygen tension during non-nutritive sucking in preterm infants. *Pediatrics, 74,* 539–542.

Paludetto, R., Robertson, S. S., & Martin, R. J. (1986). Interaction between non-nutritive sucking and respiration in preterm infants. *Biology of the Neonate, 49,* 198–203.

Pritchard, J. A. (1966). Fetal swallowing and amniotic fluid volume. *Obstetrics and Gynecology, 28,* 606–610.

Roman, C. (1966). Nervous control of peristalsis in the esophagus. *Journal of Physiology (Paris), 58,* 479–506.

Ross, M. G., Sherman, D. J., Ervin, M. G., Day, L., & Humme, J. (1989). Stimuli for fetal swallowing: Systemic factors. *American Journal of Gynecology and Obstetrics, 161,* 1559–1565.

Ross, M. G., Sherman, D. J., Ervin, M. G., Day, L., & Humme, J. (1990). Fetal swallowing: Response to systemic hypotension. *American Journal of Physiology, 258,* R130–R134.

Sarosiek, J., Bilski, J., Murty, V. L. N., Slomiany, A., & Slomiany, B. L. (1988). Role of salivary epidermal growth factor in the maintenance of physicochemical characteristics of oral and gastric mucosal mucus coat. *Biochemical and Biophysical Research Communications, 152,* 1421–1427.

Shapiro, J., & Healy, G. B. (1988). Dysphagia in infants. *Otolaryngologic Clinics of North America, 21,* 737–741.

Shiere, F. R., & Manly, R. S. (1952). The effect of the changing dentition on masticatory function. *Journal of Dental Research, 31,* 526–534.

Shipp, T., Deatsch, W. W., & Robertson, K. (1970). Pharyngo-esophageal muscle activity during swallowing in man. *Laryngoscope, 80,* 1–16.

Sondheimer, J. M. (1983). Upper esophageal

sphincter and pharyngeal motor function in infants with and without gastroesophageal reflux. *Gastroenterology, 85*, 301–305.

Vakil, N. B., Kahrilas, P. J., Dodds, W. J., & Vanagunas, A. (1989). Absence of an upper esophageal sphincter response to acid reflux. *American Journal of Gastroenterology, 84*, 606–610.

Vanderhoof, J. A., Rappaport, P. J., & Paxon, C. L. (1978). Manometric diagnosis of lower esophageal sphincter incompetence in infants: Use of a small, single lumen perfused catheter. *Pediatrics, 62*, 805–808.

Walker, W. A., Durie, P. R., Hamilton, J. R., Walker-Smith, J. A., & Watkins, J. B. (Eds.). (1991). *Pediatric gastrointestinal disease.* Philadelphia: B. C. Decker.

Weaver, L. T. (1991). Anatomy and embryology. In W. A. Walker, P. R. Durie, J. R. Hamilton, J. A. Walker-Smith, & J. B. Watkins (Eds.), *Pediatric gastrointestinal disease* (pp. 195–216). Philadelphia: B. C. Decker.

Welch, R. W., Luckmann, K., Ricks, P. M., Drake, S. T., & Gates, G. A. (1979). Manometry of the normal upper esophageal sphincter and its alteration in laryngectomy. *Journal of Clinical Investigation, 63*, 1036–1041.

Welch, R. W., & Gray, J. E. (1982). Influence of respiration on lower esophageal pressure recordings in humans. *Gastroenterology, 83*, 590–594.

Widstrom, A. M., Marchini, G., Matthiesen, A. S., Werner, S. Winberg, J., & Uvnas-Moberg, K. (1988). Non-nutritive sucking in tube fed preterm infants: Effects on gastric motility and gastric contents of somatostatin. *Journal of Pediatric Gastroenterology and Nutrition, 8*, 517–523.

Williams, P. L., & Warwick, R. (Eds.). (1984). *Gray's anatomy* (p. 1320). London: Churchill Livingstone.

Winans, C. S. (1972). The pharyngoesophageal closure mechanism: A manometric study. *Gastroenterology, 63*, 768–777.

Wolfe, P. H. (1968). The serial organization of sucking in the young infant. *Pediatrics, 42*, 943–956.

Issues Surrounding the Development of Feeding and Swallowing

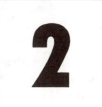

2

CHAPTER

Rhonda S. Walter, M.D.

Growth is the process whereby a child gains in size and matures in function; it requires an adequate supply of energy derived from nutritional intake. In the absence of pathology, growth is dependent on the oral intake of food via the feeding process. Milla (1991) summarizes several factors that affect feeding: structure and function of foregut, overall development, early behavior patterns, and parental influence. Feeding not only accomplishes the nutritional intake necessary to sustain growth, but provides a context in which the child becomes socialized to others and an environment for the acquisition of speech skills (Morris & Klein, 1987; Ottenbacher, Bundy, & Short, 1983; Stevenson & Allaire, 1991). The development of normal feeding and swallowing can be viewed as a dynamic process dependent on an orderly sequence of acquisition of skills precedent on reflex emergence and timed extinction, mediated by learning from others, and paralleling physical, cognitive, and social/emotional milestones.

Concept of Critical or Sensitive Period

The unfolding of the developmental milestones of feeding is based on progressive mastery of skills, from basic to more complex. In the healthy infant without physical or emotional barriers, the mechanical process of feeding is "regularly and consistently paired with feelings of satiety, pleasure, security, and relaxation" (Singer, 1990, p. 60). How an infant "learns" a specific pattern of behavior, the crucial timing for introduction of such information, and the translation of feeding information into functional feeding skills has often been speculated on (see, for example, Bosma, 1986; Morris & Klein, 1987; Stevenson & Allaire, 1991).

Perhaps the most quoted theoretical perspective relevant to feeding development is that of the critical or sensitive period, first elaborated by Illingworth and Lister (1964). Borrowing from prior work in animal models and observations, Illingworth reviewed the concept of critical periods, fairly well delineated times when a specific stimulus must be applied to produce a particular action. This is, he noted, closely coupled with the optimal time for application of a given stimulus (i.e., the "sensitive period"). In the strict interpretation, a given behavior pattern cannot be "learned" after the critical period. Additionally, it is more difficult to learn the pattern after the sensitive period has passed (Illingworth, as summarized in Stevenson & Allaire, 1991).

Illingworth and Lister (1964), and subsequent others, speculated that some common problems of infant feeding appear to be related to these concepts, taking the perhaps intuitive position that: "If children are not given solid food to chew at a time when they are first able to chew, troublesome feeding problems may occur" (p. 847).

Although these concepts are unproven from a "hard science" standpoint, they offer an interesting explanation for feeding delays and deviant feeding behavior in children, which can be viewed as arising from a missed or a variant timing in the introduction of a given feeding skill. Hence, an absent or inappropriate response occurs to the stimulus of food introduction (i.e., disordered feeding and swallowing).

The Concept of Conditioned Dysphagia

Difficulties with food acceptance and feeding may result from an aversion to swallowing, the so-called "conditioned dysphagia" described by DiScippio and Kaslon (1982) and DiScippio, Kaslon, and Ruben (1978). Basically, conditioned dysphagia is a learned disorder, acquired and maintained through a behavioral conditioning process that occurs when a noxious stimulus is paired with the act of swallowing. Examples are suctioning of the mouth and/or nasopharynx, nasogastric tube passage, and various medical procedures such as bronchoscopy, upper endoscopy, radiographic contrast studies, and tracheostomy (Tuchman, 1991). When the intrusive act (stimulus) is paired with swallowing, the patient may respond by conditioned avoidance to swallowing, including food refusal and/or ultimate suppression of swallowing. Persistence of food refusal and impaired swallowing behaviors beyond the termination of the aversive stimulus leads to maladaptive habits. For example, DiScippio and Kaslon (1982) found that about 40% of children with cleft palate continued to have conditioned dysphagia even after corrective pharyngeal flap surgery. As noted by Tuchman (1991), the continued avoidance of stimuli (noxious or innocuous) can reduce sensory input to the oral cavity. The avoidance behavior becomes self-perpetuating, and pathology persists secondary to aberrant behaviors and perhaps reversion to primitive oromotor patterns.

Multiple etiologies can disorder the feeding process (see Chapter 4). Children "at risk" for feeding difficulties are those who experience interruption in the developmentally appropriate timing of introduction of food either on a mechanical, behavioral, or social interactive basis. Table 2–1

TABLE 2–1. Pediatric population at risk for feeding and swallowing difficulties.

Neurologic problems
Cerebral palsy
Traumatic brain injury
Neurodegenerative disease

Congenital anomalies
Genetic or chromosomal entities: Down's syndrome, spina bifida, cleft lip and/or cleft palate syndromes

Metabolic disorders
PKU
Other inborn errors of metabolism

Cognitive or behavioral limitations
Mental retardation
Autism
"Difficult temperament"

Psychosocial
Vulnerable child
Parental stress and deprivation

Chronic illness
Cystric fibrosis
Malignancies
BPD

GI disorders
Inflammatory bowel disease
Reflux esophagitis
Supplemental tube dependence
Prematurity and low birth weight

Source: Adapted from Singer, L. (1990). When a sick child won't — or can't — eat. *Contemporary Pediatrics, 12,* p. 67.

lists groups of children at risk for feeding and swallowing difficulties. Early identification of these children may facilitate and maximize intervention strategies.

In children, as distinct from adults, the progression of feeding skills and acceptance of the feeding process is clearly intertwined with developmental phases (both physical and cognitive) and existent reflex patterns available from which to progress. "Normal" timing of introduction of feeding stimuli and acquisition of feeding developmental milestones are discussed in the following section.

Oral Motor Reflexes and the Development of Feeding

The oral pharyngeal reflexes that are present at birth are the underpinnings for future feeding and swallowing maturation. As noted by Ogg (1975), the infantile reflexes may be evaluated individually, but their significance is related to the coordinated sequence of their action as the child learns to eat. Individual reflexes present at birth which are summarized in Table 2–2 include the suck-swallow, root, bite, gag, Babkin's, and palmomental. The newborn infant has a repertoire of automatic oral motor movements, and feeding and swallowing can be considered "reflex-bound" (Stevenson & Allaire, 1991). These primitive oral reflexes (much like their correlates in gross and fine motor streams of development) will extinguish or modify within the first 6 months of life, yielding to more mature patterns and enabling transition to higher feeding textures.

The rooting reflex or reaction which allows the infant to localize the source of food, either breast or bottle nipple, appears soon after birth (Morris & Klein, 1987). Bosma (1986) notes that, once the infant is in a feeding ready state (i.e., arousal state), touch stimulation in the perioral area elicits rooting and the mouth is moved toward the nipple or stimulating object. The rooting reflex, then, is a stereotypic response to stroking around the mouth of movement of the head toward the source

TABLE 2–2. Infantile oral-motor reflexes.

Reflex	Description	Time of Extinction
Rooting	Stroking around mouth elicits movement of head toward source of stimulus and "latching on" to nipple.	3–4 months
Suck-Swallow	Stroking anterior third of tongue or center of lips elicits suck/swallow movements.	6 months (evolution to mature sucking)
Biting	Stroking gum elicits rhythmic vertical biting motion of the jaw.	6 months
Gag	The stimulus to the posterior three fourths of the tongue or pharyngeal wall elicits constriction and elevation of the pharynx.	Sensitivity shifts to back one quarter of the tongue and the pharyngeal wall by adulthood
Babkin's	Stroking of the palm of the hand elicits mouth opening, eye closing, head moving forward and midline.	3–4 months
Palmomental	Stroking of the palm of the hand elicits wrinking of the mentalis muscle.	Can persist to adulthood

Source: Adapted from Morris, S. E., & Klein, M. D. (1987). Pre-feeding skills. *A comprehensive resource for feeding development.* And Stevenson, R. D., & Allaire, J. H. (1991). The development of normal feeding and swallowing. *Pediatric Clinics of North America, 38*(6).

of stimulus, allowing the infant to latch onto the nipple. It generally extinguishes by 3 to 4 months, perhaps later in breast-fed infants (Stevenson & Allaire, 1991).

As with rooting behavior, the suck-swallow reflex is present in the newborn, and phases out by 3 to 4 months. At birth, light touch to the face of a full-term infant may elicit reflexive sucking. In several days, the sucking response is more specifically elicited when stimuli are applied to the mouth area (Morris & Klein, 1987). The term suck-swallow reflex itself is used to refer to the suck-swallow response elicited by stroking the anterior third of the tongue or center of the lips. Suckling and sucking are phases of suck that occur in infant development. The two are distinguished as follows: Suckling is the earliest pattern, describing an extension-retraction pattern of the tongue with loose approximation of the lips (Bosma, 1986; Morris & Klein, 1987). This is the so-called "lick suck." This rhythmical backward and forward pattern of the tongue combines with opening and closing of the jaw to draw liquid into the mouth. In the mature or "true" suck, the tongue, lips, mandible, and hyoid move together in alternating directions. The lips approximate more firmly, and the total effect is increased negative pressure and a greater pull of liquid (and/or soft food) into the mouth (Milla, 1991). The infant utilizes a mixture of the suck and suckle until approximately 6 months of age, when the more efficient suck pattern begins to predominate (Stevenson & Allaire, 1991).

The biting reflex in the infant differs from the more mature, or adult, functional bite used in mastication. The infantile reflex pattern refers to the automatic (stereotyped) rhythmic vertical bite and release pattern that is elicited by stroking or pressure on the anterior and lower aspects of the upper and lower gums (Milla, 1991). This antecedent reflex pattern of vertical bite to pressure stimulus persists until approximately 6 months of age. It is then integrated into the mature pattern of volitional, lateral, and rotatory movements of

the jaw seen in chewing (Ogg, 1975). A prolonged or persistent biting reflex — the so called "tonic bite" — is pathologic. It may be seen in children with cerebral palsy, and its presence may inhibit food acceptance or progression to higher textures.

The gag is a reflex that is present in the newborn and persists to adulthood, albeit with some modification. In the infant, a stimulus applied to the back three fourths of the tongue elicits a gag, with forceful movement of the tongue and subsequent reverse peristaltic movement of the pharynx (Morris & Klein, 1987). By 6 to 9 months, the stimulus sensitive area moves to the posterior third of the tongue (Stevenson & Allaire, 1991), and some elements of volitional control emerge by adulthood. The gag reflex, including constriction and elevation of the pharynx, clearly serves a protective role as a mechanism by which the pharynx can help seal off the lower aspects of the digestive tract from unwanted elements. Thus, its persistance into adulthood and incorporation into the mature feeding and swallowing process makes teleologic sense (at least to this author).

A recently described primitive reflex is swallowing in response to a puff of air administered to an infant's face — the so-called "Santmyer swallow" (Orenstein, Bergman, Proujansky, Kacoslis, & Giarusso, 1992; Orenstein, Santmeyer, Varusso, Proujansky, & Kocoslis, 1988). The response produced is a primary peristaltic sequence with motility characteristics similar to those of a spontaneous swallow, occurring within seconds after the puff of air is administered. The reflex is thought to require a stimulation of the perioral area, via the maxillary and/or mandibular branches of the trigeminal nerve (Orenstein et al., 1992). The Santmyer reflex is noted to be present in both premature and full-term infants, but not present in normal older children (more than 1–2 years old) or adults. It does implicate the removal of cortical inhibitory control (i.e., frontal release allowing a primitive reflex to surface). Clinicians who work with the cerebral palsy population have relied on variance of this reflex for years — utilizing a puff of air to the face to "force" children to swallow and thus break a temper tantrum surrounding feeding, aid in videofluoroscopy, or pass a nasogastric tube (Linda Miller-Schuberth, personal communication). Although the relevance of this reflex to the development of feeding is speculative, it does point out the complex neurologic and functional interactions existent in the feeding and swallowing processes.

Evolution of Mature Feeding Patterns

The feeding reflexes present at birth evolve, with modification over time, into adultlike patterns by approximately 3 years of age. Ottenbacher, Bundy, and Short (1983)

summarized the refined patterns as including coordinated breathing and swallowing, rotary chewing, and precise tongue and lip movements (pointing, flattening, and bunching) that allow for sucking and swallowing with minimal jaw movements.

It is beyond the scope of this chapter to fully discuss prefeeding skills and the various assessment and treatment tools available to the clinician. The reader is referred to the work of Bosma (1986) for theoretical discussion and Morris and Klein (1987) for theory in practice applications. It is, as Stevenson and Allaire (1991) pointed out, useful to view the development of skills as paralleling the types of food eaten, manner of presentation, and age at time of progression. Table 2–3 summarizes the stages of oral pharyngeal motor activity utilized in feeding and food transition.

Tasks of maturation of feeding include progression from breast/bottle to assisted

TABLE 2–3. Stages of oral motor activity utilized in feeding progression.

Age (in months)	Food Type	Oral Motor Activity	Method of Food Presentation
Birth–6	milk, liquids	suckling — progression to suck on bottle/breast	bottle/breast
4–6	cereals, pureed foods	maturation sucking/swallowing	spoon
5–7	liquid, purees, teething biscuits	diminishing bite/suck reflexes cleaning spoon with lips emergence munch/chew	spoon
8–12	ground, junior, mashed, finger foods, introduction of chopped fine	active upper lip in spoon feeding lateralization of tongue begins, with movement of food to teeth biting on objects	cup introduced
12–15	chopped fine	refinement of tongue lateralization emergence of munching with rotary chewing licking food off lips	bottle/breast weaning cup spoon
15–24	"table food"	decrease drooling increased maturity of rotary chew internal jaw stability in cup drinking tongue tip elevation for swallowing	cup spoon fork

Sources: Adapted from Milla, P. J. (1991). Feeding, tasting, and sucking. In W. A. Walker et al. (Eds.), *Pediatric gastrointestinal disease — Pathophysiology, diagnosis, management* (pp. 217–233). Philadelphia: B. C. Decker; and Stevenson, R. D., & Allaire, J. F. (1991). The development of normal feeding and swallowing. *Pediatric Clinics of North America, 38*(6), 1439–1453.

spoon feeding combined with finger feeding, and ultimately to independent cup drinking and utensil use (Ogg, 1975). The child must learn how to manipulate and process increasing higher textures of foods and safely coordinate respiration with swallowing activities. Transitional feeding is the term used to describe the intermediary steps from sucking to chewing, and encompasses the process of taking purees from a spoon (Stevenson & Allaire, 1991).

Stolovitz and Giesel (1991) described circumoral behaviors in normal children during the oral phase of ingestion. They summarized maturation of feeding behavior as characterized by better lip control, increased mobility of the tongue, and decreased involvement of the circumoral structures in swallowing. They examined the eating behaviors of 143 children aged 6 months to 2 years for responses to three different food textures (solid, viscous, and purees) by videotape and data analysis. They described circumoral structures during anticipation of food, removal of food from a spoon, and during initiation of chewing and swallowing.

The changes in oral motor patterns noted in feeding maturation are dependent on developmental changes in the central nervous system, a process referred to by Bosma (1986) as the encephalization of feeding. This is the mechanism "by which suprabulbar mechanisms become capable of utilizing the coordination resources of the medulla to accomplish qualitatively different performances" (p. 214). Feeding competence is achieved as sensory inputs to feeding are extended (via concomitant brain development) into midbrain, cerebellum, thalamus, and ultimately the cerebral cortex. The child thus acquires the capability to evaluate the physical character of food involuntarily ingested. Sensory input is utilized for the volitional phases of intraoral food preparation, sizing of the swallow, and initiation of swallow (Bosma, 1986). The physical apparatus of swallowing matures as well. This is extensively discussed in Chapter 1. Ultimately, physical growth, along with the eruption of teeth,

further allows the refinement of biting and chewing necessary to break food down into a manageable bolus.

Parallels to Motor Developmental Milestones

As many clinicians in the field of pediatric feeding and swallowing disorders have noted, development of a child's oral motor and feeding skills parallels general physical development, especially in the gross motor and fine motor spheres (Morris & Klein, 1987; Ogg, 1975; Ottenbacher et al., 1983). It is imperative for the clinician to assess the child's overall motor level, degree of mobility of upper extremities, and neurologic integrity of oral motor apparatus prior to evaluating a "feeding and swallowing" problem. The reader interested in theoretical perspective on "the connection between the mouth and body" is referred to Morris and Klein (1987) for an extensive discussion on the concepts of whole body stability and mobility, separation of movement planes, and midline development.

Although a full discussion of gross motor development and milestone acquisition is beyond the scope of this chapter (see Capute & Acardo, 1991), a review of a few general principles is warranted. Milestones are achieved through an orderly sequential unfolding of development, underscored by central nervous system maturation. Infants are born with a repertoire of "primitive" reflexes — stereotyped automatisms that are massive involuntary functional units. Over time, these primitive reflexes break down with maturation, giving way to postural reactions. These are best thought of as small units of patterned movement. The patterns work, through various recombinations and with emerging elements of volitional control, to sustain and support voluntary movement and activity. Regarding oral pharyngeal function and its relations to eating, Ogg (1975) summarized that the presence of whole body reflexive mechanisms denotes the level of development of the central nervous system of the child.

> With growth and the child's ability to assume an upright position, these reflexive responses fade and the child is able to participate voluntarily and actively in the event of eating. Abnormal persistence of primitive reflexes, however, interferes with the child's ability to eat normally (p. 240).

An evolution must take place from the infants' semi-recumbent flexed position with head in neutral position to an upright sitting position (approximately 6 months), and finally to unassisted stable chair sitting, for feeding to take place safely and efficiently (i.e., utilizing the forces of gravity in protecting the airway).

Perhaps the most important development related to motor function is control of the head and trunk (Ottenbacher et al., 1983). Feeding therapists have long noted that postural variation of the body, head, and neck affect the flow of food and liquid through the oropharynx (Fox 1990; Chapter 7). Poor postural alignment can exaggerate the expession of gross motor primitive reflex patterns and potentially interfere with progression of feeding skills. Head and trunk positioning can also impinge on expression of a child's muscle tone (see below), with implications for relationship of structures within the pharyngeal cavity (Fox, 1990).

The Role of Muscle Tone in Feeding Development

Muscle tone is an entity perhaps more easily described clinically than precisely quantified or defined. "Normal" muscle tone and general muscle integrity is, however, critical to feeding and swallowing tasks. Abnormality of muscle tone such as hypertonus, hypotonus, or fluctuating muscle tone can affect a child's ability to open and close the mouth, swallow, or maintain an upright position to take food

(Ogg, 1975). Ottenbacher et al. (1983) noted that, to qualify as "normal," muscle tone "must be high enough to allow the individual to resist gravity, but low enough that the individual can move through it" (p. 10). Most clinicians would agree that there is a continuum of muscle tone from too low to too high, with normal falling somewhere in the middle.

Oral motor dysfunctions common to all abnormalities of muscle tone include drooling, poor oral exploration and/or selective movement, the inability to initiate, grade, or sustain oral patterns, and potential impingement on breathing coordination (Ottenbacher et al., 1983). Specifically, children with hypertonus tend toward marked extensor patterns involving the head, trunk, and extremities. Such patterns and resultant spasms can limit oral movements and/or be associated with abnormal oral motor patterns, including jaw and tongue thrusting and lip retraction. These would result in inefficient chewing and swallowing processes. The facial expression of a child with hypertonicity changes slowly, may be restricted in range, and is often exaggerated in its final state (e.g., the "hung up" or "ear to ear" smile of the spastic child) (Ogg, 1975). Children with fluctuating tone (e.g., athetoid individuals) may have a more mobile facial expression, but they may be unable to balance respiration with feeding, grade jaw movements, coordinate sucking, swallowing, biting, and chewing (Ottenbacher et al., 1983). Hypotonic individuals may lack the ability to maintain head and trunk postural stability, impinging on respiratory ability. Low tone may also impinge as well on ability to initiate or sustain suck-swallow and subsequent food manipulation.

The Role of Tactile Sensitivity

Feeding patterns and the learning of skills necessary for progression of food manipulation can be influenced by sensation and sensory feedback. As Stevenson and Al-laire (1991) noted, this aspect of the learning experience involves processing of information related to proprioception, touch, pressure, food temperature, and taste. Normal sensory processes can be thought of as combining appropriate ability of sensory organs to receive input, appropriate "gating" of the information that is being processed by the brain, and the brain's ability to interpret and act on the received sensory message (Morris & Klein, 1987). Deviations from these areas can disrupt the feeding process, as exemplified in children who exhibit tactile hypersensitivity and feeding aversion.

In "normal" development, early exploratory mouthing of feet, hands, and toys may help set the stage for later feeding experiences (Stevenson & Allaire, 1991). Such exploration can act to appropriately "desensitize" the child to later incoming stimuli (i.e., food) and diminish the potential for a child to react aversively as higher textures are introduced. According to Ottenbacher, Bundy, and Short (1983), the oral structures most likely involved in sensory play are the tongue and lips. Tactile hypersensitivity in children may be manifested as a strong and negative reaction to stimuli on the face and in the mouth. It has been postulated that there is a stronger reaction, a "hyperreaction," to a specific stimuli than would be expected (Morris & Klein, 1987). A hypersensitive child may be viewed as having a lowering of the sensory threshold. The multiple stimuli inherent in the feeding and swallowing process can then create an uncomfortable experience for such a child, whose system cannot cope with too much sensory information.

Tactile hypersensitivity is seen with significant frequency in children with multiple handicaps, especially those with physical and cognitive impairments that might lead to a lack of oral experience. Certainly, many clinicians who care for infants who are exclusively supplemental tube fed (and hence lack in oral feeding experience) report exaggerated oral tactile sensitivity (Milla, 1991). Perhaps, as Stevenson and Allaire (1991) implied, lack of early mouthing exploratory activity in some children with motor disabilities (physically unable to bring objects to their mouth or locomote to furniture) causally relates to their oral hypersensitivity. Whether such children exhibit tactile hypersensitivity secondary to an aberrant feeding experience or a "missed timing" during a critical period is an intriguing, but rather unprovable, line of speculation.

References

Bosma, J. F. (1986). Development of feeding. *Clinical Nutrition, 5,* 210–218.

Capute, A. S., & Accardo, P. J. (1991). *Developmental disabilities in infancy and childhood.* Baltimore: Paul H. Brookes.

DiScippio, W., Kaslon, K., & Ruben, R. (1978). Traumatically acquired conditioned dysphagia in children. *Annals of Otology, Rhinology, and Laryngology, 87,* 509.

DiScippio, W., & Kaslon, Kr. (1982). Conditioned dysphagia in cleft palate children after pharyngeal flap surgery. *Psycho Medicine, 44,* 247.

Fox, C. A. (1990). Implementing the modified barium swallow evaluation in children who have multiple disabilities. *Infants and Young Children, 3*(2), 67–77.

Illingworth, R. S., & Lister, J. (1964). The critical or sensitive period, with special reference to certain feeding problems in infants and children. *The Journal of Pediatrics, 65*(6), 839–848.

Milla, P. J. (1991). Feeding, tasting, and sucking. In W. A. Walker et al. (Eds.), *Pediatric gastrointestinal disease — Pathophysiology, diagnosis, management* (pp. 217–233). Philadelphia: B. C. Decker.

Morris, S. E., & Klein, M. D. (1987). Pre-feeding skills. *A comprehensive resource for feeding development.* Tucson, AZ: Therapy Skill Builders.

Ogg, H. L. (1975). Oral-pharyngeal development and evaluation. *Physical Therapy, 55*(3), 235–241.

Orenstein, S. R., Bergman, I., Proujansky, R., Kocoslis, S., & Giarusso, V. S. (1992). Swallowing reflex: Facial receptor distribution and stimulus characteristics. *Dysphagia, 7,* 150–154.

Orenstein, S. R., Santmeyer, Varusso, V., Proujansky, R., & Kocoslis, S. (1988). The Santmeyer swallow: A new and useful infant reflex. *Lancet, i,* 345–346.

Ottenbacher, K., Bundy, A., & Short, M. A. (1983). The development and treatment of oral-motor dysfunction: A review of clinical research. *Physical and Occupational Therapy in Pediatrics, 3*(2), 1–13.

Singer, L. (1990). When a sick child won't — or can't — eat. *Contemporary Pediatrics, 12/90,* 60–76.

Stevenson, R. D., & Allaire, J. H. (1991). The development of normal feeding and swallowing. *Pediatric Clinics of North America, 38*(6), 1439–1453.

Stolovitz, P., & Giesel, E. G. (1991). Circumoral movements in response to three different food textures in children 6 months to 2 years of age. *Dysphagia, 6,* 17–25.

Tuchman, D. (1991). Oro-pharyngeal and esophageal complications of enteral tube feeding. In S. S. Baker, R. D. Baker, & A. Davis (Eds.), *Pediatric enteral nutrition.* Boston: Andover Medical Publishers.

Neurology of Deglutition

3

CHAPTER

Rebecca N. Ichord, M.D.

The neurologic substrate for feeding behavior involves virtually all neuronal systems in a highly integrated manner which evolves from instinct-driven reflexive behavior in the newborn to socially sensitive, highly modulated behavior in the adult. The neurologic basis for ingestion, chewing, and swallowing comprises an essential core for more complex feeding behaviors, and will be the focus of this chapter, which reviews the structure and function of the neurologic systems controlling deglutition and discusses how neurologic and neuromuscular disorders in infants and children disrupt these systems, leading to feeding disorders. The neurologic evaluation of children with feeding and swallowing disorders will be described.

Neuroanatomic Substrate of Deglutition

Deglutition is best understood as a specialized example of motor control. It is composed of three phases: oral, pharyngeal, and esophageal (Miller, 1986). The exercise of this system involves a dynamic interplay of descending motor tracts (afferent) and ascending sensory tracts (efferent) which are integrated or modulated at mul-

tiple sites en route (Figure 3–1). Corticospinal and corticobulbar (pyramidal) tracts carry inputs from cortical motor centers in the frontal lobe, subject to continual modulation from basal ganglia and cerebellum via the thalamus. In the case of deglutition, descending motor tracts converge on central pattern generators in the lower brainstem, which integrate activity in multiple cranial nerve motor nuclei to effect ingestion, chewing, sucking, and swallowing in proper synchrony with respiration. The motor cranial nerves (CNs) participating in deglutition include: motor trigeminal (CN V) for muscles of mastication; facial (CN VII) for oral and buccal muscles; glossopharyngeal (CN IX) and vagus (CN X) for muscles of the palate, pharynx, esophagus, larynx, and respiratory control centers; and hypoglossal (CN XII) for the intrinsic muscles of the tongue. Cortical and subcortical motor systems such as cerebellum and basal ganglia play an important role in maintaining postural stability and head position through the spinal accessory nerve (CN XI) and cervical spinal cord segments controlling neck muscles.

Ascending sensory tracts reflexively evoke motor programs via the central pattern generator and provide continual feedback to modulate the descending motor

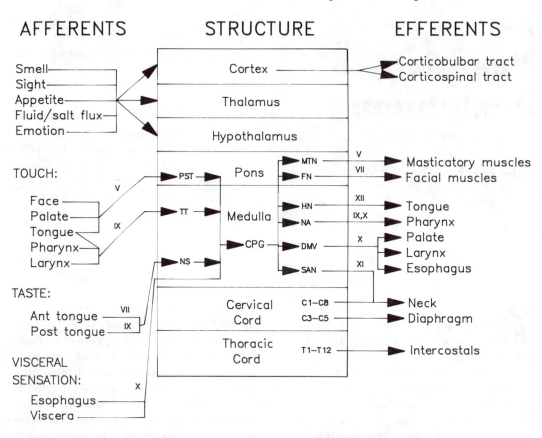

FIGURE 3-1. Neuroanatomy of deglutition. PST, principal sensory nucleus of the trigeminal nerve; TT, tract of the trigeminal nerve; NS, nucleus solitarius; CPG, central pattern generator for swallowing; MTN, motor nucleus of the trigeminal nerve; FN, facial nucleus; HN, hypoglossal nucleus; NA, nucleus ambiguus; DMV, dorsal motor nucleus of the vagus; SAN, spinal accessory nucleus.

systems. Sensation from the face and anterior tongue travels via the trigeminal nerve to the spinal trigeminal tract in the upper cervical cord and main trigeminal sensory nucleus in the pons. Sensation from the posterior tongue, palate, pharynx, larynx, and viscera travels via the glossopharyngeal and vagus nerves. Taste sensation is conducted by the trigeminal and glossopharyngeal nerves to the nucleus solitarius in the medulla. Sensory inputs also arise from neck muscles and joints, via cervical segmental pathways, and from vestibular organs via the brainstem to provide information regarding head position. Head posture is critical in maintaining orientation toward the food source, optimizing swallow efficiency, and allowing for airway protection. Ad-

ditional influences on the threshold for reflexively evoked deglutition derive from visceral sensations, via the autonomic nervous system, and from hypothalamic centers which regulate appetite and homeostatic functions (thirst, hunger, temperature, fluid/salt balance).

Neurophysiology of Deglutition

In general, the execution of movement patterns involves integration of sensory and motor pathways in a hierarchy of circuits which expands as the complexity of the task grows. The most elementary integration occurs at the level of motor neurons, where excitatory and inhibitory inputs converge, combining the effects of simple reflex arcs with those of more distant modulating centers. In the case of deglutition, considerable integration occurs in the brainstem. Data from animal and human clinical studies support the existence of central pattern generators (CPG) for swallowing (Dodds, 1989; Kennedy & Kent, 1988). These groups of interneurons located on each side of the medulla, in the vicinity of the nucleus solitarius and nucleus ambiguous, generate the complex sequence of semiautomatic movements that constitute the "program" for swallowing. There are likely several components of the CPG, each specializing in a different phase of swallowing, including the oral, pharyngeal, and esophageal phases. The CPG generates reflexively initiated swallowing as a result of stimulation of specific sensory fields and integrates voluntary or learned patterns of feeding behavior arising from higher cortical centers. The CPG is located in close proximity to respiratory control centers in the medulla, which allows for synchrony among initiation of swallowing, closure of the glottis, and inhibition of respiration during the pharyngeal phase of swallowing.

Deglutition begins with the oral or preparatory phase. In the newborn and young infant, this is reflexively driven through stimulation of rooting and suckling behaviors. In older infants and children, the oral phase comes under voluntary control from higher cortical centers and involves mastication and more complex learned patterns of jaw, tongue, and mouth movement in preparing the food bolus for swallowing. As chewing is completed, the jaw is stabilized; and the tongue in coordination with the soft palate propels the bolus toward the pharynx, initiating the "program" for swallowing. Timing of the pharyngeal phase of swallowing depends in part on sensory input from the posterior tongue, palate, and tonsillar pillars. The pharyngeal phase is a complex sequence of semiautomatic movements which accomplishes several things: closure of the mouth and nasal and laryn-

geal passages to prevent aspiration, opening the upper esophageal sphincter by elevation and anterior displacement of the larynx, and generating a pressure gradient to propel the bolus toward the esophageal opening.

The esophageal phase involves another complex sequence of now almost entirely automatic movements (Dodds, 1989; Miller, 1986). At rest, the upper esophageal sphincter (UES) tone is maintained by continuous background central neural input, whereas lower esophageal sphincter (LES) tone is based primarily on intrinsic smooth muscle activity. Swallowing involves a wave of inhibition resting sphincter tone, followed by an orderly march of peristaltic contraction. Relaxation of the UES is believed to involve an inhibition of background central neural inputs to the pharyngeal and upper esophageal constrictor muscles, whereas relaxation of the LES is believed to involve activation of local autonomic neurons which release a hyperpolarizing neurotransmitter, thereby inhibiting the intrinsic tone of the smooth muscle. Esophageal motility during swallowing is comprised of primary and secondary components. Primary peristalsis is activated as part of the centrally regulated swallowing program. Secondary peristalsis is initiated and sustained by the presence of a bolus in the esophagus, and is believed to be mediated by a combination of intrinsic contractile properties of esophageal smooth muscle and central modulation via autonomic sensory feedback circuits.

Cortical inputs are critical in controlling the sequential interaction of facial, tongue, sucking, and chewing movements with the CPG for swallowing to achieve functional feeding behavior. Cortical inputs, such as might occur when experiencing hunger, or the sight or smell of food, also modify the threshold of reflexively evoked swallowing.

Reflexively initiated swallowing may be elicited from a variety of receptive fields, with stimulus-response characteristics specific to each field, and thus each phase of swallowing (Miller, 1986). Stimulation of the posterior tongue, oropharynx, pharynx, and larynx can all evoke swallowing. Slowly adapting pressure receptors predominate in the tongue and oropharynx, which allows for initial management of size, shape, and texture of the food bolus necessary during the oral phase of deglutition. While gustatory receptors predominate in the pharynx, the initiation of the pharyngeal phase of swallowing is heavily dependent on sensory feedback relaying information about pressure and muscle activity during the oral phase. Cortical inputs influence the threshold for the pharyngeal phase of swallowing, but are less important during this more automatic movement pattern than during the oral phase. In the larynx, water receptors are most sensitive in eliciting swallowing. Thus salivary output influences the threshold for swallowing. The esophageal phase of swallowing follows almost automatically from the pharyngeal phase, but its duration and intensity are dependent on continuous sensory feedback as to the size, texture, and location of the bolus in the esophagus. Combining stimuli over several receptive fields and in varied modalities enhances the effectiveness of eliciting swallowing.

The development of the neurophysiologic mechanisms for deglutition is poorly understood. Animal studies suggest that the stimulus-response characteristics of the central pattern generators evolve gradually, beginning prenatally and maturing postnatally (Miller, 1976). Human fetal studies have shown that feeding behavior in the newborn, although appearing to be reflexive, is in fact a complex motor program built from more elementary fragments (Humphrey, 1964). Cutaneous stimulation around the face and mouth of a fetus elicits fragments of movement — head orientation, jaw opening, lip closure, tongue movement, and swallowing — in a manner dependent on fetal maturity and the exact site and intensity of the stimulus. These "local reflexes" can be seen as early as 8 weeks of fetal life. It is not until near

term that local reflexes are integrated into the smoothly functioning sequences we recognize as rooting, sucking, and swallowing in proper synchrony with respiration. The timing and nature of cortical influences on deglutition during postnatal development are even less well understood. There appears to be a gradual transition during the first 3 years of life from primitive, reflexively driven suckling patterns to more complex, learned voluntary chewing patterns, particularly for the oral phase of deglutition (Bosma, 1985; Sheppard & Mysak, 1984).

Neurochemistry of Deglutition Pathways

Recent animal studies have shed some light on neurochemical regulatory mechanisms in brainstem regions involved in swallowing and respiration (Bieger, 1991; Sessle & Henry, 1989). Glutamate is the predominant excitatory neurotransmitter in the mammalian CNS. It occurs in high concentrations in the region of the nucleus solitarius (NS) and may serve as a neurotransmitter for primary afferent neuron projections to reflex interneurons and respiratory neurons. As such, it may mediate rapid-onset, short-duration afferent sensory signals important in reflexively initiated deglutition. Gamma-aminobutyric acid (GABA) is the most widely distributed inhibitory neurotransmitter and has been found in the region of the NS. It has been proposed that GABA neurons produce a tonic inhibition of deglutitive neurons in the central pattern generator, release from which allows initiation of the swallow synergy. GABA has also been implicated in the inhibition of respiration and other vegetative reflexes produced by muscle afferent fibers involved in deglutition, and by inhibitory hypothalamic inputs.

Central catecholaminergic pathways (dopamine and norepinephrine) appear to have a predominantly facilatory effect on central control centers for swallowing. Studies of serotonin suggest it plays a complex role, mediating activation of central swallowing centers from distant projections in one set of neurons, while producing negative modulation perhaps through local inhibitory interneurons. Acetylcholine plays an obvious critical role as the major transmitter at the neuromuscular junction, postganglionic transmission in the parasympathetic nervous system, and preganglionic transmission in both sympathetic and parasympathetic systems. Furthermore, cholinergic neurons have been shown to participate in the vagal motor efferents for swallowing arising in the region of the brainstem central pattern generator, and may be particularly active during the esophageal phase of swallowing.

A large number of neuropeptides have been found in the region of the NS. Substance P, a neuropeptide found in high concentrations in the NS, produces a delayed-onset, prolonged excitatory response in reflex interneurons. It is thought to act as a regulator of sensory afferent transmission in the medullary centers controlling swallowing and respiration. Opioid peptides, somatostatin, oxytocin and vasopressin are also present and active in central deglutitive mechanisms. Although their precise roles remain to be defined, their abundance and variable effects attest to a high degree of complexity in the brainstem regulatory mechanisms subserving deglutition and respiration.

The neurochemistry of central deglutitive pathways provides clues for the as yet unexplored problem of the clinical neuropharmacology of dysphagia. There are few examples of dysphagia in childhood which might shed some light on this problem. However, a number of adult disorders illustrate the possible relevance of neurochemical mechanisms in swallowing disorders. Dopaminergic antagonism produced by neuroleptics has been associated with a significant incidence of oral dyskinesia and dysphagia, lending support to the notion that dopamine plays a role in deglutition.

Patients with Parkinson's disease, in which there is a loss of dopaminergic neurons, frequently complain of dysphagia. Benzodiazepines, such as nitrazepam and clonazepam, which are GABA agonists, are known to depress swallowing activity, supporting a role for GABA-mediated inhibitory neurotransmission. The importance of opioid peptides is suggested by the altered swallowing and respiratory function resulting from acute morphine administration, and in morphine-dependent subjects. The neurochemistry of deglutition, particularly in known pathologic conditions, should continue to provide avenues of study with important pharmacotherapeutic implications.

Neurologic Disease in Childhood Causing Feeding Disorders

The neurologic basis of feeding disorders in childhood poses a multiplicity of problems for the clinicians caring for children with these disorders. First, in the case of the child with a known neurologic disorder, an understanding of the neurology may assist the clinician in analyzing the causes and designing treatment for the feeding problem. In the case of the child who presents with a feeding problem, in whom no specific neurologic disorder has been diagnosed, an understanding of the neurologic conditions that may present in this way may lead to a specific etiologic diagnosis and effective treatment. The following sections review neurologic and neuromuscular disorders in childhood that may cause disordered feeding and deglutition. These disorders are summarized in Table 3–1.

Diffuse Cortical Injury

Diffuse or multifocal dysfunction of the cerebral hemispheres has a multitude of causes and a wide spectrum of severity. These children may manifest a spectrum of neuro-

TABLE 3–1. Neurologic conditions of childhood associated with feeding disorders.

A. Diffuse or bilateral dysfunction of cortex or basal ganglia
　1. Static encephalopathy with neuromotor deficits
　　a. Prenatal onset: brain dysgenesis, in utero infections, in utero intoxications, chromosomal defects, cerebrovascular accidents
　　b. Perinatal onset: hypoxia-ischemia, hypoglycemia, complicated prematurity, CNS infection, cerebrovascular accidents
　　c. Postnatal onset: trauma, hypoxia-ischemia, CNS infection, hypoglycemia, intoxications, cerebrovascular accidents
　2. Progressive encephalopathy with neuromotor deficits
　　a. Metabolic: inborn errors of metabolism, Wilson's disease
　　b. Infectious/Post-infectious: SSPE, HIV
　　c. Demyelinating: multiple sclerosis
　　d. Other: juvenile Huntington's, Pelizeus-Merzbacher, post-irradiation, vasculitis, drug-induced movement disorders (neuroleptics, dilantin, reglan)
B. Brainstem
　1. Congenital CNS anomalies: Arnold-Chiari malformation, syringomyelia, Mobius anomaly, congenital varicella infection
　2. Skeletal dysplasias: dwarfism with foramen magnum stenosis, osteopetrosis, some craniosynostoses
　3. Malignancy: tumors of brainstem or posterior fossa
　4. Metabolic: mitochondrial encephalomyopathy
　5. Trauma: diffuse axonal injury
　6. Vascular: cerebrovascular accident, arteriovenous malformations
　7. Infection: brainstem encephalitis
　8. Demyelinating: multiple sclerosis
C. Cranial nerves
　1. Trauma: basilar skull fracture
　2. Motor neuron disease: spinal muscular atrophy, poliomyelitis, juvenile amyotrophic lateral sclerosis, progressive bulbar paralysis of childhood, facio-scapulohumeral neurogenic atrophy, congenital hypomyelination neuropathy)
　3. Tumors: schwannoma (neurofibromatosis)
　4. Demyelinating: Guillian-Barré syndrome (acute & chronic)
　5. Toxins: diphtheria, heavy metals
D. Neuromuscular junction
　1. Myasthenia gravis
　2. Drugs/Intoxications: botulism, organophosphate poisoning, tetanus, streptomycin, neomycin, kanamycin, bacitracin, polymyxin, colistin, Mg, beta blockers, phenothiazines, trimethaphan, methoxyflurane
E. Muscle
　1. Congenital: myotonic dystrophy, congenital muscular dystrophy, congenital myopathies
　2. Inflammatory: dermatomyositis, polymyositis
　3. Familial or metabolic: facioscapulohumeral dystrophy, mitochondrial encephalomyopathy, ocular muscular dystrophy, inborn errors of metabolism affecting muscle
　4. Endocrine: Hyper-, hypothyroidism; steroid myopathy
F. Esophageal motility
　1. Associated with CNS dysfunction: incoordination of pharyngeal and esophageal phases of swallowing, deficient central regulation of esophageal peristalsis
　2. Induced by reflux esophagitis
　3. Drug-induced: beta adrenergics, anticholinergics, muscle relaxants
　4. Associated with myopathies

motor, cognitive and behavioral deficits with highly variable effects on feeding and deglutition. Neuromotor impairment from cerebral cortical dysfunction may disturb the feeding and swallowing apparatus at multiple levels:

1. Damaged corticobulbar and corticospinal pathways, interfering with the careful orchestration of voluntary facial, oral, tongue and chewing movements necessary for the oral phase of swallowing;

2. Abnormal cortical modulation of reflexively initiated components of deglutition, leading, for example, to hyperactive or hypoactive gag and airway protective reflexes;

3. Failure of inhibition by cortical centers of maladaptive tone patterns and primitive reflexes, interfering with the postural control necessary for efficient feeding;

3. Failure of modulation of voluntary movement by extrapyramidal systems (basal ganglia, cerebellum), leading, for example to bradykinesia, rigidity, or intrusive involuntary movements such as chorea and dystonia.

Cerebral palsy encompasses children with a static disorder of brain function causing deficits in the control of movement and posture. Severe neuromotor impairments in the child with handicapping cerebral palsy present obvious problems for feeding, which may affect any or all phases of deglutition (Kenny, Casas, & McPherson, 1989; Morris, 1989). Most often there are multiple deficits, including poor postural control of head position; defective or delayed patterns of oral, buccal and lingual elements of the oral phase; poor timing and sequencing of the pharyngeal phase; and esophageal dysmotility.

Many children with mild neuromotor dysfunction of a static, developmental nature, present with feeding disorders that pose management challenges (Mathisen, Reilly, & Skuse, 1992; Mathisen, Skuse, Wolke, & Reilly, 1989). Typically, their abnormalities in deglutition are less pervasive, and are more apparent in the complex, learned voluntary patterns of the oral phase. The spectrum of mild neuromotor dysfunction includes infants with mild motor developmental delays and a mildly abnormal neuromotor exam. In some cases, feeding and respiratory problems predominate in the early months. Over time, the tone problems often improve, although motor development may continue to be delayed, and with this the feeding problems improve. It is likely that many of these children have deficiencies in the cortical inputs to the voluntary or learned components of oral, pharyngeal and laryngeal control which manifest early as delays and inefficiencies in feeding skills. Such infants often later have delays and inefficiencies in speech-motor function. The precise etiology of the cortical dysfunction has little direct bearing on the course of the feeding disorder. The timing of the insult and the capacity for recovery of preexisting functions and for resumption of normal development are more important in determining prognosis (Christensen, 1989). For example, in trauma or tumor-related compression there is a greater chance for functional recovery than in the irreversible cell death or disruption of development which accompanies hypoxia-ischemia, hypoglycemia, or a highly dysgenic brain. Similarly, an acquired postnatal injury occurring in late infancy is much more likely to be followed by recovery of premorbid feeding skills than an early prenatal injury, where only the most rudimentary functions have developed and progress will be painfully slow.

There are rare conditions among children which cause progressive impairment of cortical or basal ganglia mechanisms of deglutition. Inborn errors of metabolism account for most neurodegenerative conditions in children. The precise biochemical defects are known for many of these conditions, and may be grouped as disorders of amino acid, urea cycle, peroxisomal, lysosomal, carbohydrate, fatty acid, and intermediate metabolism. Other neurodegenerative diseases are less well characterized. Those with prominent movement disorders are more likely to affect feeding and deglutition. These include Pelizeius-Merzbacher, dystonia muscularum deformans, juvenile Parkinson's disease, Halloverden-Spatz, juvenile-onset Huntington's chorea, and Wilson's disease. HIV encephalopathy is increasingly recognized as a cause of both static and progressive encephalopathy, and may evolve to spasticity, rigidity, or an extrapyramidal syndrome, usually with cognitive impairment. Multiple sclerosis is a chronic, progressive demyelinating condition with prominent involvement of brainstem and cerebellar tracts causing significant dysphagia, especially in advanced stages. It occurs rarely in childhood.

Drug-induced movement disorders that impair deglutition are important to identify because they are potentially reversible. The child with underlying neurologic dysfunction is more likely to develop such a complication, making diagnosis somewhat difficult. Drugs linked with the occurrence of movement disorders include neuroleptics (dystonia, oral-buccal-lingual dyskinesias), phenytoin (chorea, hyperkinesias), and metoclopramide (dystonias, Parkinsonism).

Brainstem Disorders

Neurologic disorders that predominantly affect the brainstem are relatively uncommon. The most common of these conditions encompass the myriad of brainstem and cervical cord abnormalities that occur in children with myelodysplasia. The majority of children with myelomeningocele can be shown to have an Arnold-Chiari malformation. This is a complex group of brainstem malformations which includes caudal displacement of the medulla and cerebellar tonsils through the foramen magnum. The most significant effects are dysphagia and apnea due to compression of the medullary centers and cranial nerves subserving swallowing and respiration. Many of these children develop syringomyelia (syrinx), which is expansion of the central canal of the spinal cord, sometimes extend-

ing into the lower brainstem. A syrinx may further compromise brainstem and lower cranial nerve dysfunction in a child with an Arnold-Chiari anomaly. Decompensated hydrocephalus in children with myelomeningocele may cause a latent Arnold-Chiari malformation and/or syrinx to become overtly symptomatic. Other congenital anomalies of brainstem cranial nerve nuclei involved in deglutition include Mobius anomaly (absent CN VI and VII) and congenital varicella.

Skeletal dysplasias are known to cause high cervical cord compression and, in some cases, to lower medullary compression because of bony stenosis. The combination of mechanical and neurogenic abnormalities in oropharyngeal and respiratory control may lead to feeding, swallowing and respiratory symptoms in children with achondroplasia and other dwarfism syndromes.

Disorders of brainstem function may be caused by variety of pathogenic events. Stroke or arteriovenous malformations, diffuse axonal injury due to trauma, viral encephalitis or postinfectious demyelinating disorders have all been described. Certain forms of mitochondrial encephalopathies, formerly known as Leigh's disease, have a predilection for the highly energy-dependent nuclei in the brainstem, producing prominent dysphagia and abnormalities in respiratory control. The majority of primary brain tumors in children occur in the subtentorial compartment. Masses in the cerebellum or fourth ventricle compromise brainstem function to a variable degree depending on the site and degree of compression. Intrinsic brainstem tumors are more ominous because they are less amenable to surgical excision, and they directly invade important functional centers.

Cranial Nerve Disorders

Disorders that selectively impair cranial nerves are relatively rare causes of dysphagia in children. Trauma leading to basilar skull fracture, although relatively common, only infrequently involves the jugular foramen (CN IX, X, XI) or hypoglossal canal (CN XII). The jugular foramen syndrome (Vernet's syndrome) is characterized by ipsilateral trapezius and sternocleidomastoid paresis and atrophy (CN XI), dysphonia, dysphagia, depressed gag reflex, ipsilateral palatal and vocal cord weakness, ipsilateral loss of taste on the posterior third of the tongue, and ipsilateral anesthesia of the posterior third of the tongue, soft palate, uvula, pharynx, and larynx (CN IX and X). Tumors may selectively invade cranial nerves, primarily schwannomas in patients with neurofibromatosis. These may be solitary, as in acoustic neuromas affecting the eighth cranial nerve with some secondary mass effects on cranial nerves V and VII in the region of the cerebellar-pontine angle; or multiple and bilateral anywhere along the brainstem. Demyelinating disease in the form of Guillain-Barre syndrome may, in its more fulminant form, affect cranial nerves and autonomic nerves subserving swallowing. Toxins that selectively impair peripheral nerves leading to dysphagia, among other symptoms of neuropathy, include diphtheria and heavy metal ingestion. Congenital hypomyelination neuropathy is a rare condition presenting at birth with diffuse weakness and areflexia, in which bulbar dysfunction dominates the early course. The pathological findings are distinguished by the absence of myelin around cranial and peripheral nerves.

Diseases that affect motor neurons predominantly are important causes of dysphagia in adults. Although uncommon in children, they are important to identify because of their progressive or familial features. The most important of these disorders affecting children is spinal muscular atrophy, a progressive degeneration of anterior horn cells causing flaccid weakness and muscle atrophy and fasciculations. The infantile forms usually have their onset before 6 months of age and progress relentlessly to ultimately involve cranial motor nerves subserving deglutition. Less severe forms of spinal muscular atrophy, often with a later onset and slower progression, may not include feeding problems prominently in their symptomatology.

Several other degenerative disorders of motor neurons have been described in children. A juvenile form of amyotrophic lateral sclerosis with onset in adolescence produces progressive lower motor neuron degeneration, particularly of lower brainstem cranial nerves and cervical cord, along with corticospinal tract degeneration (Nelson & Prensky, 1972). Bulbar dysfunction is a prominent part of the symptomatology, beginning early in the course of this disease. Progressive bulbar paralysis of childhood (Fazio-Londe disease) is a degenerative disorder of cranial motor neurons, predominantly affecting cranial nerves VII and XII (Alexander, Emery, & Koerner, 1976). It is probably genetically determined, with variable age of onset and course. The pathology resembles spinal muscular atrophy (SMA), and it is viewed by some as a variant of SMA. Facioscapulohumeral neurogenic atrophy is a familial disorder causing lower motor neuron weakness and atrophy in the distribution of the face, neck and shoulders. Poliomyelitis causes bulbar paralysis in a minority of patients infected, and still deserves consideration in populations lacking complete primary immunization (Buchholz & Jones, 1991).

Diseases of Muscle and Neuromuscular Junction

Disorders of the neuromuscular junction fall under the general clinical category of myasthenic syndromes. A variety of inherited or autoimmune-mediated defects in cholinergic (Ach) transmission in striated muscle leads to use-related weakness. Although uncommon in children (1% of myasthenics are children), its recognition may lead to definitive treatment and in some cases nearly complete remission of symptoms. There are forms with neonatal and juvenile onset. Transient neonatal myasthenia gravis occurs in infants of mothers with autoimmune myasthenia, due to the presence of circulating maternal anti-AChreceptor antibodies, and resolves in weeks to months. Persistent neonatal myasthenia develops within hours to days of birth, and may be due to an acquired autoimmune mechanism (anti-ACh-receptor antibodies) or a nonautoimmune hereditary defect in acetylcholine metabolism. Patients with neonatal myasthenic syndromes have generalized weakness, prominent ptosis and ophthalmoplegia, with weak suck, dysphagia, and respiratory insufficiency dominating the clinical problems. Juvenile myasthenia gravis is most often immune-mediated, with onset after age 5 years. Weakness is patchy and variable, most commonly including ptosis, ophthalmoplegia, and facial weakness, but sparing pupillary responses. Dysphagia is a troubling symptom at the peak of symptomatology. A variety of systemic conditions have been reported in patients with acquired myasthenia gravis. These include hyper- and hypothyroidism, rheumatoid arthritis, lupus erythematosus, leukemia, neuroblastoma, and trimethadione administration.

Botulism is produced by a bacterial toxin that blocks acetylcholine release at the neuromuscular junction. Onset of symptoms may be rapid or insidious, characterized by progressive bulbar and spinal lower motor neuron weakness. Although generalized weakness is present, it is usually the occurrence of progressive feeding and swallowing dysfunction and respiratory insufficiency that brings an infant or young child to medical attention. Careful examination usually demonstrates more pervasive evidence of neuromuscular junction dysfunction, including ptosis, ophthalmoplegia, pupillary abnormalities, and symmetric facial weakness. The treatment is supportive and recovery is variable over a period of months.

A number of drugs have been reported to induce a myasthenic syndrome of weakness (see Table 3–1). There is bulbar and peripheral weakness, including pupillary responses, with variable dysphagia,

dysarthria, and respiratory insufficiency. The onset of anesthetic-related myasthenic syndromes often occurs postoperatively, following the use of neuromuscular blocking anesthetic agents (succinylcholine, tubocurarine). In contrast to true myasthenia, intravenous calcium administration is most effective in treating these conditions.

Primary muscle diseases with congenital or infantile onset frequently cause feeding and swallowing problems. Myotonic dystrophy (neonatal onset), congenital myopathies, and congenital muscular dystrophies present in the newborn period with generalized hypotonia and weakness. Bulbar weakness leading to weak suck, dysphagia, and respiratory insufficiency is a prominent part of the clinical symptomatology in cases with a severe neonatal onset. Less common variants of these myopathies may present later in infancy or childhood, with less severe feeding and respiratory problems. In most cases, the course is one of gradual improvement; in others it is static or slowly progressive. Central nervous system abnormalities frequently coexist with congenital muscle disease, giving rise to cognitive deficiency and seizures which may further complicate the acquisition of feeding and swallowing skills. The classic muscular dystrophies of childhood, X-linked Duchenne's and Becker's muscular dystrophy, usually spare oropharyngeal musculature so that feeding difficulties do not appear until late in the course of the disease.

A large number of metabolic muscle diseases have been described in which inborn errors of metabolism involve the lysosomal, cytosolic, or mitochondrial enzymes necessary for efficient energy production. The age of onset and spectrum of clinical signs are protean in these diseases. Many follow a stuttering or relentlessly downhill course, and may affect central nervous systems as well. Dysphagia and feeding difficulties will be most prominent in cases with a generalized neonatal onset or rapid progression during infancy. Inflammatory muscle diseases (dermatomyositis, polymyositis) occasionally cause dysphagia in combination with progressive limb girdle and axial weakness, muscle pain, and evidence of autoimmune disease in other organ systems (skin, joints, kidneys). These diseases may occur within the context of some other primary connective tissue disease, such as rheumatoid arthritis or systemic lupus erythematosus.

Esophageal Motility Disorders

Disorders of esophageal motility may exist with or without more generalized nervous system or striated muscle disease. Pharyngeal and esophageal manometry have been used in attempts to classify esophageal dysmotility in adults in whom subjective symptoms dominate the clinical picture (DiPalma & Meyer, 1987). This approach is limited in children by the technical difficulties of performing manometry (Tuchman, 1989) and inability to define subjective symptoms beyond global behaviors (regurgitation, irritability, food refusal, anorexia). It is further confounded by the variability in the normal development of esophageal motility and esophageal sphincter function during infancy. Nonetheless, studies over the past 10 years have yielded important observations.

Disorders of esophageal motility frequently coexist with gastroesophageal reflux, which may further be complicated by reflux esophagitis (Cucchiara et al., 1986). The disturbed lower esophageal motility associated with reflux esophagitis resolves with treatment of the esophagitis in infants with intact or minimally abnormal CNS function. In children with moderate-to-severe CNS abnormalities, esophageal dysmotility may persist after esophagitis resolves and may involve incoordination of pharyngeal and esophageal phases or deficient central regulation of the esophageal peristalsis (Staiano, Cucchiara, De Vizia, Andreotti, & Auricchio, 1987; Staiano, Cucchiara, Del Giudice, Andreotti, & Minella, 1991). The frequent occurrence of chronic lung disease or severe spasticity in these patients may further confound the picture because of the effects of drugs used to treat the lung disease (beta adrenergics, anticholinergics) or spasticity (muscle relaxants). Children with myopathies may have disordered swallowing because of direct involvement of esophageal smooth muscle, as well as esophageal striated muscle elements which initiate the esophageal phase of deglutition.

Neurologic Evaluation of Children with Feeding and Swallowing Disorders

Goals

The broad goals of the neurologic evaluation of children with feeding and swallowing disorders center on assessment of the integrity of nervous system's function and state of development. If a neurodevelopmental abnormality is found, the next steps are to determine where in the neuraxis the deficiencies exist ("where is the lesion?") and under what circumstances the problem arose. Determining these factors provides the basis for a rational approach to diagnosing the cause(s) for the disorder and describing the specific mechanisms by which the deglutitive apparatus might be disturbed. Specific neurologic and developmental diagnoses then allow a rational approach to treatment. In some cases, a definitive neurologic treatment is available, such as decompression of an Arnold-Chiari malformation or pharmacologic treatment for myasthenia gravis. In other cases, comprehensive neurodevelopmental diagnosis forms the basis for a comprehensive educational and habilitation program, which addresses feeding and swallowing in the context of overall function. The existence of a neurodevelopmental disorder strongly increases the probability of coexisting gastroesophageal reflux and esophagitis, which has distinct diagnostic and treatment implications. Finally, a specific neurodevelopmental diagnosis allows for rational family counseling as to long-term prognosis. Prognostic factors should play a role in decisions regarding technologically complex, life-prolonging, or medically risky therapies, which may commit the family and society to extreme financial burdens, or expose the child to pain or risk of further morbidity or mortality.

History

The history should include a detailed chronology of feeding and swallowing in the context of overall developmental skill acquisition. Detailed techniques for eliciting and analyzing neurodevelopmental history are available elsewhere, and are beyond the scope of this chapter. From the developmental and feeding history it should be possible to formulate several critical points:

1. Was the onset prenatal, perinatal, or postnatal?

2. If postnatal, is the course static or progressive?

3. If postnatal, was the onset attributable to a known process, such as head trauma, or not clearly caused by a known CNS injury?

4. If postnatal and of unknown cause, are there clues in the history pointing to a general category of disease?

Such clues may help to define the localization of the process. For example, the presence of seizures or cognitive deficits point to cortical involvement; the presence of involuntary movements with sparing of intelligence points to the basal ganglia; the occurrence of use-related fatigue and true weakness point to a disorder in the neuromuscular junction.

Other clues in the history may help define the nature of the process. For example, unremitting, progressive headache points to an intracranial space-occupying lesion; bulbar paralysis following an acute meningoencephalitis or other febrile illness should suggest an infectious etiology or postinfectious demyelinating process; acute unexplained encephalopathy with variable recovery and with unusual metabolic symptoms (e.g., hyperammonemia, ketosis, hypoglycemia) should raise the possibility of inborn errors of metabolism.

5. What is the developmental level of function in each of the major streams of development (cognitive, motor)?

This information is necessary for describing the nature (cognitive, motor) and severity of developmental handicaps, and has a direct bearing on treatment strategies for feeding disorders (see subsequent chapters on diagnosis and management).

The family history is important in identifying disorders with known patterns of inheritance (e.g., autosomal dominant myotonic dystrophy), and in identifying other family members whose examination may shed light on the diagnosis. A full three-generation pedigree is warranted in cases of undefined encephalopathies or suspected peripheral neuromuscular disease.

Examination

The history sets the stage for the physical examination. The general physical examination may provide clues to specific etiologies of neurologic abnormalities, such as multiple congenital anomalies or evidence of multisystem connective tissue disease. In the neurologic examination, the examiner should attempt to verify hypotheses raised by the history as to localization of neurologic disorders causing feeding and swallowing disorders. A simplified approach to localization is to try to determine if the dysfunction can be classified as (a) primarily motor, sensory, or both; and (b) if motor, primarily upper motor neuron (above the level of the primary motor neuron) or lower motor neuron (involving the motor neuron, neuromuscular junction, or muscle). In addition, particular attention should be given to examination of each of the cranial nerves subserving swallowing.

Assessment of cortical function is determined by age and developmental level of function. Level of consciousness, cognition, language, behavioral regulation, and visual fields should all be assessed. Evaluation of central motor control systems includes the evaluation of pyramidal tract function, which is primarily responsible for finely modulated voluntary movements, and extrapyramidal tract function, which is more involved with semiautomatic control of speed, direction, and the postural base for movement. Pyramidal tract dysfunction in children may manifest as a paucity of well-modulated, voluntarily directed movement, especially involving the limbs, along with spasticity, exaggerated deep tendon reflexes, and failure of inhibition of primitive reflexes. Extrapyramidal tract dysfunction may manifest as rigid hypertonicity; a paucity of well-modulated postural adaptations to voluntary movement; or the intrusion of involuntary movements such as chorea, tremor, and athetosis. Localizing dysfunction in the central motor control systems is possible if there are coexisting deficits pointing to a specific level in the neuraxis, for example, a visual field cut pointing to a cortical injury or multiple pontine cranial nerve deficits pointing to a brainstem lesion. In most cases of severe, static neuromotor dysfunction in children, the site of the neurologic injury is in fact extensive, involving multiple cortical and subcortical central motor systems.

Isolated brainstem abnormalities should suggest a different set of entities (see preceding section). Careful cranial nerve examination allows assessment of each level of the brainstem: CNs III and IV, the midbrain; CNs V, VI, VII, and VIII, the pons and ponto-medullary junction; CNs IX, X, XI, and XII, the medulla. The cranial nerves subserving deglutition deserve special attention. The trigeminal nerve (CN V) is assessed by testing touch and pain sensation in each of the major divisions (ophthalmic,

maxillary, mandibular) and muscles of mastication (chewing and jaw movement). The facial nerve (CN VII) is assessed by observing facial movement: brow elevation, eyelid closure, labial movement during emotional expression, and lip closure and buccal movement during feeding and speech. The glossopharyngeal nerve is best tested by eliciting the gag reflex with tactile stimulation on each side of the pharynx. In the older cooperative patient, taste can be tested over the anterior (CN VII) and posterior (CN IX) aspects of the tongue.

Motor function of the vagus nerve (CN X) may be assessed by observing the resting position and elicited movement of the palate, and observing the phonation and airway protective reflexes (the efferent arc of the gag reflex and coughing) in addition to direct examination of the pharyngeal and esophageal phases of swallowing. The spinal accessory nerve (CN XI) is tested by evaluating neck flexors (sternocleidomastoid) and shoulder elevation. Unilateral sternocleidomastoid weakness will cause weakness of turning the head with chin toward the opposite side. Hypoglossal nerve (CN XII) lesions cause the tongue to protrude toward the weak side. A nuclear or lower motor neuron lesion of the hypoglossal nerve causes marked tongue atrophy, weakness, and fasciculations; whereas an upper motor lesion leads to a paucity, or poor modulation, of the complex sequences of tongue movement necessary for speech and for the oral phase of deglutition, without causing atrophy.

A more general disturbance of medullary function may lead to a lack of integration of the multiple sensory and motor elements necessary for deglutition. This may be evident on simple bedside observation of voluntary oropharyngeal movements such as speech, cough, or swallow. Precise analysis of the deficits in integration or the impact of multiple cranial nerve abnormalities on deglutition requires good videofluoroscopy with a specialist trained in the developmentally specific patterns of oropharyngeal function in infants and children.

Examination for signs of muscle disease should focus on observation of functional skills. Ptosis and deficits in eye movements are common in diseases of muscle and neuromuscular junction that produce dysphagia. Facial weakness may be apparent as a paucity of emotional expression, inability to bury the eyelashes on eye closure, weakness of pursing the lips or of maintaining a tight seal of the lips against forced air expulsion. Truncal musculature can be assessed by watching the child's ability to maintain posture against gravity, either spontaneously or with provocative maneuvers such as pull-to-sit or prone suspension. Limb weakness is best detected by observation of spontaneous movement. An infant with true limb weakness will have difficulty generating sufficient power to lift the limbs against gravity from a supine position. Older children may be unable to match the power of the examiner in maintaining arms abducted and elevated, or in performing a wheelbarrow maneuver (weight-bearing on outstretched arms while the examiner holds the feet). Proximal hip girdle weakness may be evident in the difficulty a child has in rising to stand from a low seated position or in coming to a stand from supine. The gait may be waddling and slow. Muscle bulk may be normal, diminished, or show pseudohypertrophy. Deep tendon reflexes are usually present although diminished in muscle disease, whereas they are absent in neuropathies.

Supplementary Studies

The use of laboratory and x-ray studies should be guided by clinical data on an individualized basis. History and physical findings should generate a reasonably limited list of probable diagnoses as to localization in the neuraxis and etiology. In some cases, the cause and localization are very clear, such as in the case of post-traumatic or post-hypoxic-ischemic diffuse brain injury. In these cases, extensive neuroimaging or laboratory testing adds very little to management or prognosis. If a developmental brain anomaly, tumor, Arnold-Chiari malformation, or neurodegenerative disease is suspected, neuroimaging studies should be done. In cases of static encephalopathy of presumed perinatal onset, neuroimaging may demonstrate unsuspected prenatal-onset developmental anomalies. This information may be helpful to parents searching for complete answers and prognosis, but will have little direct practical effect on managing the feeding or swallowing problems.

Magnetic resonance imaging (MRI) will be the study of choice in most cases for several reasons: (1) it is more sensitive to subtle developmental anomalies such as pachygyria; (2) it is the only way to clearly define brainstem, posterior fossa and cervicomedullary junction; and (3) it is superior to CT in defining white matter abnormalities associated with degenerative diseases or perinatal injury. Its disadvantage is the need for deep sedation for a study taking 20 to 30 minutes, as compared to 10 to 15 minutes for computerized tomography. Children with dysphagia may be particularly at risk for airway or respiratory compromise with this kind of sedation, so appropriate precautions must be taken to monitor and support these children during and after the study. Children with neuromuscular disease may have marginal pulmonary reserve at best, and could decompensate with sedation. If neuromuscular disease is being considered for a given child, it would be prudent to perform the appropriate diagnostic studies for muscle disease before subjecting a child to sedation for an MRI. Laboratory studies should also be tailored to specific diagnostic hypotheses raised by the history and physical examination. The studies one does for mental retardation of probable prenatal onset would be quite distinct from those for suspected inborn errors of metabolism. A full discussion of the laboratory work-up of childhood neurologic diseases is beyond the scope of this chapter, and may be found in more comprehensive texts.

The use of electrophysiologic studies in evaluating children with feeding and swallowing disorders is central to the diagnosis of diseases of peripheral nerve, neuromuscular junction and muscle. Electromyography (EMG) and nerve conduction studies (NCV) are very challenging to perform and interpret in children, particularly in infants, even in the best of hands. In the ideal circumstance, the electrophysiologist would be a clinician skilled in evaluating neuromuscular disease in infants and children and would determine, based on a clinical evaluation, which studies to perform and how to interpret them. EMG of the muscles of deglutition is rarely available outside of a research setting, and rarely is necessary to determine that neuromuscular disease is the cause of the swallowing disorder. In some cases of suspected neuromuscular disease in an infant, electrophysiologic study of family members may be definitive. In many cases of suspected peripheral nerve or muscle disease, a nerve and muscle biopsy is necessary for definitive diagnosis. This should be given strong consideration in cases with potentially definitive, although risky, treatments (steroids for inflammatory myopathies), or lethal outcomes (spinal muscular atrophy).

Brainstem auditory evoked responses (BAER) are sometimes considered in children with suspected brainstem dysfunction. The usefulness of BAERs in studying dysphagia is limited by the fact that they sample only auditory pathways, which traverse above the cranial nerve and swallowing centers in the medulla. These studies may be useful in defining other sites of white matter lesions not detected clinically or by MRI in cases of suspected multiple sclerosis. Outside of this application, and in the assessment of auditory function, BAERs add little to the evaluation of children with disorders of deglutition. Similarly, the electroencephalography (EEG) is useful in evaluating seizure disorders and some cases of suspected neurodegenerative diseases, but does not have a direct role in the evaluation of children with feeding and swallowing disorders.

References

Alexander, M. P., Emery, E. S., & Koerner, F. C. (1976). Progressive bulbar paresis in childhood. *Archives of Neurology, 33,* 66–68.

Bieger, D. (1991). Neuropharmacologic correlates of deglutition: Lessons from fictive swallowing. *Dysphagia, 6,* 147–164.

Bosma, J. F. (1985). Postnatal ontogeny of performances of the pharynx, larynx, and mouth. *American Review of Respiratory Disease, 131,* S10–S15.

Buchholz, D., & Jones, B. (1991). Dysphagia occurring after polio. *Dysphagia, 6,* 165–169.

Christensen, J. R. (1989). Developmental approach to pediatric neurogenic dysphagia. *Dysphagia, 3,* 131–134.

Cucchiara, S., Staiano, A., Di Lorenzo, C., D'Ambrosio, R., Andreotti, M. R., Prato, M., De Filippo, P., & Auricchio, S. (1986). Esophageal motor abnormalities in children with gastroesophageal reflux and peptic esophagitis. *Journal of Pediatrics, 108,* 907–910.

DiPalma, J. A., & Meyer, G. W. (1987). A rational clinical approach to esophageal motor disorders. *Dysphagia, 2,* 97–108.

Dodds, W. J. (1989). Physiology of swallowing. *Dysphagia, 3,* 171–178.

Humphrey, T. (1964). Some correlations between the appearance of human fetal reflexes and the development of the nervous system. *Progress in Brain Research, 4,* 93–135.

Kennedy, J. G., & Kent, R. D. (1988). Physiological substrates of normal deglutition. *Dysphagia, 3,* 27–34.

Kenny, D. J., Casas, M. J., & McPherson, K. A. (1989). Correlation of ultrasound imaging of oral swallow with ventilatory alterations in cerebral palsied and normal children: Preliminary observations. *Dysphagia, 4,* 112–117.

Mathisen, B., Reilly, S., & Skuse, D. (1992). Oral-motor dysfunction and feeding disorders of infants with Turner syndrome. *Developmental Medicine and Child Neurology, 34,* 141–149.

Mathisen, B., Skuse, D., Wolke, D., & Reilly, S.

(1989). Oral-motor dysfunction and failure to thrive among inner-city infants. *Developmental Medicine and Child Neurology, 31,* 293–302.

Miller, A. J. (1976). Characterization of the postnatal development of superior laryngeal nerve fibers in the postnatal kitten. *Journal of Neurobiology, 7,* 483–494.

Miller, A. J. (1986). Neurophysiological basis of swallowing. *Dysphagia, 1,* 91–100.

Morris, S. E. (1989). Development of oral-motor skills in the neurologically impaired child receiving non-oral feedings. *Dysphagia, 3,* 135–154.

Nelson, J. S., & Prensky, A. L. (1972). Sporadic juvenile amyotrophic lateral sclerosis. A clinicopathological study of a case with neuronal cytoplasmic inclusions containing RNA. *Archives of Neurology, 27,* 300–306.

Sessle, B. J., & Henry, J. L. (1989). Neural mechanisms of swallowing: Neurophysiological and neurochemical studies on brain stem neurons in the solitary tract region. *Dysphagia, 4,* 61–75.

Sheppard, J. J., & Mysak, E. D. (1984). Ontogeny of infantile oral reflexes and emerging chewing. *Child Development, 55,* 831–843.

Staiano, A., Cucchiara, S., De Vizia, B., Andreotti, M. R., & Auricchio, S. (1987). Disorders of upper esophageal sphincter motility in children. *Journal of Pediatric Gastroenterology and Nutrition, 6,* 892–898.

Staiano, A., Cucchiara, S., Del Giudice, E., Andreotti, M. R., & Minella, R. (1991). Disorders of oesophageal motility in children with psychomotor retardation and gastrooesophageal reflux. *European Journal of Pediatrics, 150,* 638–641.

Tuchman, D. N. (1989). Cough, choke, sputter: The evaluation of the child with dysfunctional swallowing. *Dysphagia, 3,* 111–116.

Suggested Readings

Cranial Nerve Testing

Swaiman, K. F. (1989). *Pediatric Neurology. Principles and Practice* (pp. 18–23). Baltimore: Mosby.

Myasthenia Gravis in Infants and Children

Fenichel, G. M. (1988). *Clinical Pediatric Neurology. A Signs and Symptoms Approach* (pp. 160–161). Philadelphia: Saunders.

Arnold-Chiari Malformation and Dysphagia

Pollack, I. F., et al. (1992). Neurogenic dysphagia resulting from Chiari malformations. *Neurosurgery, 5,* 709–719.

Benzodiazepines and Swallowing

Wyllie, E., Wyllie, R., & Cruse, R. (1986). The mechanism of nitrazepam induced drooling and aspiration. *New England Journal of Medicine, 314,* 35–38.

Disorders of Deglutition

CHAPTER 4

David N. Tuchman, M.D.
Rhonda S. Walter, M.D.

In the pediatric population, feeding and swallowing problems rarely present as isolated events but occur mainly in individuals with multiple impairments or as part of an underlying disorder. Unfortunately, accurate prevalence data for swallowing disorders in infants and children are not available. Underlying conditions which predispose to impaired swallowing in the pediatric population include central and peripheral nervous system disorders, diseases of muscle, and structural abnormalities of the oral cavity, pharynx, and esophagus (Table 4–1). The spectrum of pediatric swallowing disorders has been reviewed in detail by others including Bosma (1986), Cohen (1983), Fisher, Painter, & Milmoe (1981), Illingworth (1969), Kramer (1985), Shapiro and Healy (1988), Tuchman (1988, 1989), and Weiss (1988). During evaluation and treatment of pediatric patients, a number of clinical considerations unique to this age group should be considered (Table 4–2) (Tuchman, 1988). These issues and their importance to the approach and management of pediatric patients with impaired feeding and swallowing are reviewed in this and other chapters throughout the book.

The processes of deglutition and feeding differ, although both are complex and interrelated. Deglutition, or swallowing, functions to transport materials from the oral cavity to the stomach without allowing entry of substances into the airway. Deglutition is a motor event that, to be successful, requires intact and functioning central and peripheral nervous systems and the intricate coordination of actions of multiple muscles of the oral cavity, pharynx, and esophagus (Miller, 1982). Feeding, defined as the overall process whereby the infant or child ingests food, involves the act of deglutition but is also influenced by developmental, behavioral, and social factors (Milla, 1991) (Figure 4–1).

In clinical practice, the terms dysphagia, impaired swallowing, and dysfunctional swallowing are frequently used interchangeably. The word dysphagia is derived from the Greek words *dys*, translated as "with difficulty," and *phagia*, "to eat." *Dysphagia* is used to describe the subjective symptom of difficulty in swallowing. Patients describe that food may "get stuck" or "not go down easily" while eating. Another commonly used term, especially by clinicians caring for adult patients, is *trans-*

TABLE 4–1. Conditions associated with impaired swallowing in the pediatric age group.

I. Prematurity

II. Upper Airway-Foodway Anomalies

    A. Nasal and nasopharyngeal
        1. Choanal atresia and stenosis
        2. Nasal and sinus infections
        3. Septal deflections
        4. Tumors

    B. Oral cavity and oropharynx
        1. Defects of lips and alveolar processes
        2. Cleft lip and/or cleft palate
        3. Hypopharyngeal stenosis and webs
        4. Craniofacial syndromes (e.g., Pierre Robin, Crouzon, Treacher Collins, Goldenhar)

    C. Laryngeal
        1. Laryngeal stenosis and webs
        2. Laryngeal clefts
        3. Laryngeal paralysis
        4. Laryngomalacia

III. Congenital Defects of the Larynx, Trachea, and Esophagus

    A. Laryngo-tracheo-esophageal cleft

    B. Tracheoesophageal fistula/esophageal atresia

    C. Esophageal strictures and webs

    D. Vascular anomalies
        1. Aberrant right subclavian artery (dysphagia lusorum)
        2. Double aortic arch
        3. Right aortic arch with left ligamentum

IV. Acquired Anatomic Defects

    A. Trauma
        1. External trauma
        2. Intubation and endoscopy

V. Neurologic Defects

    A. Central nervous system disease
        1. Head trauma
        2. Hypoxic brain damage
        3. Cortical atrophy, microcephaly, anencephaly
        4. Infections (e.g., meningitis, brain abscess)
        5. Myelomeningocele

    B. Peripheral nervous system disease
        1. Traumatic
        2. Congenital

    C. Neuromuscular disease
        1. Myotonic muscular dystrophy
        2. Myasthenia gravis
        3. Guillain-Barré syndrome
        4. Poliomyelitis (bulbar paralysis)

    D. Miscellaneous
        1. Achalasia
        2. Cricopharyngeal achalasia
        3. Esophageal spasm
        4. Esophagitis
        5. Dysautonomia
        6. Paralysis of esophagus (atony)
        7. Tracheo-esophageal fistula/esophageal atresia-associated nerve defects
        8. Aberrant cervical thymus
        9. Conversion dysphagia, behavioral, anorexia of infancy

Sources: Adapted from Weiss, M. H. (1988). Dysphagia in infants and children. *Otolaryngologic Clinics of North America,* *21,* 727–735; and Cohen, S. R. (1983). Difficulty with swallowing. In C. D. Bluestone, & S. F. Stool (Eds.), *Pediatric otolaryngology.* Philadelphia, PA: W. B. Saunders.

fer dysphagia which is defined as difficulty transferring food voluntarily from mouth to esophagus. Transfer dysphagia generally refers to conditions that affect the region orad to the esophagus, namely, the oral and pharyngeal cavities (Castell, 1989).

In the pediatric population, especially in patients with cognitive limitations, it may be difficult to obtain a history of specific subjective complaints relating to feed-

ing. Therefore, when dealing with infants and children, many clinicians use the term dysphagia in a broad sense to describe any type of difficulty with feeding or swallowing. Unless otherwise noted, the term "dysphagia" will be used to describe subjective difficulties associated with swallowing while "impaired swallowing" or "impaired deglutition" will be used to describe abnormal function of the swallowing apparatus.

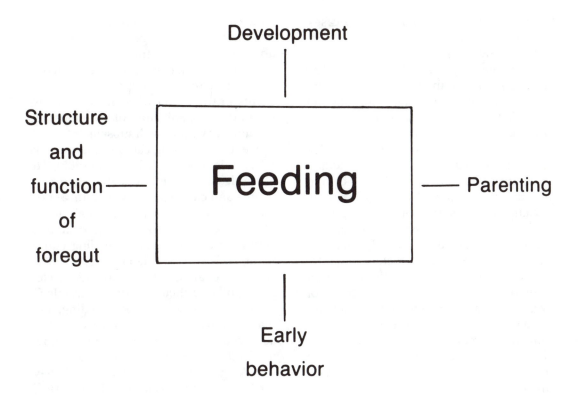

FIGURE 4-1. Factors that affect feeding (From Milla, P. J. [1991]. Feeding, tasting and sucking. In W. A. Walker, P. R. Durie, J. R. Hamilton, J. A. Walker-Smith, & J. B. Watkins [Eds.], *Pediatric gastrointestinal disease, pathophysiology, diagnosis, management* [p. 217]. Philadelphia, PA: W. B. Saunders, reprinted with permission).

TABLE 4–2. Swallowing impairment in the pediatric patient: Clinical issues to consider.

Anatomical and functional growth and development of the swallowing apparatus

Development and maturation of feeding behavior

Importance of oral feeding in the development of parent-child bonding

Importance of swallowing function in providing nutritional adequacy for growth

Altered or poor cognitive ability in certain patient populations resulting in inability to report symptoms and to follow therapeutic recommendations

Source: Adapted from Tuchman, D. N. (1988). Dysfunctional swallowing in the pediatric patient: Clinical considerations. *Dysphagia, 2,* 203–208.

General Approach to the Pediatric Patient with Impaired Swallowing

Successful diagnosis and management of the patient presenting with feeding or swallowing difficulties begins with a carefully obtained medical and feeding history. This process should include a clear understanding of the chief complaint, as well as major questions and concerns. In many instances, the clinical history is provided by the primary caregiver because infants and older children with cognitive impairment may be unable (or unwilling) to report symptoms.

The evaluation procedure should include a complete physical examination, including close inspection of the components of the swallowing apparatus and a neurological examination. In many cases, it is clear that the patient's underlying medical condition has resulted in an impairment of feeding or swallowing. In other instances, feeding and swallowing difficulties may be the presenting symptom and should, therefore, alert the clinician to the presence of an underlying disorder.

Table 4–1 provides a broad list of disorders associated with impaired deglutition in pediatric patients. A heterogenous group of conditions are included and grouped according to type of anomaly. Although this classification scheme may be useful as a means of reference, in clinical practice it may be preferable to characterize the degree of function (or dysfunction) for each stage of deglutition. Any or all phases of swallowing may be impaired. Classifying patients according to swallowing phase impairment may simplify diagnostic considerations and help guide assessment and management techniques, particularly in individuals with complicated disorders. However, this classification method may be too simplistic and may not adequately reflect specific pathophysiologic mechanisms or underlying etiologies. Unfortunately, descriptive definitions of feeding and swallowing dysfunction remain necessary because there is a paucity of data regarding specific and sensitive measures of swallowing function in infants and children.

The clinician should attempt to determine whether a swallowing disturbance is the result of a structural abnormality, an abnormality of function, a problem with feeding behavior, or a combination of these factors. Examples of structural abnormalities that may result in impaired swallowing include cleft palate, laryngeal cleft, or tracheoesophageal fistula. An abnormality of swallowing function may be characterized as incoordination of the swallowing apparatus. Abnormalities of swallowing function may occur in patients with cerebral palsy, where muscles of the oral cavity and pharynx move in a poorly coordinated manner. Impaired feeding, which clinically may present as impaired swallowing, may be due to a behavioral distur-

bance. It is important to recognize that, in an individual patient, general categories of abnormality may overlap.

An abnormal swallow may function adequately due to compensatory movements of the swallowing muscles. However, decompensation of an impaired swallow may occur with subsequent development of significant clinical consequences (Buchholz, Bosma, & Donner, 1985). For example, in the infant with Down syndrome and cleft palate, a structural abnormality is present which may impair deglutition and result in feeding difficulty. Although use of adaptive feeding equipment, such as a modified nipple, may successfully deal with the problems of cleft palate, other difficulties such as muscle fatigue may intervene during feeding. This may lead to a functional disturbance characterized by discoordination of swallowing leading to ineffective feeding.

A significant change in feeding behavior, even in the patient with known swallowing impairment, should alert the clinician to a possible change in underlying clinical status. For example, a change in feeding behavior may develop in a previously stable child with cerebral palsy and impaired swallowing. Diagnostic considerations may include deterioration of neurologic function resulting in further swallowing difficulties, deleterious effect of medication on swallowing function, development of reflux esophagitis leading to refusal to feed, or onset of an emotional disorder such as depression with associated somatic symptoms such as disinterest in eating.

Clinical Clues to an Abnormality of Phase of Deglutition

Oral Dysfunction

The occurrence of respiratory difficulties in relation to the onset of a swallow has been used as a clue to suggest the abnormal phase of deglutition (Logemann, 1983). History of gagging, choking, or coughing prior to a pharyngeal swallow may suggest oral dysfunction characterized by poor oral control of the bolus. Abnormalities in the oral stage should also be suspected when there is a history of sialorrhea or drooling, difficulties with speech (either dysfluencies or articulation difficulties), facial asymmetry (possibly indicative of underlying cranial nerve damage), or external physical stigmata of malformed or maldeveloped craniofacial structures.

Pharyngeal Dysfunction

Coughing, gagging, or choking during a pharyngeal swallow suggests an abnormality in the pharyngeal phase of deglutition (Logemann, 1983). In the developmentally impaired child, it may be difficult to distinguish between oral and pharyngeal dysfunction based solely on the timing of symptoms relative to the swallow. Additional diagnostic tests, such as a videofluoroscopic study, may be required to examine oral and pharyngeal structure and function. History of recurrent pulmonary infections such as aspiration pneumonia or recurrent episodes of bronchospasm (particularly without a family history of atopy) suggest that oral contents are being aspirated secondary to abnormal function of the pharyngeal mechanism. Chronic or recurrent pulmonary disease is not a specific finding for pharyngeal impairment because chronic lung disease may also be found in the setting of oral and esophageal phase abnormalities. The absence of gagging, choking, and coughing during deglutition does not exclude aspiration of oral contents. "Silent" aspiration, or entry of materials into the airway without pulmonary symptoms, is a well-documented phenomenon in the adult patient with impaired deglutition (Linden & Siebens, 1983) and may also be seen in the pediatric patient, particularly in those with multiple disabilities.

Esophageal Dysfunction

History of gagging and choking that occur following a pharyngeal swallow may suggest esophageal disease (Logemann, 1983).

In pediatric patients, a history of food "getting stuck" in the chest or at the region of the suprasternal notch is an unusual complaint and should always prompt clinical evaluation. In general, there is poor correlation between actual location of esophageal disease (upper, mid, lower esophagus) and localization of symptoms by the patient. For example, reflux esophagitis primarily affects the distal esophagus; however, patients may report dysphagia localized to the region of the suprasternal notch. Although the symptom of dysphagia usually suggests esophageal disease, other etiologies, such as impairment of the other stages of deglutition and disorders of the central nervous system, must be considered. The differential diagnosis of dysphagia includes a functional disturbance, such as an esophageal motility disorder, and anatomical abnormalities, such as an esophageal stricture. Children with reflux esophagitis may experience dysphagia based on a disturbance in esophageal motility and/or in the presence of an esophageal stricture (Cucchiara et al., 1986). Clues to aid in distinguishing causes of esophageal dysphagia are outlined in Table 4–3.

The Clinical Setting

In most instances, the underlying medical diagnosis will suggest the etiology of the swallowing difficulty. For example, the child with neuromuscular disease such as cerebral palsy will most likely have incoordination of the stages of deglutition. Similar problems may exist in the individual following traumatic brain injury. A structural abnormality of the swallowing mechanism should be suspected in the neurologically intact newborn or infant who presents with chronic cough or episodes of cyanosis during feeding. An abnormal videofluoroscopic study, which demonstrates swallowing dysfunction with or without aspiration, should prompt a search for neuromuscular or anatomic disorders. A behavioral feeding disorder should be suspected if there are no objective findings

TABLE 4–3. Esophageal dysphagia.

	Mechanical Narrowing (tumors, strictures)	Motor Disorders (achlasia, scleroderma)
Onset	Gradual or sudden	Usually gradual
Progression	Often	Usually not
Type I bolus	Solid	Solids and/or liquids
Temperature dependent	No	Worse with cold liquids, may improve with warm liquids
Response to bolus impaction	Often must be regurgitated	Can usually be passed with repeated swallowing or washing it down with fluids

Source: Pope, C.E. (1989). Heartburn, dysphagia and other esophageal symptoms. In M. H. Sleisinger & J. S. Fortran (Eds.), *Gastrointestinal disease — Pathophysiology, diagnosis, management* (pp. 200–203). Philadelphia, PA: W.B. Saunders, used with permission.

of abnormal swallowing function based on history, physical examination, or diagnostic testing. The presence of tantrums and self-injurious behavior also suggests a behavioral component to the feeding difficulty.

Specific Clinical Entities

In the following section, disorders of deglutition are organized by general diagnostic category as outlined in Table 4–1. Each section includes a discussion of specific clinical entities.

Prematurity

Anatomic and functional development of feeding and swallowing in the preterm infant are reviewed in Chapter 1.

Upper Airway/Foodway Anomalies

Nasal and Nasopharyngeal

Choanal Atresia and Stenosis

Neonates are almost totally dependent on nasal respiration. Mouth breathing begins to evolve between 4 and 6 weeks of age

and is firmly established by 4 months. With feeding, the infant with airway obstruction may have a normal arousal reflex, begin to suck eagerly, but soon show symptoms of aspiration including stridor, coughing, choking, and cyanosis (Cohen, 1990). The inability of small infants with congenital nasal obstruction to separate the route of feeding and respiration is usually obvious, and often acutely severe, at the first feeding (Belenky, 1990; Logan & Bosma, 1967).

The most common congenital nasal anomaly is choanal atresia with reported incidences ranging from 1 in 5000 to 1 in 8000 live births. The atresia may be complete or incomplete, with approximately 90% of atresia plates composed of bone and 10% being membranous (Hengerer & Newburg, 1990). Unilateral choanal atresia is found more commonly (2:1) than bilateral. Unilateral atresia is rarely a significant problem at birth, but respiratory and feeding difficulties may present later in life if the other nasal choana develops obstruction (e.g., via trauma, significant infection, foreign body, etc.). Given their obligate nasal breathing, infants with bilateral choanal atresia present in acute respiratory distress (Belenky, 1990), with inspection and auscultation revealing no breath sounds over the nares. Assessment of airway patency reveals inability to easily pass a catheter (No. 8 French is recommended in full-term infants) through the nose into the nasopharynx (Cohen, 1990). Further diagnosis and evaluation is confirmed by horizontal computed tomography in a plane paralleling the posterior hard palate (Slovis, as quoted in Belenky, 1990). Because bilateral choanal atresia may cause complete nasal obstruction, treatment involves immediate oral airway placement and institution of gavage feedings. Tracheotomy is rarely necessary if no other anomalies exist (Hengerer & Newburg, 1990). Surgical approach is necessary for correction, and at least one major pediatric otolaryngology text advocates transpalatal approach to establish-tablishing adequate choanal passage (Hengerer & Newburn, 1990).

Once the diagnosis of congenital choanal atresia has been established, careful attention should be paid to the remaining physical examination, because up to 50% of patients with bilateral atresia may have associated congenital anomalies. According to *Smith's Recognizable Patterns of Human Malformation* (Jones, 1988), "Choanal Atresia appears to be nonrandomly associated with multiple anomalies in patients with normal chromosomes" (p. 606). A spectrum of associations can include the CHARGE syndrome (coloboma of eye, heart disease, atresia choanae, retarded growth and development, genital anomalies, and ear anomalies and/or deafness) (Jones, 1988).

Nasal and Sinus Infection

Rhinitis and sinusitis (both acute and chronic) comprise infections of the upper respiratory tract that may be troublesome to the pediatric population with impaired swallowing. These conditions may lead to the production of increased secretions and result in significant obstruction in the neonate or older child and, hence, compromise swallowing abilities. In the child with known swallowing dysfunction secondary to neurologic or anatomic disorders, a su-

perimposed infection may alter the mechanisms of compensation and lead to clinical decompensation of the swallow. For example, purulent discharge may interfere with breathing/swallowing rhythms in the young infant. In older children, viscous secretions may interfere with bolus preparation in the oral cavity. Thick secretions, which pool in the pharynx, may lead to abnormalities of the pharyngeal propulsive phase.

Viruses are the primary cause of infectious rhinitis, with myxovirus and paramyxo virus, adenovirus, picornavirus, and coronavirus comprising the major offending agents (Wald, 1990). Nasal discharge and congestion are prominent symptoms of infection and may compromise air movement through the nasal passage. This, in turn, can force mouth breathing, and potentially interfere with suck/swallow in infants and mastication in older children. Bacterial rhinitis in older children may be caused by group A streptococcal infection (especially in children under 3 years of age), pertussis, diphtheria, and the early stages of chlamydia trachomatis (Wald, 1990). Foreign body should be excluded if purulent nasal discharge is persistent, unilateral, or particularly foul-smelling. Allergic rhinitis should be considered if symptoms are seasonal, the patient is atopic, and/or a strong family history of atopy exists.

Sinusitis arises when secretions are retained in the paranasal sinuses and superinfection (generally bacterial) occurs. A detailed discussion of acute and chronic sinusitis is beyond the scope of this text. The reader is referred to Wald (1990) or Lusk, Lazar, and Muntz (1989) for discussion of pathogenesis, diagnosis, and treatment concerns. Briefly, sinusitis arises from any combination of obstruction of the sinus ostia, reduction in the number of cilia, or abnormalities in the viscosity of secretions. Sinus radiographs are useful in confirming the diagnosis, with computerized tomography or magnetic resonance imaging usually reserved for complicated cases that potentially involve intracranial or intraorbital sites or patients with persistent infection refractory to medical therapy. One of the authors (RSW) has also found computerized tomography to be helpful in the diagnosis of sinusitis in children under 6 years of age, microcephalic patients (where plain radiographs do not often clearly demonstrate anatomic delineation of sinuses), and in the multiply handicapped population with chronic upper respiratory infections and persistent low-grade fever of unclear origin. Lusk, Lazar, and Muntz (1989) based on experience at St. Louis Children's Hospital, noted that plain radiographs may over- and underestimate the degree of sinus disease present, especially as it relates to misdiagnosis of ethmoid involvement in chronic sinusitis. Etiologic agents of acute sinusitis (as summarized by Wald, 1990) include streptococcus pneumonia, moraxella catarrhalis, and hemophilus influenza. Treatment includes appropriate antimicrobial agents in acute cases, with drainage procedures reserved for patients refractory to medical therapy.

Septal Deflections

The nasal septum has osseous and cartilaginous components, and is subject to deflection on a congenital or acquired basis. Fairbanks (1990) noted that asymmetry may affect any part of the septum, with a common area of deflection along the articulation between the vomer and the perpendicular plate of the ethmoid. Nasal septal deviation does not often result in obstruction severe enough to interfere with deglutition (Weiss, 1988). However, severe trauma to the nose with septal deflection can produce dysphagia and, thereby, mandate correction (Cohen, 1990). Of interest is that approximately 80% of humans have some deformity of the nasal septum (Fairbanks, 1990) with a seemingly trivial deformity (e.g., secondary to childhood injury) becoming more prominent during accelerated growth in adolescence. Referral to an otolaryngologist and ultimately surgical correction is reserved for cases involving compromise of the airway passage or swallowing function.

Tumors

Extensive review of the tumors of the nose, paranasal sinuses, and nasopharynx is beyond the scope of this chapter. The reader is referred to standard pediatric otolaryngologic texts (Grundfast, 1989; Stanievich & Lore in Bluestone & Stoole, 1990) or pediatric oncology texts. It is necessary, however, to include such tumors in the discussion of disorders of deglutition, because rhinonasal disease can produce serious clinical signs and symptoms of impaired swallowing. Initially, obstruction of nasal passages may occur, with nasal phonation (and/or mouth breathing) as well as nasal discharge and epistaxis. Progressive symptoms such as facial numbness, otalgia, and hearing and visual disturbances may herald a tumor of the nose, nasal pharynx, or paranasal sinuses (Stanievich & Lore, 1990). Disturbances of feeding can arise from tumor mass impinging on the swallowing apparatus as well as infiltration or obstruction of cranial nerves with resultant trismus, alteration of sensation such as hypesthesia, and discoordination of neural control of phases of swallowing.

The most common benign nasal tumors in children are hemangiomas, nasal polyps, and squamous papillomas (Stanievich & Lore, 1990). Hemangiomas are classified by level of tissue involvement or histology. Those with rapid growth in the first 6 months of life can produce airway obstruction and/or difficulty feeding. Treatment may involve a combination of observation (wait for regression), steroid therapy (intralesional or systemic), laser therapy for superficial lesions, or surgical excision for deeply invasive or life-threatening conditions.

Nasal polyps are benign, pedunculated tumors with a characteristic wet, glistening, grape-like appearance which, if large in size or multiple in number, may completely obstruct the nasal passage. Cystic fibrosis is one of the most common causes of nasal polyposis (Doershuk & Boat, 1983). A sweat chloride test should be performed in any child under 12 years of age presenting with nasal polyps (Stanievich & Lore, 1990). Etiologic factors accounting for the development of nasal polyps in older children include allergies and chronic infection. The most effective treatment is surgical removal, although precedent trials of steroids and decongestants have also been reported. Nasal papillomas include tumors of the nasal vestibule that are exophytic, pedunculated growths requiring surgical excision and close follow-up, given their tendency for reoccurrence (Stanievich & Lore, 1990).

Malignant neoplasms of the head and neck represent 5% of malignancies in the pediatric population. It must be noted, however, that more than 50% of tumors found are lymphomas (Hodgkins and non-Hodgkins) and soft-tissue sarcomas (including rhabdomyosarcomas) (Bonilla & Healy, 1989). Early diagnosis is imperative and prompt referral to an otolaryngologist of dysphagic patients with enigmatic painless cervical masses, otorrhea unresponsive to medical therapy, progressive nasal obstruction, or unexplained facial paralysis is essential (Bonilla & Healy, 1989).

Malignant tumors of the nose are noted to be rare in children and hence do not figure prominently in the differential diagnoses of pediatric feeding and swallowing disorders. The most common malignant nasal tumor in childhood is rhabdomyosarcoma. Malignant sinus tumors also include undifferentiated carcinomas. These lesions may present as erythematous, tender facial swellings that have characteristic bone destruction on radiographic examination.

Oral Cavity and Oropharynx Defects of Lips and Alveolar Processes

Serious impairment of feeding and swallowing may occur when the lips, mouth, and oropharynx are involved by either a congenital or an acquired anatomic defect (Cohen, 1990). Physical examination may disclose the majority of oral cavity abnormalities; barium swallow or videofluoroscopy may further elucidate underlying anatomic sources of difficulty. The primary

inability to form a seal, at the level of the lips and palate, and create the forces necessary to suck is most debilitating for infants who rely on the "normal piston-in-cylinder sucking reflex that initiates swallowing" (Cohen, 1990). Oral cavity and oropharyngeal abnormalities in older children may present as gradual or acute problems in bolus formation and propulsion. Oropharyngeal entities that may interfere with deglutition include congenital syndromes with or without micrognathia (see discussion below); mechanical problems such as those related to macroglossia; traumatic lesions; and infections of the oral cavity.

Specific defects of lips and alveolar processes that interfere with swallowing include infections or inflammatory processes that may extend to tongue, tonsils, and buccal mucosa. A list of such conditions is discussed by Gluckman (1991). Inflammation and/or infection can painfully disrupt the oral transit of food and interfere with acceptance and/or propulsion to the pharynx. The lips themselves can be affected by clefting (see below), congenital tumors such as hemangiomas, and a peculiar entity known as "double lip," which Parkin (1991) described as a redundancy of mucosal lining.

Disruption in feeding also can occur with macroglossia or enlargement of the tongue. Macroglossia may be the result of overdevelopment of tongue musculature or occur secondary to other causes such as pituitary gigantism, hypothyroidism, and a host of congenital malformation syndromes (see Jones, 1988). The most well known of the latter includes Down syndrome (trisomy 21) and Beckwith-Weideman syndrome (exomphalos, macroglossia, gigantism syndrome) (Jones, 1988). Mechanically, the large tongue can actually be obstructive to the airway and, in general, is less effective with regard to food acceptance, bolus preparation, and propulsion.

Craniofacial Syndromes

Craniofacial syndromes involving the oropharyngeal structures are discussed extensively in pediatric otolaryngology texts and reviews (Parkin, 1991; Poole & Redford-Badwal, 1991), as well as genetic references (Jones, 1988). Poole and Redford-Badwal (1991), in a review of craniofacial complex and congenital malformations, noted that 3 to 7% of live births have at least one congenital abnormality, with 75% of the defects affecting the cranial vault, face, neck, and oral cavity. Some of the more common entities will be discussed here.

Pierre-Robin syndrome is characterized by micrognathia, glossoptosis (closure of the airway by the tongue), and cleft of the palate (usually midline). The tongue is located posteriorly with early mandibular retrognathism thought to be the primary anomaly (Jones, 1988). The degree of mandibular hypoplasia may vary; the abnormal posterior position of the tongue makes it susceptible to negative pressure forces during swallowing and can lead to obstruction of the upper airway with subsequent choking (Paradise, 1991).

Mandibular hypoplasia with relative glossoptosis and associated feeding and respiratory problems are noted in the Treacher Collins syndrome. There is a wide variance in expression of this syndrome, with salient features including malar hypoplasia, downslanting palpebral fissures, defects of lower lids (coloboma), and malformation of the external ear (Jones, 1988). The majority of these patients have normal intelligence (mental retardation present in less than 10%). Surgical intervention may include glossopexy and tracheostomy as well as cosmetic surgery such as reconstruction of the external and middle ear (Parkin, 1991).

Choking during feeding from partial airway occlusion can also be evidenced (albeit to a lesser degree) in craniofacial dysostosis, or the Crouzon syndrome, which consists of maxillary hypoplasia, shallow orbits, and premature craniosynostosis (Jones, 1988). Transmitted via an autosomal dominant pattern, the defect lies in the ossification process of the developing fetus and involves varying degrees of premature fusion of the coronal, sagittal, and lambdoidal sutures of the skull. Conductive hearing loss may occur, and mental retardation may be associated (Parkin, 1991).

Cleft Lip and/or Cleft Palate

The ability of the oral cavity to form a sealed compartment depends on intact labial and palatal competence. Cleft lip and palate are the most common cranial facial deformities of the head and neck (Bardach, 1990) and may potentially compromise feeding and swallowing. In the first few weeks of life, sucking efficiency is impaired given the involved palate's inability to separate (seal) the nasal cavity and nasal pharynx, oral cavity, and oral pharynx. Potential exists for nasal regurgitation and choking episodes (Paradise, 1991). This can give rise to less than adequate feeding experiences for parent and child from both a nutritional and nurturing standpoint.

Clefting encompasses a spectrum of severity, varying from simple cleft lip to complete cleft of lip and palate (Kaufman, 1991). The malformations occur in structures normally developed by the end of the 9th to 12th week of intrauterine life (McWilliams, 1990). These include the maxillary processes that fuse to form the upper lip and alveolus by the 7th week and the palatal processes that fuse to form the secondary palate by week 12. Cleft lip occurs when the premaxilla fails to fuse with the alveolus during embryologic development; cleft palate arises from poor fusion of the horizonal palatal segments (Parkin, 1991). Multiple hypotheses exist regarding etiology of the disruption of palatal fusion. General consensus, however, is that clefts result from multifactorial causation, including genetic and environmental factors, a theory that allows for the known association between teratogens and clefting (Kaufman, 1991; McWilliams, 1990).

Incidence and prevalence statistics draw on multiple studies of frequency of various forms of clefting and, hence, often present disparate background figures. A conservative figure suggests an overall incidence of 1 in 750 live births (McWilliams, 1990), with incidences in clefting varying among races and nations (Bardach, 1990). Clefting is statistically higher in North American Indians and Japanese (Bardach, 1990), and is noted to be 1.5 times greater in Orientals than Caucasians and 2.1 times greater in Caucasians than Negroes (Kaufman, 1991). Clefts of both lip and palate occur more often in males than females; however, palatal only involvement is more common in females (McWilliams, 1990). Unilateral clefts outnumber bilateral (Kaufman, 1991, reported 73% versus 27%; Bardach, 1990, reported a ratio 1.0:2.0), with most unilateral clefts occurring on the left side. Classification systems for cleft palate have been set forth by the American Cleft Palate Association but tend to vary with modifications from author to author, based on degree of clefting (complete, incomplete, or submucous), laterality, and proposed embryologic derivation (McWilliams, 1990).

Individuals with cleft lip and/or palate require a multidisciplinary team approach for diagnosis, treatment, and subsequent therapies. Goals and management include primary aesthetic surgical repair, satisfactory facial growth, control of middle ear disease, and minimization of consequent hearing impairment and production of "normal" speech patterns by school age (Bardach, 1990; Cooper, 1979; Kaufman, 1991; McWilliams, 1990; Paradise, 1991). The reader is referred to previously cited sources for discussion of timing of lip and/or palatal repair, dental intervention, and discussion of social/emotional sequelae on cleft lip and palate.

Most sources agree that clefts which involve both lip and palate result in primary inability to sustain intraoral pressure and interfere with successful feeding (Kaufman, 1991). Children with cleft lip alone or small isolated clefts of the soft palate may not experience much difficulty in feeding because the infant can use the breast or bottle to generate enough negative intraoral pressure to feed fairly efficiently. For pa-

tients with a significant cleft palate, compensatory feeding devices include those that permit direct expression of milk into the infant's mouth. Several sources favor cleft palate nursers consisting of compressible plastic bottles with soft rubber crosscut nipples (Paradise, 1991) which allow control of milk volume and flow rates (Kaufman, 1991). Breast feeding is not contraindicated for children with cleft lip or partial palate of clefts, and may, in the opinion of some authorities, help facilitate "the emotional bond between mother and child" (Cooper, 1979). However, close attention must be paid to weight and nutritional gains, and supplemental devices utilized if inadequate growth ensues.

Hypopharyngeal Stenosis and Webs

Cumming, Akhtar, Ferentzi, and Feteih (1986) reported an infant presenting with coughing and choking during feeding as a result of obstruction by a fibroblastic ring at the level of the hypopharynx. Contrast studies demonstrated a filling defect at the cricopharyngeus, and biopsies of the lesion showed replacement of muscle bundles with well-differentiated fibroblasts.

Congenital Defects of the Larynx, Trachea, and Esophagus

Laryngo-tracheo-esophageal Cleft

Laryngo-tracheo-esophageal cleft is a rare congenital anomaly that is characterized by communication of the larynx and trachea with the esophagus through a midline defect (Burroughs & Leape, 1974; Fuzesi & Young, 1976; Glossop, Smith, & Evans, 1984; Novoselec, Dangel, & Fisch, 1973; Roth, Rose, Benz-Bohm, & Gunther, 1983; Zaw Tun, 1988). The mode of presentation and degree of disturbance generally depends on the extent of the cleft in the larynx and trachea. Formation of the cleft results from failure of the trachea to separate from the esophagus. Although the extent of the cleft varies, the larynx is always involved. Three types of clefts have been characterized by Pettersson (1969). In type I, which is the mildest form, the cleft is limited to the posterior wall of the larynx. In type II, the cleft is limited to the six proximal tracheal rings, whereas in type III it extends caudally to the carina. In severe cases, the posterior wall of the trachea and the anterior wall of the esophagus are absent allowing these structures to share a common lumen. A schematic representation of a laryngo-tracheo-esophageal cleft is shown in Figure 4–2.

The embryologic origins of this condition have been reviewed by Blumberg, Stevenson, Lemire, and Boyden (1965). In the unaffected fetus, the septum separating the foregut lumen and lung bud normally fuses by the end of the 5th gestational week while dorsal fusion of the cricoid occurs by the 7th week. In affected cases, the lung bud fails to separate completely from the foregut lumen, and there is incomplete cephalic migration and posterior fusion of the lateral folds of the foregut.

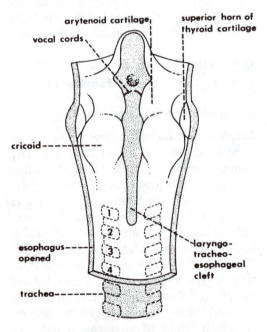

FIGURE 4-2. Schematic representation of a laryngo-tracheo-esophageal cleft (From Burroughs, N., & Leape, L. L. [1974]. Laryngotracheoesophageal cleft: Report of a case successfully treated and review of the literature [p. 517]. *Pediatrics, 53,* 516–522, reprinted with permission).

This is followed by failure of the cricoid cartilages to fuse dorsally. Failure of dorsal fusion of the cricoid may lead to cleft formation even if formation of the tracheoesophageal septum is complete.

Presentation is usually at birth or in early infancy. A cleft should be suspected in the infant with stridor, increased saliva production, and low or soundless crying. Symptoms may be intermittent, particularly in mild clefts. In some instances, the clinical picture is similar to the infant with esophageal atresia and tracheoesophageal fistula. Chest radiograph may show signs of an aspiration pneumonia. A lateral radiograph of the chest with a nasogastric tube in place may show the tube shifted ventrally into the larynx and trachea. Videofluoroscopy will demonstrate entry of contrast material into the trachea, although it may be difficult to distinguish an uncoordinated swallow from an anatomic abnormality (Delahunty & Cherry, 1969). The optimal diagnostic approach is direct visualization of the larynx by laryngoscopy. The endoscopist should have a high suspicion for this disorder since the defect may be difficult to demonstrate even on direct visualization because the edges of the defect may approximate, especially on inspiration. A probe may be necessary to demonstrate the cleft. Management is surgical repair and usually requires a tracheostomy (Evans, 1985). Although patients with mild clefts tend to do well, morbidity remains substantial for patients with more severe clefts and for those with associated disorders such as esophageal atresia and tracheoesophageal fistulae. In addition to esophageal anomalies, laryngeal cleft may be a manifestation of several syndromes including the Pallister-Hall syndrome (congenital hypothalamic hamartoblastoma, hypopituitarism, imperforate anus, and postaxial polydactyly) and the G syndrome (Tyler, 1985).

Tracheoesophageal Fistula/Esophageal Atresia

The most common congenital anomaly of the esophagus is esophageal atresia (EA) with or without a distal tracheoesophageal fistula (TEF). This condition and other esophageal anomalies have been reviewed in detail by Boyle (1982), Wright (1991), and others. There are many variations of EA and TEF, but, in general, lesions are grouped into five basic types as shown in Figure 4–3. The etiology of EA and TEF is unclear, but this lesion probably develops between the 4th and 6th week of gestation (Ingalls, 1949). Hypotheses for its development include disturbance of the blood supply to the esophagus, persistence of the obliterative phase of the esophageal lumen, defective septation of the laryngo-tracheal ridge, and localized pressure on the esophagus by vascular anomalies (Boyle, 1982).

The overall incidence of esophageal atresia is approximately 1:3000 live births (Cudmore, Rickham, Lister, & Irving, 1978). A history of polyhydramnios is seen in approximately 50% of patients (Scott & Wilson, 1957). Associated anomalies occur in 50% of patients and may include the VACTEREL (vertebral, anorectal, cardiovascular, tracheoesophageal, renal, and limb) syndrome (Baumann, Greinacher, Emmrich, & Spranger, 1976; Quan & Smith, 1973). EA and TEF may also occur as part of trisomy 17 and 18 (Rabinowitz, Moseley, Mitty, & Hirschorn, 1967).

Clinical presentation includes respiratory distress with feeds (usually the first feed), excessive oral secretions, and chronic regurgitation. Once the diagnosis is suspected, passage of a nasogastric tube should be attempted with documentation of passage into the stomach by radiograph. In cases where EA is present, air in the abdomen generally indicates the presence of a distal fistula. Use of contrast studies to confirm the diagnosis are controversial because of the risk of aspiration (Boyle, 1982). An isolated TEF (H-type) may present at a later age and rarely even in adulthood. Patients with this type of fistula may have a history of recurrent pneumonia and complain of coughing and/or choking with feeding. Diagnosis of an isolated fistula (H-type) may be difficult due to the small size of the fistula and its oblique position. The radiologist should be alerted to the possibility of an isolated fistula so that a specialized contrast study may be considered. Because a routine barium esophagram may not clearly demonstrate the fistula, a naso-esophageal tube may be required to deliver small volumes of contrast material directly into the esophageal lumen. In some instances, bronchoscopy is necessary to directly visualize the fistula by using a dye

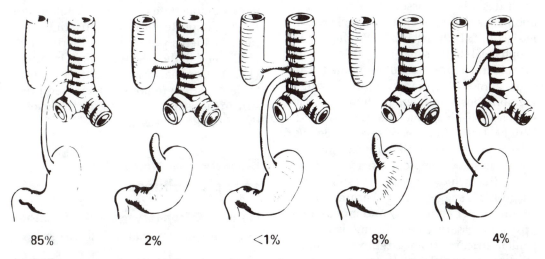

85%   2%   <1%   8%   4%

FIGURE 4-3. Types and incidence of esophageal atresia with or without and tracheo-esophageal fistulae (From Wright, V. M. [1991]. The esophagus, congenital anomalies. In W. A. Walker, P. R. Durie, J. R. Hamilton, J. A. Walker-Smith, & J. B. Watkins [Eds.], *Pediatric gastrointestinal disease, pathophysiology, diagnosis, management* [p. 367]. Philadelphia, PA: W. B. Saunders, reprinted with permission).

technique (Andrassy, Ko, Hanson, Kubota, Hays, & Mahour, 1980).

Treatment is surgical and includes ligation of the fistula, direct anastomosis of the proximal and distal portions of the esophagus, and placement of an enteral feeding (gastrostomy) tube. In some cases, the distance between the esophageal segments is too great to attempt an anastomosis during infancy. In these patients, the esophageal "gap" is bridged in stages and various esophageal lengthening procedures may be used including colonic interposition (German & Waterston, 1976), creation of a gastric tube (Anderson & Randolph, 1978), or mechanical elongation (Gwinn & Lee, 1971). Potential problems following surgical repair include persistence of the fistula, esophageal dysmotility complicated by gastroesophageal reflux, and chronic pulmonary disease.

Esophageal Strictures and Webs

Congenital esophageal strictures and webs are extremely rare, being much less common than acquired esophageal strictures that arise as a result of acid injury secondary to gastroesophageal reflux. Esophageal stenosis presenting at birth occurs at a frequency of 1 in 25,000 to 50,000 and has been described in association with other anomalies (Nihoul-Fekete, DeBacker, Lortat-Jacob, & Pellerin, 1987; Wright, 1991). Esophageal stenosis may be associated with ectopic tracheobronchial remnants (cartilage, glands, respiratory epithelium), a membranous diaphragm, or fibromuscular stenosis (Nishina, Tsuchida, & Saito, 1981; Wright, 1991). In cases of severe stenosis, infants present with difficulty swallowing liquids. In some, symptoms do not occur until the diet includes ingestion of solid food. Diagnosis is suggested by a barium esophagram. Upper endoscopy and mucosal biopsy is necessary to help distinguish a congenital stricture from a reflux associated stricture. In patients with ectopic remnants, treatment generally requires esophageal resection and end-to-end esophageal anastomosis. Esophageal dilatation may be successful in patients with a membranous diaphragm or muscular stenosis (Wright, 1991).

Vascular Anomalies

Aberrant Right Subclavian Artery (Dysphagia Lusorum)

Vascular anomalies in the thorax, particularly anomalies of the aortic arch, may compress the trachea and esophagus and result in significant respiratory distress and/or feeding difficulties. The most common aortic arch anomaly is an aberrant right subclavian artery which occurs in 0.5 to 1.8% of the population (Edwards, 1953). In this condition, the right subclavian artery arises from the left side of the aortic arch and externally compresses the esophagus. The term used to describe difficulty swallowing in association with an aberrant right subclavian artery is dysphagia lusorum. Although this lesion may be present at birth, it usually does not become clinically significant until middle age. There have been reports of dysphagia lusorum occurring in the pediatric patient (Martin, Rudolph, Hillemeier, & Heyman, 1986; Orenstein, 1984). The usual method of diagnosis is a barium esophagram which on lateral view demonstrates an oblique filling defect in the posterior esophagus. In the series of patients presented by Martin et al. (1986) and in the case report by Orenstein (1984), esophageal manometry was used to demonstrate regions of increased pressure in the esophageal lumen at the level of the anomalous vessel.

Motility Disorders of the Esophagus

Isolated Cricopharyngeal Dysfunction and Cricopharyngeal Achalasia

The term *achalasia* is strictly defined as "failure to relax." In the clinical setting, a diagnosis of cricopharyngeal achalasia implies dysfunction of the cricopharyngeus muscle resulting in obstruction or impairment to intraluminal flow at the level of the hypopharynx. However, nonrelaxation of the sphincter resulting from primary cricopharyngeal disease differs from nonopening of the sphincter due to weak propulsive forces generated in the proximal pharynx (Hellemans, Agg, & Pelemans, 1981). Therefore, when the diagnosis of cricopharyngeal dysfunction or achalasia is considered, the clinician should exclude impaired pharyngeal function characterized by an inability to propel the bolus through a relaxed, but unopened, sphincter.

Isolated cricopharyngeal dysfunction or achalasia is an uncommon disorder in infants and children and is usually associated with a more global disorder of deglutition involving the oral phase and other non-sphincteric-related aspects of pharyngeal function (Bishop, 1974; Reichert et al., 1977; Staiano et al., 1987). Patients with cricopharyngeal achalasia generally present at birth with feeding difficulties, although some may present as late as 6 months. Utian & Thomas (1969) described cricopharyngeal incoordination in two infants with small mandibles which opened poorly. Contrast studies demonstrated functional obstruction at the level of the cricopharyngeus with dilatation of the pharynx. Histologic section of the upper third of the esophagus demonstrated nerve fibers but no ganglion cells. It is unclear whether this histologic finding is a primary process analogous to Hirschsprung's disease (aganglionosis) or secondary to long-standing obstruction and incoordination. At autopsy, a dilated pharyngeal cavity was noted with hypertrophy of pharyngeal constrictor muscles.

The diagnosis of isolated cricopharyngeal dysfunction may be suggested by radiographic contrast studies. However, a horizontal bar ("cricoid bar") in the proximal esophagus representing the cricopharyngeus muscle may be seen in up to 5% of adults undergoing radiographic examinations for all indications and may also be a normal radiologic sign in infants (Seaman,

1966; Gideon & Nolte, 1973). Esophageal manometric studies have demonstrated normal relaxation and decreased UES pressure in some patients with a prominent bar seen on radiographic study (Hellemans, Agg, & Pelemans, 1981; Hurwitz & Duranceau, 1978). Alternatively, manometric studies may be normal in patients with clinical or radiologic evidence of cricopharyngeal dysfunction (Dinari, 1987; Fisher, Painter, & Milmoe, 1981; Hellemans et al., 1981).

Improvement of cricopharyngeal achalasia may occur spontaneously, or following dilatation (Dinari et al., 1987; Lernau, Sherzer, Mogle, & Nissan, 1984). Surgical treatment consists of cricopharyngeal myotomy. Preoperative selection of appropriate surgical candidates requires motility and radiographic studies (Berg, Jacobs, Persky, & Cohen, 1985). Surgery is usually contraindicated in patients with gastroesophageal reflux or poor pharyngeal peristalsis.

Achalasia

Primary achalasia of the esophagus usually occurs in adulthood, but there are many series describing its occurrence in childhood and even in infancy (Berquist et al., 1983; Nurko, 1991). This esophageal motility disorder is characterized by any or all of the following:

1. increased resting pressure of the lower esophageal sphincter (LES),

2. failure of the LES to relax following deglutition, and

3. incomplete or absent peristalsis in the esophageal body.

The etiology of achalasia is unknown, although autopsy studies in patients have described degeneration of ganglion cells in the central nervous system. An inconsistent pathologic finding has been absent ganglion cells in the myenteric plexus in the dilated portion of the esophagus. These findings suggest a neurogenic abnormality in patients with achalasia (Nurko, 1991).

Other conditions associated with primary achalasia include alacrimia (absence of tears) and adrenal insufficiency secondary to ACTH insensitivity (Illgrove, Clayden, Grant, & McCaulay, 1978). Acquired causes of achalasia include infection with the organism Trypanosoma Cruzi (Chagas disease) (Csendes et al., 1985) and tumors involving the gastroesophageal junction (Tucker, Snape, & Cohen, 1978).

Individuals may present with vomiting, difficulty swallowing solids and liquids, weight loss, substernal discomfort, odynophagia (painful swallowing), and recurrent pneumonia. During mealtime, food tends to "get stuck." In fact, it is not uncommon for patients to vomit the evening meal as late as the following morning due to markedly delayed esophageal emptying. Nighttime cough is common and occurs due to aspiration of secretions retained in the esophagus. Diagnosis should be suspected on a chest radiograph if an air-fluid level is seen in the region of the mid-thorax. Barium esophagram demonstrates a dilated esophagus with significant tapering at the distal end, giving rise to the classic "beak-like" appearance. Fluoroscopic examination will demonstrate the motility disturbance, which can be confirmed by using esophageal manometry. Upper endoscopy is performed to help exclude a tumor in the region of the gastroesophageal junction.

Treatment of achalasia has been reviewed in detail by Nurko (1991) and is summarized below. In the majority of cases, the motor abnormality involving the esophageal body is not reversible; and therefore, treatment is directed at relieving the functional obstruction at the level of the LES. Forceful dilatation of the sphincter is accomplished using pneumatic dilatation. Success rates following dilatation vary from 60 to 95%, depending on the number of dilatations. Complications of dilatation include perforation (1 to 5%), bleeding (1%), and, rarely, the development of gastroesophageal reflux. Surgery is reserved for patients requiring repeated dilatations or those with a tortuous esophagus (S-shaped or sigmoid esophagus) associated with longstanding achalasia. The surgical procedure is a Heller myotomy which, in adult patients, has a success rate of 64 to 94%. Acute complications of myotomy include inadvertent perforation of the esophageal mucosa, bleeding, and phrenic nerve paralysis. Long-term complications include the development of gastroesophageal reflux, prompting some authors to suggest combining the myotomy with an anti-reflux procedure.

Other Esophageal Motor Disorders

Other esophageal motility disorders include diffuse esophageal spasm, nutcracker esophagus, and nonspecific esophageal abnormalities. Wyllie, Rothner, and Morris (1989) described an infant with psychomotor retardation who presented with irritability and posturing secondary to esophageal spasm and was treated successfully with a calcium channel blocker. However, it is unclear whether this patient had reflux esophagitis. Systemic disorders that may affect gastrointestinal motility, including the esophagus, are scleroderma, other collagen vascular diseases, and diabetes mellitus.

Drug Effects

Drug-induced dysfunction of the upper esophageal sphincter, has been reported by Wyllie et al. (1986). Two children developed drooling and aspiration following institution of nitrazepam, a benzodiazepam anti-convulsant. Manometric studies demonstrated that relaxation of the upper esophageal sphincter (cricopharyngeus muscle) was delayed by as much as 0.3 seconds after the onset of hypopharyngeal contraction. In control patients, cricopharyngeal relaxation precedes hypopharyngeal contraction.

Miscellaneous

Transient Incoordination of Swallowing Function During Infancy

Transient incoordination of swallowing function during infancy is a rare condition (Frank & Baghdassarian Gatewood, 1966; Macaulay, 1951). This disorder occurs in otherwise well full-term infants and is characterized by feeding difficulties that occur soon after birth. Other causes of impaired swallowing, including anatomic and neurologic abnormalities, should be excluded. Aspiration of oral contents is documented on videofluoroscopic study. This may be secondary to pooling of secretions in the hypopharynx spilling over into the trachea (Frank & Baghdassarian Gatewood, 1966). The clinical course includes spontaneous improvement of swallowing function, usually in a matter of weeks. Macaulay (1951) hypothesized that transient incoordination of swallowing, laryngeal movements, and breathing are secondary to immaturity of the bulbar centers in the central nervous system, a condition usually associated with prematurity. Spontaneous improvement of swallowing function in this disorder suggests a maturational defect.

Congenital Dysphagia

Arden et al. (1965) described five infants (four infants were full-term) with difficulty swallowing noted at birth. Clinical history was characterized by excessive oropharyngeal secretions, and cyanosis and choking during feeds. This condition was termed congenital dysphagia and thought to be a secondary to paresis of the pharyngeal musculature. All affected infants required nutritional support using enteral tube feeding. Swallowing impairment was persistent and coexisted with other neurological deficits. "Congenital dysphagia" probably does not represent a distinct clinical entity, and, in practice, its use should be avoided unless isolated pharyngeal dysfunction is present.

Aberrant Cervical Thymus

Bistritzer et al. (1985) described an infant presenting with difficulty feeding and dyspnea secondary to a cervical mass. On excision, this was found to be an aberrant cervical thymus. This lesion probably occurs secondary to failure of the right thymic bud to separate from its origin in the pharynx and to descend completely into the mediastinum.

Sialorrhea

Sialorrhea, or excessive drooling, is the unintentional loss of saliva and other oral contents from the mouth (Blasco et al., 1990). Drooling, which may be normal in infancy, resolves by 15 to 18 months of age as oro-motor function matures. Although occasional drooling may occur beyond this age, persistence of drooling beyond 4 years is considered abnormal (Crysdale, 1989). Drooling occurs mainly in the setting of neurologic disease complicated by motor abnormalities affecting oral motor function. Examples include disorders such as cerebral palsy, peripheral neuromuscular disease, facial paralysis, or severe mental retardation (Blasco et al., 1990). In children with drooling, the primary problem is usually related to oral motor dysfunction and not excessive production of saliva (Myer, 1989). There are a number of excellent reviews regarding this subject, including those by Blasco et al. (1990) and Bailey (1988).

Normal Saliva Production

Approximately 0.5 to 1.0 liters of saliva are produced daily in the adult. Saliva functions to lubricate the oral cavity, lubricates food and mucus membranes during swallowing, protects teeth from decay, helps prevent periodontal and gingival disease, and contains enzymes that play a role in the digestion of starches and fats (Blasco et al., 1990). In the resting state, about 90% of saliva is produced by the large paired glands: the submandibular, parotid, and sublingual glands. The minor salivary glands account for the remaining 10%. The increase in saliva flow in response to eating results mainly from the parotid glands. The viscosity of saliva produced is gland-dependent: The parotids produce watery saliva, whereas the sublingual and submandibular glands produce a more viscous secretion.

Clinical Manifestations

In children with cerebral palsy, it has been estimated that as many as 10 to 13% of individuals are affected by sialorrhea (Makhani, 1974). In these patients, impairment of the oral phase of swallowing exists secondary to poor coordination of the muscles of the tongue, palate, and face. In addition, individuals with cerebral palsy and drooling swallow less frequently than those with nondrooling cerebral palsy or control children (Sochaniwskyj et al., 1986).

Drooling may occur as an anterior oral spill, which is visible and characterized by loss of saliva onto the face. With posterior drooling, saliva pools in the pharynx with secretions spilling through the faucial isthmus. If this occurs without triggering a pharyngeal swallow, aspiration may result (Blasco et al., 1990). Other clinical complications of drooling include soaking of clothes, offensive odors, and macerated skin around the mouth and chin. As a result, drooling may be stigmatizing and interfere with interpersonal relationships. Drooling also may lead to significant loss of fluid causing dehydration and impair articulation.

Other factors which interfere with saliva clearance should be considered when evaluating patients with sialorrhea, including any conditions that cause nasal obstruction. Abnormal head position and body posture, inability to concentrate, malocclusion of the jaw, abnormal tongue, poor tongue control, and impaired sensory capability of the lips and oral cavity may contribute to drooling.

Diagnosis of Drooling

The diagnosis of drooling is made mainly by history. However, objective measures of drooling have been developed and include weighing saliva collected on a bib (Harris & Dignam, 1980), measuring drool volume in a plastic bag attached to the chin (Wilkie, 1970), or use of a collection cup and air tight vacuum pump system (Sochaniwskyj, 1982). Ekedahl and Hallen (1973) used a radioisotope, technetium 99, which is injected intravenously and secreted in saliva. Radioactivity of saliva spilled onto a bib may be measured and drool volume calculated.

Management of Sialorrhea

General

Initial treatment is directed at the underlying medical condition. Correction of nasal obstruction may alleviate a problem with drooling. This includes medical treatment of allergic rhinitis, vasomotor rhinitis, and sinusitis or, when indicated, surgical management of nasal obstruction such as adenoidectomy or nasal septal reconstruction (Guerin, 1979).

Nonmedical, Nonsurgical Techniques

The therapist must determine the degree of voluntary control and cognitive abilities of the patient regarding awareness and understanding of the problem (Bailey, 1988). Crysdale and White (1988), drawing on experience of more than 400 patients with drooling, suggested that "spontaneous improvement of drooling will occur without treatment, especially in some with good mobility and head control and lesser oral motor involvement" (p. 88). Speech therapy or physiotherapy techniques directed toward oral motor abnormalities have been used including oral prosthetic devices, bio-feedback (Koheil et al., 1987), and behavioral modification (Dunn, Cunningham, & Backman, 1987). Methods of improving jaw control such as stability and closure, increasing tongue strength and positioning, and improving lip closure may aid in reducing of drooling (Bailey, 1988). Samelstad (1988) used oral stimulation techniques to enhance sensorimotor feedback mechanisms. Unfortunately, the efficacy of these techniques in successfully treating drooling is not well-documented. Studies are plagued by incomplete response to therapy, small sample sizes, and poor quantification of drool (Ottenbacher, Bundy, & Short, 1983). Radiation therapy is not considered a useful treatment modality because of the variation of response, gland regeneration, and the possibility of inducing malignant change in the gland or surrounding tissues.

Medical Therapy

Because salivation is under parasympathetic control, anti-cholinergic medications have an inhibitory effect on salivary flow. Unfortunately, doses of anti-cholinergics required to significantly effect saliva flow and diminish drooling generally result in side effects such as blurred vision, urinary retention, and restlessness. This is due to poor selectivity against the target organ, which is the salivary gland. Camp-Bruno, Winsburg, Green-Parsons, and Abrams (1989) used benztropine (Cogentin™), a synthetic anti-cholinergic, to control drooling in children with developmental disability. Talmi, Zohar, Finkelstein, and Laurian (1988) described successful experience with transdermal scopolamine. Reddihaugh, Johnson, Staples, Hudson, and Exarchos (1990) used benzhexol (Artane™) in children with cerebral palsy and found variable success. Glycopyrrolate (Robinol™), an antimuscarinic compound that decreases secretions and has little effect on the central nervous system, may be a useful drug but requires further study (Blasco et al., 1990).

Surgical Therapy

Surgical approaches to treatment of sialorrhea are discussed in Chapter 8. In general, these techniques include interruption of the parasympathetic nerve supply to the major salivary glands, gland removal, duct ligation, and duct re-routing.

References

Anderson, K. D., & Randolph, J. G. (1978). Gastric tube interposition. A satisfactory alternative to the colon for esophageal replacement in children. *Annals of Thoracic Surgery, 25*, 521–525.

Andrassy, R. J., Ko, P., Hanson, B. A., Kubota, E., Hays, D. M., & Mahour, G. H. (1980). Congenital tracheoesophageal fistula without esophageal atresia. A 22 year experience. *American Journal of Surgery, 140*, 731–733.

Arden, G. M., Benson, P. F., Butler, N. R., Ellis, H. L., & McKendrick, T. (1965). Congenital dysphagia resulting from dysfunction of the pharyngeal musculature. *Developmental Medicine and Child Neurology, 7*, 157–166.

Bailey, C. M. (1988). Management of the drooling child. *Clinics of Otolaryngology, 13*, 319–322.

Bardach, J. (1990). Plastic and reconstructive surgery of the head and neck. In C. D. Bluestone, S. S. Stool, & M. D. Scheetz (Eds.), *Pediatric otolaryngology* (2nd ed., pp. 694–717). Philadelphia, PA: W. B. Saunders.

Baumann, W., Greinacher, I., Emmrich, P., & Spranger, J. (1976). Vater syndrome. *Klin Paediatric, 188*, 328–337.

Belenky, W. M. (1990). Nasal obstruction and rhinorrhea. In C. D. Bluestone, S. S. Stool, & M. D. Scheetz (Eds.), *Pediatric otolaryngology* (2nd ed., pp. 657–671). Philadelphia, PA: W. B. Saunders.

Berg, H. M., Jacobs, J. B., Persky, M. S., & Cohen, N. L. (1985). Cricopharyngeal myotomy: A review of surgical results in patients with cricopharyngeal achalasia of neurogenic origin. *Laryngoscope, 95*, 1337–1340.

Berquist, W. E., Byrne, W. J., Ament, M. E., Fonkalsrud, E. W., & Euler, A. R. (1983). Achalasia: Diagnosis, management and clinical course in 16 children. *Pediatrics, 71*, 798–805.

Bishop, H. C. (1974). Cricopharyngeal achalasia in childhood. *Journal of Pediatric Surgery, 9*, 775–778.

Bistritzer, T., Tamir, A., Oland, J., Varsano, D., Manor, A., Gall, R., & Aladjem, M. (1985). Severe dyspnea and dysphagia resulting from an aberrant cervical thymus. *European Journal Pediatrics, 144*, 86–87.

Blasco, P. A., Allaire, J. H., Hollahan, J., Blasco, P. M., Edterton, M. T., Bosma, J. F., Nowak, A. J., Sternfeld, L., McPherson, K. A., & Kenny, D. J. (1990). *Consensus statement of the Consortium on Drooling,* Charlottesville, Virginia.

Blumberg, J. B., Stevenson, J. K., Lemire, R. J., & Boyden, Q. A. (1965). Laryngotracheoesophageal cleft, the embryonic implications: Review of the literature. *Surgery, 57,* 559–566.

Bonilla, J. S., & Healy, G. B. (1989). Management of malignant head and neck tumors in children. *Pediatric Clinics of North America, 36*(6), 1443–1448.

Bosma, J. F. (1986, February). Oral-pharyngeal interactions in feeding. Presented at Symposium on Dysphagia, Johns Hopkins University.

Boyle, J. T. (1982). Congenital disorders of the esophagus. In S. Cohen, & M. D. Soloway (Eds.), *Diseases of the esophagus* (pp. 97–120). New York: Churchill Livingstone.

Buchholz, D. W., Bosma, J. F., & Donner, M. W. (1985). Adaptation, compensation, and decompensation of the pharyngeal swallow. *Gastrointestinal Radiology, 10,* 235–239.

Burroughs, N., & Leape, L. L. (1974). Laryngotracheoesophageal cleft: Report of a case successfully treated and review of the literature. *Pediatrics, 53,* 516–522.

Camp-Bruno, J. A., Winsberg, B. G., Green-Parsons, A. R., & Abrams, J. (1989). Efficacy of benztropine therapy for drooling. *Developmental Medicine and Child Neurology, 31,* 309–319.

Castell, D. O. (1989). Dysphagia: A general approach to the patient. In D. W. Gelfand & J. E. Richter (Eds.), *Dysphagia: Diagnosis and treatment* (pp. 3–9). New York: Igaku-Schoen.

Cohen, S. R. (1990). Difficulty with swallowing. In C. D. Bluestone & S. F. Stool (Eds.), *Pediatric otolaryngology* (pp. 843–849). Philadelphia, PA: W. B. Saunders.

Cooper, H. K. (1979). Historical perspectives and philosophy of treatment. In S. S. Spencer (Ed.), *Cleft palate and cleft lip: A team approach to clinical management and rehabilitation of the patient* (p. 15). Philadelphia, PA: W. B. Saunders.

Cucchiara, S., Staiano, A., DiLorenzo, C., D'Ambrosio, R., Andreotti, M. R., Prato, M., DeFilippo, P., & Auricchio, S. (1986). Esophageal motor abnormalities in children with gastroesophageal reflux and peptic esophagitis. *Journal of Pediatrics, 108,* 907–910.

Crysdale, W. S. (1989). Management options for the drooling patient. *Ear, Nose and Throat Journal, 68,* 820–830.

Crysdale, W. S., & White, A. (1989). Submandibular duct relocation for drooling. A 10-year experience with 194 patients. *Otolaryngology Head and Neck Surgery, 101,* 87–90.

Csendes, A., Smok, F., Braghetto, I., Ramirez, C., Velasco, N., Henriquez, A. (1985). Gastroesophageal sphincter pressure and histologic changes in distal esophagus in patients with achalasia of the esophagus. *Digestive Diseases and Sciences, 30,* 941–945.

Cudmore, R. E., Rickham, P. P., Lister, J., & Irving, I. M. (Eds.) (1987). *Neonatal surgery* (2nd ed., p. 192). London: Butterworths.

Cumming, W. A., Akhtar, M., Ferentzi, C., & Feteih, W. (1986). Cricopharyngeal ring. A case report. *Pediatric Radiology, 16,* 152–153.

Delahunty J. E., & Cherry, J. (1969). Congenital laryngeal cleft. *Annals of Otology, Rhinology and Laryngology, 78,* 96–106.

Dinari, G., Danziger, Y., Mimouni, M., Rosenbach, Y., Zahavi, I., Grunebaum, M. (1987). Cricopharyngeal dysfunction in childhood: Treatment by dilatations. *Journal of Pediatric Gastroenterology and Nutrition, 6,* 212–216.

Doershuk, C. D., & Boat, T. F. (1983). Cystic fibrosis. In R. E. Behrman & V. C. Vaughan (Eds.), *Nelson textbook of pediatrics* (12th ed., p. 1098). Philadelphia, PA: W. B. Saunders.

Dunn, K. W., Cunningham, C. E., & Backman, J. E. (1987). Self-control and reinforcement in the management of a cerebral-palsied adolescent's drooling. *Developmental Medicine and Child Neurology, 29,* 305–310.

Edwards, J. E. (1953). Malformations of the aortic arch system manifested as "vascular rings." *Laboratory Investigations, 2,* 56–75.

Ekedahl, C., & Hallen, O. (1973). Quantitative measurement of drooling. *Otolaryngology, 75,* 464–469.

Evans, J. N. (1985). Management of the cleft larynx and tracheoesophageal clefts. *An-*

nals of Otology, Rhinology and Laryngology, 94, 627–630.

Fairbanks, D. N. (1990). Embryology and anatomy. In C. D. Bluestone, S. S. Stool, & M. D. Scheetz (Eds.), Pediatric otolaryngology (2nd ed., pp. 807–815). Philadelphia, PA: W. B. Saunders.

Fisher, S. E., Painter, M., & Milmoe, G. (1981). Swallowing disorders in infancy. Pediatric Clinics of North America, 28, 845–853.

Frank, M. M., & Baghdassarian Gatewood, O. M. (1965). Transient pharyngeal incoordination in the newborn. American Journal of Diseases of Childhood, 111, 178–181.

Fuzesi, K., & Young, D. G. (1976). Congenital laryngotracheoesophageal cleft. Journal of Pediatric Surgery, 11, 933–937.

Gengerer, A. S., & Newburg, J. A. (1990). Congenital malformations of the nose and paranasal sinuses. In C. D. Bluestone, S. S. Stool, & M. D. Scheetz (Eds.), Pediatric otolaryngology (2nd ed., pp. 718–728). Philadelphia, PA: W. B. Saunders.

German, J. C., & Waterston, D. J. (1976). Colon interposition for replacement of the esophagus in children. Journal of Pediatric Surgery, 11, 227–234.

Gideon, A., & Nolte, K. (1973). The non-obstructive pharyngo-esophageal cross roll. Annals of Radiology, 16, 129–135.

Glossop, L. P., Smith, R. J., & Evans, J. N. (1984). Posterior laryngeal cleft: An analysis of ten cases. International Journal of Pediatric Otorhinolaryngology, 7, 133–143.

Gluckman, J. L. (1991). Inflammatory diseases of the mouth and pharynx. In C. D. Bluestone, S. S. Stool, & M. D. Scheetz (Eds.), Pediatric otolaryngology (2nd ed., pp. 807–815). Philadelphia, PA: W. B. Saunders.

Grundfast, K. M. (Ed.). (1989). Recent advances in pediatric otolaryngology. Pediatric Clinics of North America, 36, 6.

Guerin, R. L. (1979). Surgical treatment of drooling. Archives of Otolaryngology, 105, 535–537.

Gwinn, J. L., & Lee, F. A. (1971). Esophageal elongation in esophageal atresia. Annals of Radiology, 14, 279–283.

Harris, M. M., & Dignam, P. F. (1980). Non-surgical method of reducing drooling in cerebral-palsied children. Developmental Medicine and Child Neurology, 22, 293–299.

Hellemans, J., Agg, H. O., & Pelemans, W. (1981). Pharyngoesophgeal swallowing disorders and the pharyngoesophgeal sphinc-

ter. Medical Clinics of North America, 65, 1149–1171.

Hurwitz, A. L., & Duranceau, A. (1978). Upper-esophageal sphincter dysfunction. Pathogenesis and treatment. Digestive Diseases, 23, 275–281.

Illgrove, H., Clayden, G. S., Grant, D. B., & McCaulay, J. C. (1978). Familial glucocorticoid deficiency with achalasia of the cardia and deficient tear production. Lancet, 1, 1284.

Illingworth, R. S. (1969). Sucking and swallowing difficulties in infancy: Diagnostic problem of dysphagia. Archives of Diseases of Childhood, 44, 655–665.

Illingworth, R. S., & Lister, J. (1964). The critical or sensitive period, with special reference to certain feeding problems in infants and children. Journal of Pediatrics, 65, 839–848.

Ingalls, T. H., & Pringle, R. A. (1949). Esophageal atresia with tracheoesophageal fistula. Epidemiologic and teratologic implications. New England Journal of Medicine, 240, 987–994.

Jones, K. L. (1988). Smith's recognizable patterns of human malformation (4th ed.). Philadelphia, PA: W. B. Saunders.

Kaufman, F. L. (1991). Managing the cleft lip and palate patients. Pediatric Clinics of North America, 38(5), 1127–1145.

Kramer, S. S. (1985). Special swallowing problems in children. Gastrointestinal Radiology, 10, 241–250.

Koheil, R., Sochaniwskyj, A. E., Bablich, K., Kenny, D. J., & Milner, M. (1987). Biofeedback techniques and behavior modification and the conservative remediation of drooling by children with cerebral palsy. Developmental Medicine and Child Neurology, 29, 19–26.

Lernau, O. Z., Sherzer, E., Mogle, P., & Nissan, S. (1984). Congenital cricopharyngeal achalasia treatment by dilatations. Journal of Pediatric Surgery 1984, 19, 202–203.

Linden, P., & Siebens, A. (1983). Dysphagia: Predicting laryngeal penetration. Archives of Physical Medicine and Rehabilitation, 64, 281–284.

Logan, W. J., & Bosma, J. F. (1967). Oral and pharyngeal dysphagia in infancy. Pediatric Clinics of North America, 14, 47.

Logemann, J. A. (1983). Evaluation and treatment of swallowing disorders. San Diego, CA: College-Hill Press.

Lusk, R. P., Lazar, R. H., & Muntz, H. (1989). The diagnosis and treatment of recurrent sinusitis in children. *Pediatric Clinics of North America, 36*(6), 1411–1421.

Macaulay, J. C. (1951). Neuromuscular incoordination of swallowing in the newborn. *Lancet, 1,* 1208.

Makhani, J. S. (1974). Dribbling of saliva in children with cerebral palsy and its management. *Indian Journal of Paediatrics, 41,* 272–277.

Martin, G. R., Rudolph, C., Hillemeier, C., & Heyman, M. B. (1986). Dysphagia lusorum in children. *American Journal of Diseases of Children, 140,* 815–817.

McWilliams, B. J. (1990). Multiple speech disorders (cleft palate and cerebral palsy speech). In C. D. Bluestone, S. S. Stool, & M. D. Scheetz (Eds.), *Pediatric otolaryngology* (2nd ed., pp. 1402–1414). Philadelphia, PA: W. B. Saunders.

Milla, P. J. (1991). Feeding, tasting and sucking. In W. A. Walker, P. R. Durie, J. R. Hamilton, J. A. Walker-Smith, & J. B. Watkins (Eds.), *Pediatric gastrointestinal disease: Pathophysiology, diagnosis, management.* Philadelphia, PA: B. C. Decker.

Miller, A. J. (1982). Deglutition. *Physiological Reviews, 62,* 129.

Myer, C. M. (1989). Sialorrhea. *Pediatric Clinics of North America, 36,* 1495–1500.

Nihoul-Fekete, C., DeBacker, A., Lortat-Jacob, S., & Pellerin, D. (1987). Congenital esophageal stenosis. A review of 20 cases. *Pediatric Surgery International, 2,* 86–92.

Nishina, T., Tsuchida, Y., & Saito, S. (1981). Congenital esophageal stenosis due to tracheobronchial remnants and its associated anomalies. *Journal of Pediatric Surgery, 16,* 190–193.

Novoselac, M., Dangel, P., & Fisch, U. (1973). Laryngotracheoesophageal cleft. *Journal of Pediatric Surgery, 8,* 963–964.

Nurko, S. (1991). The esophagus: Motor disorders. In W. A. Walker, P. R. Durie, J. R. Hamilton, J. A. Walker-Smith, & J. B. Watkins (Eds.), *Pediatric gastrointestinal disease,* (pp. 393–416), Philadelphia, PA: B. C. Decker.

Orenstein, S. R. (1984). Manometric demonstration of aberrant right subclavian artery associated with dysphagia. *Journal of Pediatric Gastroenterology and Nutrition, 3,* 634–636.

Ottenbacher, K., Bundy , A., & Short, M. A. (1983). The development and treatment of oral-motor dysfunction: A review of clinical research. *Physical and Occupational Therapy in Pediatrics, 3,* 147–160.

Paradise, J. L. (1991). Primary care of infants and children with cleft palate. In C. D. Bluestone, S. S. Stool, & M. D. Scheetz (Eds.), *Pediatric otolaryngology* (2nd ed., pp. 860–866). Philadelphia, PA: W. B. Saunders.

Parkin, J. L. (1991). Congenital malformations of the mouth and pharynx. In C. D. Bluestone, S. D. Stool, & M. D. Scheetz (Eds.), *Pediatric otolaryngology* (2nd ed., pp. 850–859). Philadelphia, PA: W. B. Saunders.

Pettersson, G. (1969). Laryngo-tracheo-oesophageal cleft. *Zeitschrift Fur Kinderchirurgie, 7,* 43.

Poole, A. E., & Redford-Badwal, D. A. (1991). Structural abnormalities of the craniofacial complex and congenital malformations. *Pediatric Clinics of North America, 38*(5), 1089–1126.

Pope, C. E. (1989). Heartburn, dysphagia and other esophageal symptoms. In M. H. Sleisinger & J. S. Fortran (Eds.), *Gastrointestinal disease — Pathophysiology, diagnosis, management* (pp. 200–203). Philadelphia, PA: W. B. Saunders.

Quan, L., & Smith, D. W. (1973). The VATER association. *Journal of Pediatrics, 82,* 104–107.

Rabinowitz, J. G., Moseley, J. E., Mitty, H. A., & Hirschorn, K. (1967). Trisomy 18, esophageal atresia, anomalies of the radius, and congenital hypoplastic thrombocytopenia. *Radiology, 89,* 488–491.

Reddihaugh, D., Johnson, H., Staples, M., Hudson, I., & Exarchos, H. (1990). Use of benzhexol hydrochloride to control drooling of children with cerebral palsy. *Developmental Medicine and Child Neurology, 32,* 985–989.

Reichert, T. J., Bluestone, C. D., Stool, S. E., Sieber, W. K., & Sieber, A. M. (1977). Congenital cricopharyngeal achalasia treatment by dilatations. *Annals of Otology, Rhinology and Laryngology, 86,* 603–610.

Roth, B., Rose, K. G, Benz-Bohm, G., & Gunther, H. (1983). Laryngo-tracheo-oesophageal cleft. Clincial features, diagnosis and therapy. *European Journal of Pediatrics, 140,* 41–46.

Samelstad, K. M. (1988). Treatment techniques to encourage lip closure and decrease drooling in persons with cerebral palsy. *Occupational Therapy Journal of Research, 8,* 164–175.

Scott, J. S., & Wilson, J. K. (1957). Hydramnios

as an early sign of esophageal atresia. *Lancet, 2,* 569–572.

Seaman, W. B. (1966). Cineroentgenographic observation of the cricopharyngeus. *American Journal of Radiology, 96,* 922–931.

Shapiro, J., & Healy, G. B. (1988). Dysphagia in infants. *Otolaryngologic Clinics of North America, 21,* 737–741.

Sochaniwskyj, A. E. (1982). Drool quantification: Noninvasive technique. *Archives of Physical Medicine and Rehabilitation, 63,* 605–607.

Sochaniwskyj, A. E., Koheil, R. M., Bablich, K., Milner, M., & Kenny, D. J. (1986). Oral motor functioning, frequency of swallowing and drooling in normal children and in children with cerebral palsy. *Archives of Physical Medicine and Rehabilitation, 6,* 866–874.

Staiano, A., Cucchiara, S., De Vizia, B., Andreotti, M. R., & Auricchio, S. (1987). Disorders of upper esophageal sphincter motility in children. *Journal of Pediatric Gastroenterology and Nutrition, 6,* 892–898.

Stanievich, J. F., & Lore, J. M. (1990). Tumors of the nose, paranasal sinuses, and nasopharynx. In C. D. Bluestone, S. D. Stool, & M. D. Scheetz (Eds.), *Pediatric otolaryngology* (2nd ed., pp. 780–792). Philadelphia, PA: W. B. Saunders.

Talmi, Y. P., Zohar, Y., Finkelstein, Y., & Laurian, N. (1988). Reduction of salivary flow with scopoderm TTS. *Annals of Otology, Rhinology, and Laryngology, 97,* 128–130.

Tuchman, D. N. (1988). Dysfunctional swallowing in the pediatric patient: Clinical considerations. *Dysphagia, 2,* 203–208.

Tuchman, D. N. (1989). Choke, cough, sputter: The evaluation of the child with dysfunctional swallowing. *Dysphagia, 3,* 111–116.

Tuchman, D. N. (1991). Disorders of Deglutition. In W. A. Walker, P. R. Durie, J. R. Hamilton, J. A. Walker-Smith, & J. B. Watkins (Eds.), *Pediatric gastrointestinal disease* (pp. 359–366), Philadelphia, PA: B. C. Decker.

Tucker, H. J., Snape, W. J., & Cohen, S. (1978). Achalasia secondary to carcinoma: Manometric and clinical features. *Annals of Internal Medicine, 89,* 315–318.

Tyler, D. C. (1985). Laryngeal cleft: report of eight patients and a review of the literature. *American Journal of Medical Genetics, 21,* 61–75.

Utian, H. L., & Thomas, R. G. (1969). Cricopharyngeal incoordination in infancy. *Pediatrics 43,* 402–406.

Wald, E. R. (1990). Rhinitis and acute and chronic sinusitis. In C. D. Bluestone, S. S. Stook, & M. D. Scheetz (Eds.), *Pediatric otolaryngology* (2nd ed., pp. 729–744). Philadelphia, PA: W. B. Saunders.

Weiss, M. H. (1988). Dysphagia in infants and children. *Otolaryngologic Clinics of North America, 21,* 727–735.

Wilkie, T. F. (1970). Surgical treatment of drooling: follow-up report of five years experience. *Plastic and Reconstructive Surgery, 45,* 549–554.

Wright, V. M. (1991). The esophagus: Congenital anomalies. In W. A. Walter, P. R. Durie, J. R. Hamilton, J. A. Walker-Smith, & J. B. Watkins (Eds.), *Pediatric gastrointestinal disease,* (pp. 367–370), Philadelphia, PA: B. C. Decker.

Wyllie, E., Syllie, R., Rothner, A. D., & Morris, H. H. (1989). Diffuse esophageal spasm: A cause of paroxysmal posturing and irritability in infants and mentally retarded children. *The Journal of Pediatrics, 115*(2), 261–263.

Wyllie, E., Wyllie, R., Cruse, R. P., Rothner, A. D., & Erenberg, G. (1986). The mechanism of nitrazepam induced drooling and aspiration. *New England Journal of Medicine 314,* 35–38.

Zaw-Tun, H. I. (1988). Development of congenital laryngeal atresia and clefts. *Annals of Otology, Rhinology and Laryngology, 97,* 353–358.

Behavioral Feeding Disorders

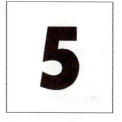

Roberta L. Babbitt, Ph.D.
Theodore A. Hoch, Ed.D.
David A. Coe, M.A.

Feeding problems have been described as absence of adequate oral consumption due singly or in combination with neuromotor dysfunction, obstructive lesions, and psychosocial factors (Palmer & Horn, 1978). Feeding problems are not a specific disease entity, but rather are the result of a cluster of related medical, environmental, nutritional, and social variables. Behavioral feeding problems are those that are at least partially attributable to motivational problems or skill deficits. Motivational problems can include food refusal or selectivity brought about by deficient caregiver skills or a lack of hunger/satiety cycle brought about by supplemental tube feeding. Skill deficits can include inability to self-feed, chew, swallow, or consume an age-appropriate texture. The multiple etiology of feeding problems dictates assessment and treatment encompassing each aspect.

The purpose of this chapter is to provide a review of the pediatric behavioral feeding literature and to acquaint the reader with basic behavioral assessment, treatment, and follow-up procedures as well as the rationales behind them. Other approaches, such as occupational therapy-based assessment and treatment, target other physiological feeding issues and are complementary to behavioral assessment and treatment practices in some cases. Behavioral assessment and treatment of feeding problems is a component of the larger field of Behavioral Medicine or Behavioral Pediatrics. An exhaustive discussion of this field is beyond the scope of this chapter. For further information, the reader is referred to Gross and Drabman (1990); Krasnegor, Cataldo, and Arasteh (1986); Luiselli (1989); and Routh (1988).

Prevalence

A wide range of prevalence statistics has been reported for feeding problems that are either totally or partially behavioral in nature. Inadequate intake has been cited as resulting in 20% of all childhood dietary insufficiencies (Palmer & Horn, 1978). Feeding problems occur frequently in handicapped children (Thompson & Palmer, 1974) and are generally reported to be more prevalent among developmentally disabled individuals. In a previous review of the literature, Jones (1982) reported a prevalence range of 19% to 61% for behavioral feeding problems among mentally retarded people. Perske, Clifton, McClean, and Stein (1977) reported that 80% of individuals with developmental disabilities exhibit maladaptive feeding behaviors that can lead to undesirable consequences for physical, social, or vocational/educational development. Feeding problems are estimated to occur in 33% of mentally retarded individuals in residential placements (Palmer & Horn 1978).

Etiology

As noted earlier, serious feeding problems frequently are precipitated by multiple factors (Hyman et al., 1987; Illingworth & Lister, 1964; Iwata, Riordan, Wohl, & Finney, 1982; Palmer & Horn, 1978; Palmer, Thompson, & Linscheid, 1975). Such factors include behavioral mismanagement, which encompasses failure to introduce solids at the appropriate age, forced feeding, excessive parental anxiety during meals, increased attention through coaxing, or removal from the feeding situation (Palmer, Thompson, & Linscheid, 1975; Singer, Nofer, Benson-Szekely, & Brooks, 1991); physiological abnormalities, such as structural physiological defects; metabolic disorders, most notably neurochemical alterations in serotonin, which is responsible for mediation of satiety (Brown, Davis, & Flemming, 1979; Christophersen & Hall, 1978; Hyman et al., 1987; Illingworth & Lister, 1964; Linscheid, 1978; Palmer & Horn, 1978; Palmer et al., 1975; Singer et al., 1991); and food intolerance due to allergies (Linscheid, 1978). Palmer and associates (1975) attributed 21% of feeding problems primarily to behavioral mismanagement. The remaining 79% of problems were attributed to neuromotor dysfunction (74%) or mechanical obstruction (5%) (Palmer et al., 1975). Budd and her colleagues (1992) classified

the etiologies of feeding problems of the 50 children in their sample as 26% organic in nature, 40% primarily organic, 24% primarily nonorganic, and 10% nonorganic. Cupoli, Hallock, and Barnes (1980) reported that feeding problems or improper feeding techniques occurred in 50 to 80% of nonorganic failure-to-thrive cases.

Children with primarily medically based problems are at risk for additional behavioral feeding problems unless the original problem is remedied quickly (Christophersen & Hall, 1978; Linscheid, 1978; Palmer & Horn, 1978). For example, rumination or vomiting may first occur as a result of physical illness, but come under control of the self-stimulatory reinforcers that it produces (Christophersen & Hall, 1978; Starin & Fuqua, 1987).

Clearly, behavioral factors have to be considered during assessment and treatment of most children with feeding problems, whether or not the problem originated as a behavioral one. Behavioral factors to consider include the child's learning history related to eating, caregivers' feeding skills, or child or caregiver skill deficits.

In cases where extreme food refusal produces acute malnutrition and dehydration, or oral motor dysfunction renders oral feeding unsafe, nasogastric or gastrostomy tube feedings are essential. Unfortunately, such medical management carries with it great potential for disrupting or even preventing development of oral feeding. Vogel (1986) described a possible learning history that could bring about food refusal and absence of swallowing (conditioned dysphagia) in tube-fed children, and reported that children who receive enteral feedings are likely to develop oral hypersensitivity and other feeding aversions. Avoidance of food often persists well after it has ceased to be adaptive (Ylvisaker & Weinstein, 1989). In general, great difficulty is often experienced in establishing oral feeding in children who have received enteral feedings. These children often fight, cry, gag, vomit, or otherwise engage in avoidant behavior when feeding is attempted (Blackman & Nelson, 1987; Geertsma, Hyams, Pelletier, & Reiter, 1985; Illingworth, 1969; Illingworth & Lister, 1964; Vogel, 1986).

The reason most often cited for difficulties in establishing oral feeding in tube-fed children is that oral feeding experiences did not occur during the child's "critical period." Although many authors have cited the seminal work of Illingworth and Lister (1964) who originally described the critical period (Blackman & Nelson, 1987; Geertsma et al., 1985; Linscheid, 1978; Tuchman, 1988; Vogel, 1986), this concept has not been empirically validated. Illingworth and Lister (1964) described the critical period for development of feeding skills as a period of physiological development (between 6 and 7 months of age) at which acquisition of oral food consumption skills is most likely and beyond which oral feeding will either not be established, or be established only with great difficulty. Deductive evidence for this concept provided by Illingworth and Lister (1964) consisted of case studies describing four children for whom solid food introduction was greatly delayed, first occurring at ages 15 months, 18 months, 2 years, and 6 years, respectively. Despite each child's attaining other developmental milestones, oral food consumption did not emerge when foods were presented (Illingworth & Lister, 1964).

Parent-child interactions are important for all aspects of early child development (Budd et al., 1992; Tuchman, 1988). Parents of a handicapped child often experience anxiety and guilt over the child's handicapping condition. Consequently, parents may overcompensate by being either too strict or too lax (Finney, 1986; Palmer & Horn, 1978). For example, at one extreme a parent may physically restrain a child and force consumption, while at the other a parent may terminate all attempts to feed conditional on crying or whining.

Types of interactions surrounding feeding that can contribute to feeding problems are numerous. A parent may provide atten-tion contingent on behaviors such as crying, throwing food, spitting, turning the head to avoid food, clenching teeth, pushing food away, inducing vomiting, and so forth. These behaviors may nurture parental anxiety, thus affecting the parent-child relationship, especially around feeding times, thereby creating a vicious cycle (Forsyth, Leventhal, & McCarthy, 1985). Meals may be terminated because the child engages in frequent or extremely inappropriate behaviors. A parent may provide preferred foods contingent on inappropriate behaviors or refusal to eat (Iwata, et al., 1982). Purees and "junior" foods may be presented exclusively to a child who is capable of consuming higher textures but refuses to do so (Christophersen & Hall, 1978). Alternatively, chronic inappropriate diet selection by parents may result in food selectivity (Christophersen & Hall, 1978). Forced feeding, either informally by parents or as part of food refusal treatment, has also been cited as another form of behavioral mismanagement that contributes to feeding problems (Riordan et al., 1980). The existence of physical problems often provides an opportunity for parental and medical mismanagement of feeding contingencies (Iwata et al., 1982). Therefore, even though a feeding problem may not be purely behavioral, it may be alleviated or lessened by proper behavioral intervention (Linscheid, 1978).

Types of Feeding Problems

Feeding problems have been classified based on apparent etiologies, physical topographies, or associated behaviors (Brown, Davis, & Flemming, 1975; Budd et al., 1992; Christophersen & Hall, 1978; Hyman, 1987; Illingworth & Lister, 1964; Linscheid, 1978; Palmer & Horn, 1978; Palmer et al., 1975; Singer et al., 1991). Such classifications can be useful in focusing initial treatment efforts. However, to develop effective behavioral treatments, attention must also be paid to specific behavioral topographies and their functions. Two main divisions, based on function, are problems that are motivationally based versus skill-deficit based.

Motivationally and Skill-Deficit Based Problems

Problems that are motivationally based are those in which behaviors are maintained by faulty reinforcement practices or occur under inappropriate circumstances. The child may possess normally functioning feeding and swallowing physiology and all behaviors needed for adequate intake, but still have inadequate intake. Food refusal, selectivity, or numerous other feeding problems may occur and be maintained by consequences such as parental attention, escape from meals, access to more preferred (and less nutritional or lower texture) foods, and so forth. Addressing these con-

sequences and arranging more beneficial ones may remedy the problems.

Skill-deficit based problems are those in which the child's feeding and swallowing physiology functions normally, but is underdeveloped from lack of experience. This condition has been described by many authors when discussing the concept of "critical period" (Blackman & Nelson, 1987; Geertsma et al., 1985; Linscheid, 1978; Tuchman, 1988; Vogel, 1986). This type of problem differs from motivational problems in that the child typically does not possess the necessary behaviors to consume food. These problems require treatment methods that shape the target behaviors, in addition to arranging motivational variables to strengthen them. A list of articles on pediatric behavioral feeding organized by problem behavior and treatment reference is presented in Table 5–1.

TABLE 5–1. Survey of common behavioral feeding problems.

Problem	References
Food refusal (partial/total)	Blackman & Nelson (1985); Budd et al. (1992); Dahl & Sundelin (1986); Duker (1981); Geertsma et al. (1985); Hoch, Babbitt, Knell, & Hackbent (in press); Iwata et al. (1982); Koepke & Thyer (1985); Luiselli & Gleason (1987); Palmer & Horn (1978); Singer et al. (1991); Ylvisaker & Weinstein (1989)
Food selectivity by type or texture	Christophersen & Hall (1978); Finney (1986); Illingworth & Lister (1964); Iwata et al. (1982); Palmer & Horn (1978); Palmer, Thompson, & Linscheid (1975); Thompson & Palmer (1974)
Tube dependence	Blackman & Nelson (1985); Geerstma et al. (1985); Vogel (1986); Ylvisaker & Weinstein (1989)
Swallowing skill deficit	Budd et al. (1992); Greer et al. (1991); Lamm & Greer (1988); Palmer & Horn (1978); Vogel (1986); Ylvisaker & Weinstein (1989)
Self-feeding skill deficit	Christophersen & Hall (1978); Iwata et al. (1982); Palmer & Horn (1978)
Mealtime tantrums and disruptive behavior	Finney (1986); Iwata et al. (1982); Palmer & Horn (1978); Thompson & Palmer (1974)
Excessive meal duration	Finney (1986)
Adipsia and polydipsia	Luiselli (1989); Palmer & Horn (1978)
Rumination and vomiting	Budd et al. (1992); Christophersen & Hall (1978); Clauser & Scibak (1990); Dahl & Sundelin (1986); Foxx, Snyder, & Schroeder (1979); Iwata et al. (1982); Starin & Fugua (1987)

Assessment

Behaviors alone do not reveal whether the problem is motivationally or skill-deficit based in nature. The environmental influences that currently maintain the feeding problem also must be isolated. To do so requires consideration of the child's feeding history and direct observation and functional analysis of the child's and caregivers' current behaviors. Steps in this process include an initial interview, preliminary assessment of child and caregiver interaction, measurement of anthropometries, and repeated measures of baseline feeding behaviors (Luiselli, 1989).

Before proceeding with behavioral assessment, information is often needed from other treating disciplines. A behavioral feeding therapist needs to know whether a child may safely consume foods and liquids orally and what textures. Physiological components to vomiting and rumination must be ruled out before they can be treated behaviorally. Excluding or medically treating gastroesophageal reflux can determine the course of behavioral treatment for a child who refuses food and also vomits. Presence or absence of food allergies or medication interactions must be documented. In addition to these physiological variables, caregiver psychological or social variables must sometimes be addressed prior to effectively treating a child's feeding problem. Marital conflict, caregiver depression, poverty, and other social problems can contribute greatly to a child's feeding problem and will affect any attempt to treat it. Given the multidisciplinary scope of these needs, a multidisciplinary approach is essential in both assessment and treatment of behavioral feeding problems.

Interview

Behavioral assessment frequently begins with an interview in which caregivers detail the child's behavioral and medical histories. The goal of the interview is to pro-

vide basic information to guide subsequent information and data collection. Information is gathered on the natural course of the child's feeding problems, the current status of the problems, prior and ongoing strategies that have or have not helped manage the child's eating, foods and textures that are now and were previously regularly consumed or rejected, meal duration and amounts consumed, the child's daily routine and family home structure, and caregivers' reports of environment-behavior relations surrounding feeding (Luiselli, 1989; Palmer & Horn, 1978; Singer et al., 1991).

When discussing environment-behavior relations with caregivers, the therapist asks the caregivers first to identify specific behavior problems from a checklist. The parent and therapist then prioritize the problems identified, and the therapist assists the parent in operationally defining behaviors that were chosen. Next, the therapist and caregiver identify situational variables, things that occur before (antecedents) and after (consequences) the problem behavior, which are hypothesized to exert some stimulus control over the problem behavior. The emphasis here, and during direct observation and functional analysis, is not on treating symptoms and causes, but rather identifying functional relationships between the feeding problem and its solution by identifying and manipulating variables that maintain the behavior (Linscheid, 1978; Thompson & Palmer, 1974).

Direct Observation

To develop an effective treatment, objective measures of the target behaviors must be made repeatedly under baseline conditions (Kazdin, 1982). Target behaviors are operationally defined in terms of their quantifiable physical characteristics. For example, accepting a bite of food (accept) may be operationally defined as "child's mouth open such that food enters within 5 seconds of presentation." The physical characteristics of the behavior described here are topography (mouth open), extensity (open such that food enters), and latency (within 5 seconds of presentation). When conceptualized in these terms, individual responses may be recorded objectively, and considered reliable if interobserver agreement figures are high (Johnston & Pennypacker, 1980).

Repeated measures are necessary to determine stability and trend of the target behavior over time, because measurement at a single point could produce aberrant behavior (Baer, Wolf, & Risley, 1968; Iwata et al., 1982; Palmer & Horn, 1978). Determining the trend is particularly important during baseline, pretreatment observations. Repeated measures of all behaviors targeted for treatment (target behaviors) is essential during baseline assessment and each subsequent phase of treatment. A general rule of thumb is that at least three observations are needed to establish a

trend, and the direction of the trend may indicate that further observation may be needed before treatment can be implemented (Cooper, Heron, & Heward, 1987). Little information can be gained from any one observation in isolation from others because unusual circumstances occurring during that observation (transient illness, new environment, fatigue, and others) may produce aberrant performances.

Initial direct observations are made systematically, under a series of standard pretreatment baseline conditions. Some of these conditions approximate the home environment (Hoch, Babbitt, Hackbert, & Stanton-Brugman, 1992). Others more closely approximate the treatment setting and have been described in great detail elsewhere (Iwata et al., 1982; Riordan et al., 1984; Riordan, Iwata, Wohl, & Finney, 1980). Tables 5–2 and 5–3 list operational definitions for behaviors commonly targeted for self-feeding and non-self-feeding children, respectively. The baseline procedures im-

TABLE 5–2. Operational definitions for self-feeder target behaviors.

Behavior	Operational Definition
Independent bite	Child voluntarily scoops food from container and places it into his or her mouth without physical guidance.
Prompted bite	Therapist physically offers a bite of food or guides child's hand to utensil, or assists child in placing a bite in his or her mouth.
Expel	Presence of any food/drink beyond the lip or chin area that had previously been in the child's mouth.
Pack	Child holds a bite or drink in his or her mouth for more than 30 seconds.
Dawdle	Each 1-minute interval in which less than 2 bites were taken.
Gag	Gagging or choking sounds emitted or facial grimacing.
Vomit	Discharge from mouth of emesis.
Negative vocalization	Any crying, whining, screaming, or stating that one does not like the food, does not want to eat, and so forth.
Interruption	Any behavior that precludes acceptance within 5 seconds of presentation.
Inappropriate Behavior	Any behavior that disrupts feeding activity and/or poses risk of injury (e.g., aggression, elopement, throwing of food or utensils, self-injury).
Grams consumed	Food preweight minus food postweight (controlling for amount spilled, expelled, or otherwise lost).
Percent Consumed	Quotient of grams consumed to food preweight.

TABLE 5–3. Operational definitions for non-self-feeder target behaviors.

Behavior	Operational Definition
Accept	Child's mouth open such that food/drink is deposited within 5 seconds.
Expel	Presence of any food/drink beyond the lip or chin area that had previously been in the child's mouth.
Mouth clean	Presence of an amount of food less than the size of two grains of rice in the child's mouth prior to the next presentation.
Gag	Gagging or choking sounds emitted or facial grimacing.
Vomit	Discharge from mouth of emesis.
Negative vocalization	Any crying, whining, screaming or stating that one does not like the food, does not want to eat, and so forth.
Interruption	Any behavior that precludes acceptance within 5 seconds of presentation.
Inappropriate behavior	Any behavior that disrupts feeding activity and/or poses risk of injury (e.g., aggression, elopement, throwing of food or utensils, self-injury).
Grams consumed	Food preweight minus food postweight (controlling for amount spilled, expelled, or otherwise lost).
Percent consumed	Quotient of grams consumed to food preweight.

plemented for each child are individualized with relevant target behaviors chosen from among those described in Tables 5–2 and 5–3.

Analysis of Child and Caregiver Interaction

An assessment of the interaction between a caregiver's feeding and a child's eating behaviors helps to identify interpersonal variables that may be maintaining the feeding problem. Specifically, the assessment delineates caregiver responses to the child's feeding behaviors, both antecedents and consequences, that appear to maintain the feeding disorder (Linscheid, 1978; Luiselli, 1989). Data are collected on the caregiver's correct use of antecedents (e.g., providing verbal prompts to eat accompanied by the presentation of a bite), prompts (e.g., following a spoken prompt-gestural prompt-physical prompt sequence unless otherwise instructed, representing expelled food), and consequences (providing positive reinforcement, such as praise or a toy,

for accepting and/or consuming the food and providing neutral consequences following other behaviors, unless instructed to do otherwise) (Babbitt & Hoch, 1992a; Iwata et al., 1982). This interaction analysis is conducted both during and outside of mealtimes to assess the caregiver's skills using a specific treatment protocol, as well as his or her general behavior management skills (Riley, Parrish & Cataldo, 1989).

Experimental Designs

Functional analysis is "the identification of important, controllable, causal functional relationships applicable to a specified set of target behaviors for an individual client" (Haynes & O'Brien, 1990, p. 654). The beginning steps in conducting a functional analysis are to narrow the field of important variables through interview and observation, and then to systematically collect baseline data to determine the nature and extent of the problem prior to intervention. The next step is to plan and methodically carry out a treatment while maintaining systematic measurement so that functional relationships between treatment procedures and the child's behavior are demonstrated. To do so requires the use of an experimental design. Single-case experimental designs use each child as his or her own control while evaluating the efficacy of the intervention. This arrangement obviates the need for a control group and circumvents the ethical issue of withholding treatment from eligible children (Iwata et al., 1982; Kazdin, 1982; Luiselli, 1989). The three most commonly used designs have been the withdrawal (ABAB) design, multiple baseline or multiple probe design, and alternating treatments design. The reader is referred to Kazdin (1982) for detailed descriptions of these experimental designs.

Environment-Behavior Relationships

As stated previously, the emphasis in treatment based on functional analysis is not on treating symptoms and causes, but rather identifying functional relationships between the feeding problem and its solution by identifying and manipulating variables that maintain the behavior (Linscheid, 1978; Thompson & Palmer, 1974). Through careful interviewing, systematic direct observation, and manipulation of treatment interventions and other variables following an experimental design, functional relationships between the child's behavior and the events surrounding it can be identified, and then modified in a readily observable manner to benefit the child. The manner in which variables are manipulated, deleterious functional relationships disrupted, and beneficial functional relationships established is discussed later in this chapter.

Functional Reinforcer Assessment

Before discussing how treatment variables are manipulated, it is important to discuss how important motivating variables can be identified. Numerous studies have demonstrated the unreliability of verbal reports (Iwata et al., 1982). It is also sometimes the case that what one "likes" doesn't function

as a positive reinforcer (Fisher et al., 1992). Functional assessments of potential reinforcers are conducted to identify objects or events (i.e., certain foods, toys, clapping, singing, tickling, and so forth) that produce a reinforcement effect (Luiselli, 1989). For in-depth reports of such assessments, the reader is referred to Pace, Ivanic, Edwards, Iwata, and Page (1985) or Fisher and associates (1992).

Food Preference Assessment

Treatment effects may sometimes be facilitated when treatment commences with foods the child is already likely to consume. Asking the child or parents to identify these foods, however, may not produce reliable data (Parsons & Reid, 1990). Instead, it is essential to objectively assess children's food preferences (Hoch et al., 1992). Hoch and associates (1992) reported that a food preference choice assessment procedure identified more preferred foods than were named by parents for all children for whom the procedure was implemented.

From Assessment to Treatment

Behavioral assessment of a child's feeding problem is conducted from a functional perspective. That is, rather than examining just the form or topography of the behavior (e.g., pushing food away, crying, spitting food out, etc.), observation of the consequences of the behavior made in conjunction with observations of the topographies yields important information about the function of the behavior. Once problems, or target behaviors, are identified in terms of their functions, particular treatment strategies are chosen to address those functions. For example, motivationally based problems are addressed with motivational procedures (i.e., reinforcement and extinction, described below), whereas skill-deficit based problems are addressed with skill acquisition procedures (e.g., shaping, described below).

Assessments yield data regarding patterns of behavioral topographies, such as food refusal or food selectivity. The particular names given to these topographical patterns are diagnoses. However, because diagnoses are names for topographical (rather than functional) patterns of behavior, these names are useful mainly for descriptive, rather than treatment purposes.

Treatment

Previous discussions have centered on identifying functional relationships between the feeding problem and its solution through interviewing, systematic direct observation, and manipulation of treatment interventions and other variables. Individual treatment procedures are discussed in the following sections. Often, however, a particular feeding problem will be treated with different procedures or combinations of procedures.

Increasing Behavior

Some behavior problems exist because, although the child is physically capable of a given behavior and occasionally engages in the behavior, the behavior does not occur frequently enough. This is a motivational problem, and is one of faulty contingencies of reinforcement.

In *positive reinforcement*, a behavior occurs, something is added to the child's environment that was not present immediately before the behavior occurred, and the behavior either continues to occur or is more likely to occur in the future. For example, when a child accepts a bite of food (behavior), the pleasant flavor of the food (which was previously absent) is sensed (consequence added), so under the previous set of circumstances (pleasant tasting food present but not in the mouth), the child will be increasingly likely (reinforcement) to open his or her mouth and accept the food. This pattern of behavior is common to non-self-feeding children who do not have feeding problems.

In *negative reinforcement*, a behavior occurs, something is removed from the child's environment that was not present immediately before the behavior occurred, and the behavior either continues to occur under those circumstances or is more likely to occur again under those circumstances in the future. For example, when a caregiver presents a spoonful of food (regardless of previous sensory experience with the food), screaming and pushing the food away (behavior) is followed by the caregiver ending the meal (stimulus terminated). When in this situation again, the child will be increasingly likely (reinforcement) to turn, scream, and push away the spoon. This pattern of behavior is common among some children with feeding problems.

Notice that in both positive and negative reinforcement, the result is that the behavior is either maintained or increases in some way. The maintenance of or increase in the behavior is the reinforcement effect. If this effect is brought about by addition of a consequence after occurrences of the behavior, the reinforcement is positive reinforcement. If this effect is brought about by removal or termination of a previously occurring event after occurrences of the behavior, the reinforcement is negative reinforcement. One commonly made error is the belief that positive reinforcement increases behavior and negative reinforcement decreases behavior (see Palmer & Horn, 1987; Thompson & Palmer, 1974). This error is probably attributable to colloquial uses of the terms "positive" and "negative." When used as technical terms, however, "positive" and "negative" are used in their mathematical sense to modify the term "reinforcement." A case study describing selection and use of positive and negative reinforcement procedures is presented in Appendix 5–1.

Positive Reinforcement Procedures

When a child is capable of consuming adequate amounts and varieties of foods but routinely fails to do so, a motivational problem may exist. Positive reinforcement for oral acceptance and consumption of food has been demonstrated to be an effective treatment for food refusal in some children (Bernal, 1972; Finney, 1986; Hatcher, 1979; Riordan et al., 1980, 1984; Singer et al., 1991). Typically, acceptance and consumption are followed by reinforcement while competing behaviors (e.g., expulsion and disruption) receive only neutral consequences. As a result, acceptance and consumption improve, and competing behaviors decrease. Initially, positive reinforcement is usually delivered immediately following every occurrence of the target behavior. Once a high, stable rate of behavior is achieved, the frequency of reinforcement can be systematically decreased, so that high rates of behavior are maintained with little effort on the part of the feeder.

Negative Reinforcement Procedures

Behavior that functions to escape or avoid a situation or stimulus is behavior that is under control of a negative reinforcement contingency. This may present a problem when a child who has been dependent on tube feedings but is physically capable of eating orally continues to avoid oral consumption by crying, turning away, expelling food, and so forth, even though these behaviors are no longer adaptive (Vogel, 1986; Ylvisaker & Weinstein, 1989). In other situations, it is desirable for children to escape or avoid potentially harmful stimuli, as when children learn to move out of the street when a car is coming. In some situations, then, it is important for some children to learn not to avoid, whereas in others, avoidance is the most adaptive form of behavior.

Iwata and associates (1982) defined two negative reinforcement paradigms. In the first, *avoidance learning*, the therapist delays or eliminates the onset of an unpleasant event if the child responds (e.g., parents shy away from new foods or textures when a child begins to whine, turn away, and kick as the spoon nears the child's

mouth.) In the second, *escape learning*, an ongoing stimulus is terminated by the response. For example, the unpleasant taste of beets can be escaped by expelling them forcefully from the mouth (e.g., feeding is regularly terminated conditional on crying, expulsion, turning away, and so forth, resulting in great frequencies of these topographies).

Treatment procedures based on negative reinforcement alone have rarely been reported in the literature. In one reported procedure, however, escape from the feeding room was made conditional on swallowing a bite of food, for children who previously escaped feeding by expelling food or holding it in their mouths for long periods of time (Babbitt, Hoch, Krell, & Williams, 1992). Frequency of swallowing bites of food increased rapidly, latency to swallowing decreased greatly, and placement of a gastrostomy tube was avoided in one case, while in another use of the gastrostomy tube was discontinued and the tube was removed.

Prompting and Modeling Procedures

Reinforcement procedures, by definition, depend on occurrence of the target behavior (albeit at low rates) prior to treatment to be effective. When a child engages in a target behavior, but does so too infrequently for a reinforcement procedure to be effective, prompting or modeling procedures can be used to facilitate occurrence of the behavior.

Prompts usually consist of instructions, gestures, or physical guidance given to increase the probability that a child will produce a behavior, so that the behavior can be reinforced. When the behavior occurs at a stable, high rate, prompts are gradually removed (faded) by either providing less assistance or delaying prompt onset to allow more time for the child to respond on his or her own. Prompting and prompt fading have been used to teach appropriate utensil use and self-feeding skills (Iwata et al., 1982; O'Brien, Bugle, & Azrin, 1972).

Some children can learn effectively when provided with a model to imitate. Modeling procedures depend on the child's imitation skills for their success. In a typical modeling procedure, the therapist instructs the child to "do this," engages in the target behavior, and provides reinforcement if the child repeats a close approximation of the behavior. Peer modeling involves having children observe other children (confederates) behave appropriately and receive reinforcement (Greer, Dorow, Williams, McCorkle, & Asnes, 1991). Parents and peers can often improve food preferences by eating a nutritionally balanced diet (Finney, 1986), and can encourage appropriate mealtime behaviors by engaging in them themselves (Linscheid, 1978).

Decreasing Behavior

A second type of motivational problem is one in which a behavior occurs to excess. When this is the case, the goal of treatment is to reduce occurrence of the behavior. Four primary methods of reducing behavioral excesses are: extinction, differential reinforcement of other behavior, punishment, and antecedent manipulation.

Extinction

The previous discussions of positive and negative reinforcement pointed out that behavior under control of such procedures is maintained by the consequences (reinforcers) it produces. To produce behavior that is maintained when not reinforced, it is essential to gradually reduce the frequency of reinforcement. However, if one abruptly disrupts the reinforcement contingency, then the behavior is likely to cease. Extinction is the termination of an ongoing reinforcement contingency, which results in an initial increase, then decrease, and possible elimination of a behavior. For example, if a child's expulsion of food previously resulted in parents' terminating meals, continuing feeding (and re-presenting bites expelled) initially is likely to re-sult in an increase in frequency (and intensity) of expulsion and then a decrease and elimination.

Time out from positive reinforcement (Time Out) is an extinction procedure in which the child is removed from a reinforcing situation contingent on a targeted inappropriate behavior. This procedure is maximally effective when the situation from which the child is removed is reinforcing, thereby giving the child a reason to avoid removal and to earn return when removal occurs. Use of Time Out is not recommended when removal from the situation could produce escape from a situation that is used to increase a target behavior. For example, if a child refuses food by throwing it and his utensils, and a goal of treatment is to increase consumption, it would not be advisable to remove the child from the meal contingent on spoon or food throwing.

Differential Reinforcement of Other Behavior (DRO)

Although extinguishing an excessive behavior by removing its reinforcers may be effective in eliminating the behavior, it does not guarantee that a more beneficial behavior will take its place. To eliminate an excessive behavior and replace it with a more beneficial target behavior, an extinction procedure (for the behavior to be eliminated) can be combined with a positive reinforcement procedure (for the behavior to be increased). This type of procedure is called differential reinforcement of other behavior (DRO) (Iwata et al., 1982). "Positive reinforcement for alternative behaviors should always be programmed when treating any clinical problem or health threatening disorder" (Luiselli, 1989, p. 122).

For example, consider a child who has previously escaped feeding situations with excessive crying and pushing the spoon away. Routinely, these behaviors have resulted in parents terminating the meal and giving the child her bottle. When the child occasionally does accept a bite, the parents are so relieved that she is eating that they leave her alone. Two problems here are (1) excessive crying and refusal, which are apparently negatively reinforced by meal termination, and (2) deficient food acceptance and consumption, which apparently receive little positive reinforcement. To ameliorate this situation, the parents should disrupt the negative reinforcement contingency by ignoring interruption and crying (extinction); continuing the meal until they have reached a predetermined time limit, volume of food consumed, or number of bites presented (extinction); and provide lavish social attention and other reinforcers when the child accepts and consumes a bite of food.

Punishment

In a reinforcement procedure, the behavior occurs, a consequence is provided (something is either added or taken away), and the behavior increases. Punishment has the opposite effect. In a punishment procedure, the behavior occurs, a consequence is provided (something is either added or taken away), and the behavior decreases. Punishment, in its scientific sense, describes either an effect on a behavior or a procedure used to produce that effect. The majority of punishment procedures reported in the feeding literature focus on decreasing rumination and vomiting. Punishers have included: noxious tastes such as lemon juice; contingent oral hygiene with mouth wash; overcorrection, or repeating a targeted adaptive behavior numerous times contingent on occurrence of a maladaptive behavior; contingent restraint; and contingent forced feeding (Blackman & Nelson, 1987; Christophersen & Hall, 1978; Clauser & Scibak, 1990; Duker, 1981; Iwata et al., 1982; Starin & Fuqua, 1987). Punishment should be attempted only when there is direct supervision provided by trained and experienced behavior analysts, ongoing medical modeling, and positive programming.

Antecedent Manipulation

The methods for decreasing behavior discussed thus far have all dealt with chang-

ing the consequences of the behavior. It is also possible to alter the antecedents of the behavior to decrease its probability. For example, a child may be less likely to expel a nonpreferred food if its taste is masked by a preferred food (Thompson & Palmer, 1974). Selectivity by texture has been addressed by gradually increasing food texture while maintaining positive reinforcement contingencies on consumption (Finney, 1986; Luiselli & Gleason, 1987). Consumption of larger portions or more nutritious, nonpreferred foods has been addressed by making access to preferred foods contingent on complete consumption of gradually increasing portion sizes of nonpreferred foods (Finney, 1986).

Skill Acquisition

Treatments discussed thus far have involved managing contingencies to address motivational problems. Skill deficit problems require a different approach. Rather than motivating the child to perform more or less of an already existing behavior, skill acquisition procedures teach the child a new or more complex behavior.

To teach a behavior the child currently does not possess, the goal behavior can be broken down into smaller components and acquisition of these components can be systematically and cumulatively reinforced until the goal behavior is achieved (Linscheid, 1978). Such a procedure is termed "shaping." Self-feeding is a complex response made up of many less complex behaviors, and many authors have described studies in which this response has been shaped (Christophersen & Hall, 1978; Finney, 1986; Iwata et al., 1982). Linscheid (1978) provides an excellent example of a program for teaching self-feeding with utensils.

Programming Generalization

Each of the procedures described above can be effective in bringing about behavioral change in the treatment setting. One cannot assume, however, that the behavioral change in the treatment setting will generalize to other feeders, settings, foods, and so forth. Following behavioral treatment procedures closely may produce excellent performances that occur only in one specific (treatment) setting and with one specific (therapist) feeder. This, of course, is rarely the end goal of treatment.

Generalization is described as the occurrence of a previously taught behavior in the presence of a novel stimulus situation (Miller, 1980, p. 169). The ultimate goals of most feeding treatment procedures is for the child to eat well for any caregiver and in all settings (Luiselli, 1989). Therefore, it is essential to explicitly program generalization across settings, caregivers, foods, and so forth.

Before programming for generalization and introducing new elements (feeders, settings, foods, etc.), it is necessary to first establish stable responding in the controlled, clinical setting. Next, distractions (such as noises or presence of siblings) can be systematically added to the meal (in the treatment setting). Once the child's performances have adjusted to these distractions, one may systematically change the feeding setting to more closely approximate the targeted home, school, or other environments.

Parent Training

Behavioral treatment is often initially conducted with the child alone to minimize effects of inappropriate caregiver-child interactions on training. The ultimate goal of treatment, however, is for the child to eat for all caregivers in a variety of settings. Caregivers have a unique feeding history with the child that usually brings about performance decrements when the caregiver is reintroduced to feeding. Sometimes these decrements may be slight, such as a child's continuing to eat but crying throughout the meal. More often, however, the child's performance temporarily returns to baseline levels. This does not create an optimal setting in which to teach the parent to feed.

Few descriptions of caregiver training are available (Riordan et al., 1984). Linscheid (1978) described a comprehensive, competency-based caregiver training package. Therapists feed until stable treatment effects are achieved. Concurrently, caregivers observe unobtrusively (through a one-way mirror) and collect data on the meals. Outside of meals, caregivers are trained to use proper general behavior management strategies (antecedents, prompts, and consequences). Following attainment of proficient general behavior management skills, caregivers are trained to implement their child's feeding treatment protocol in a series of systematic steps. First, caregivers may be trained to give correct antecedents (e.g., verbal instructions to take a bite); next, prompts and consequences (e.g., reinforcers); and then correct antecedents, prompts, and consequences together. Training may first involve role playing with dolls or confederates substituting for the child. Once the caregiver demonstrates proficient skills under these conditions, actual feeding of the child by the caregiver is implemented. This type of training allows the caregiver to master necessary skills before introducing him or her to the actual feeding situation, thereby possibly reducing caregiver anxieties and any effects that caregiver errors might have on the child's progress (Babbitt & Hoch, 1992a, 1992b).

Procedural Fading and Follow-up

Another end goal of treatment is for the child to eat well with as few supports as are necessary. Treatment procedures described previously in this chapter may produce excellent performances but, in the absence of systematic fading, require continued adherence to the protocol. To do otherwise would result in regression to baseline performances. If treatment is faded gradually and systematically, gains can be maintained while returning mealtime to a more natural state. Treatment fading can include fading the frequency of reinforcement, transferring control to more naturally occurring reinforcers (e.g., praise instead of toy play, or preferred foods such as dessert), and fading any prompting procedures that may be in effect (Iwata et al., 1982).

Follow-up is an integral component in the treatment continuum. Palmer and Horn (1978) recommend rigorous follow-up at specified intervals immediately following discharge from treatment to ensure continued progress and reduce the probability of regression. Descriptions of follow-up procedures, however, have not been published, and minimal follow-up data have been generally reported. Optimally, follow-up services should span the course of at least 1 year following discharge. Frequency of contacts and intensity of services could be lessened as goals are maintained or new goals achieved.

Treatment Efficacy

To systematically assess treatment efficacy, it is essential to employ some sort of experimental design. The use of single-case experimental designs was previously discussed, and Kazdin (1982) is an excellent reference on this topic. When data indicate that a treatment procedure is not effective, a series of questions should be asked to pinpoint possible uncontrolled variables. Important variables to consider in treatment of behavioral feeding problems are outlined in Table 5–4. This table describes a number of variables that may produce undesirable effects and recommends courses of action for remediating them.

Conclusions and Future Directions

Behavioral assessment and treatment of medical problems is a relatively new field. Children's feeding and nutritional problems is a primary area of clinical research. The intent of this chapter has been to provide a review of the pediatric behavioral feeding literature and to acquaint the reader with basic assessment, treatment, and fol-

TABLE 5–4. Variables that may negatively influence treatment efficacy.

Variables	Potential Problems
Difficulty level of behavioral objectives	Objectives may need to be further analyzed and taught in smaller steps or in a different sequence. Alternatively, a problem that initially appeared to be motivational in nature may actually reflect a skill deficit.
Competing behaviors	These may need to be systematically targeted and changed before the initial target behavior can be addressed.
Data collection	Current behavioral measures may be inaccurate or lack utility and may need to be revised into more detailed or functional terms.
Medication regimen or illness	Medications may exert multiple effects on behavior and should be continuously monitored. Illness can also adversely affect performance. Changes in behavioral programming should not coincide with changes in medication or health status.
Reinforcement schedule	Reinforcers may not be given promptly or consistently. They may also be accessible outside of meals, limiting their effectiveness. Alternatively, satiation may have occurred, creating a need for additional reinforcers.
Behavior of caregivers or significant others	These individuals may not be following treatment procedures or may be engaging in behaviors that undermine treatment. In either event, further training and arrangement of motivating variables for caregivers may be necessary.

low-up procedures and the rationales behind them. The complex interrelationships between physiological, developmental, environmental, and social influences on these problems require multidisciplinary assessment and treatment (Koepke & Thyer, 1985; Palmer & Horn, 1978; Palmer et al., 1975; Thompson & Palmer, 1974; Tuchman, 1988; Warren & Fox, 1987). What previous authors have underestimated, and what this chapter emphasizes, is the valuable team membership role that can be served by a trained, experienced behavior analyst. The disciplines of medicine and behavior analysis naturally complement each other. Medical science provides analysis and control of physiological processes. Behavior analysis similarly provides analysis and control of behavioral processes.

Future directions of behavioral feeding treatment and research include continued development, systematic refinement, and experimental evaluation of treatments considerate of social and caregiver variables that account for or contribute to the improvement of medical variables. Development of procedures that are maximally effective within accountability constraints imposed by changes in health care systems would be essential (Babbitt, Hoch, Sestero, & Cataldo, 1991). Such work would enhance both behavioral and medical spheres of assessment, treatment, and research and expand the range of effective treatment options available for children with feeding problems.

Appendix 5–1
Increasing Behavior: Case Study Involving Positive and Negative Reinforcement Procedures

Anne was a 25-month-old girl diagnosed with severe mental retardation, caudal regression syndrome, hypertension, gastroesophageal reflux, microcephaly, colosto-my, renal insufficiency, and failure-to-thrive. Anne's history included food refusal and frequent expulsion, leading to inadequate oral intake and nasogastric tube feeding. Baseline observations confirmed a low percentage of acceptance and high percentage of expulsion. Given the apparent avoidant function of Anne's food refusal and expulsion, and lack of reinforcement for the few instances of acceptance that did occur, motivational treatment procedures were selected. A positive reinforcement procedure increased acceptance. Next, an extinction procedure was added that decreased expulsion. However, absence of expulsion did not produce increased consumption, but rather resulted in Anne escaping further presentations by holding bites in her mouth for long periods of time (packing). Escape and avoidance both appeared to be functions of Anne's packing, as meals historically had been terminated conditional on these behaviors. Given this apparent negative reinforcement function, leaving the meal situation was made contingent on Anne's swallowing the food. Once Anne was regularly swallowing her bites within a reasonable period of time, meal size was gradually increased until Anne was presented with, and consuming, whole meals. Nasogastric tube feedings were eliminated 2 weeks prior to discharge, and Anne has since received adequate nutrition and hydration orally.

Appendix 5–2
Decreasing Behavior: Case Study Involving Differential Reinforcement of Other Behavior and Antecedent Manipulation

Michael was a 4-year-old boy diagnosed with profound mental retardation, cerebral palsy, total visual impairment, profound hearing impairment, history of failure-to-thrive, pathological tongue thrust, and status posttracheostomy. Michael was admitted for assessment and treatment of solid food refusal and self-injurious behavior. At admission, Michael was completely dependent on formula feeds by bottle every 30 minutes when awake, and all attempts to introduce solid foods had been unsuccessful. During baseline sessions, Michael was presented with food by spoon, diluted purees by bottle, or a mixture of formula and purees by bottle with no consequences provided for any behaviors. When presented with food by spoon, Michael would push the food away, turn his head, cry, clamp his mouth shut, slap his face, pull his hair, and act aggressively toward the feeder. These behaviors did not occur when purees and formula were presented by bottle. Given the occurrence of the problem behaviors only in the presence of feeding by spoon, an antecedent manipulation procedure (gradually changing from bottle to spoon) was combined with differential reinforcement (reinforcing only acceptance and not other behaviors). Treatment began using Michael's most preferred food group (starches) to ensure early success and then incorporated other food groups once a stable, high percentage of acceptance was achieved. Concurrently, a push bottle (allowing the therapist to control flow of food delivery) was substituted for the standard bottle, and once acceptance again stabilized, a spoon was introduced.

Appendix 5–3
Skill Acquisition: Case Study Involving Shaping

One type of shaping involves eliciting a reflex, such as swallowing, and transferring control of the reflex to instructions, food, and reinforcers. Gina was a 16-month-old girl diagnosed with average intellectual functioning, gastroesophageal reflux, status postgastrostomy tube and Nissen fundoplication, dysphagia, and history of as-

piration. Gina was admitted for assessment and treatment of swallowing skill deficit, food refusal, and tantrums. During baseline, purees were presented by spoon and liquids by cup. Baseline observations revealed very infrequent acceptance and reliable expulsion once food was accepted. To address motivational variables in Gina's food refusal, the first treatment combined positive reinforcement for acceptance and extinction to decrease interruption, expulsion, and other inappropriate behaviors. When swallowing did not spontaneously emerge, a prompt eliciting a swallow was combined with reinforcement to first elicit a swallow reflex and follow it with reinforcement. As swallowing became more regular and stable (as determined through audiological monitoring), elicitation was faded to regular spoon presentation. Treatments addressing motivational variables increased frequency of acceptance and reduced avoidant behaviors (except for expulsion), but did not increase grams consumed. Thus, this phase determined that absence of swallowing was not motivational in nature. Treatment addressing skill acquisition produced dramatic increases in swallowing and oral consumption, and supplemental tube feedings were discontinued prior to the child's discharge.

Appendix 5–4
Programming Generalization: Case Study

Zoey was a 5-year-old girl diagnosed with moderate mental retardation, Dandy Walker malformation, cortical blindness, and a seizure disorder posttraumatic brain injury. Following her injury, she lost the suck response and stopped eating. She was subsisting by gavaging milk down her throat through an enlarged bottle nipple. This hospitalization was the fourth to address feeding, and baseline assessments revealed total solid food refusal and tantrums. A generalized compliance training (GCT) paradigm was implemented, whereby compliance to both nonfood (high probability) and food (low probability) requests was differentially reinforced, and inappropriate behaviors were placed on extinction. Increases in consumption and decreases in inappropriate behaviors did not generalize to other feeders until they had been trained. Each new feeder needed to be trained and systematically introduced into the treatment meal setting before consistently high accepts were achieved (Babbitt, Cataldo, Hoch, & McKew-Kuhn, 1991).

References

Babbitt, R. L., Cataldo, M. F., Hoch, T. A., & McKew-Kuhn, K. (1991, May). *The treatment of food refusal using a generalized compliance training paradigm.* Poster presented at the Convention for the Association for Behavior Analysis, Atlanta, GA.

Babbitt, R. L., & Hoch, T. A. (1992a, May). *Behavioral assessment of pediatric feeding disorders.* Paper presented at the Conference of the International Society for Infant Studies, Miami, FL.

Babbitt, R. L., & Hoch, T. A. (1992b, May). *Parent training in a pediatric medical setting.* Paper presented at the Convention of the Association for Behavior Analysis, San Francisco, CA.

Babbitt, R. L., Hoch, T. A., Krell, D., & Williams, K. (1992, May). *Exit criterion: Treating motivational absence of swallowing.* Poster presented at the Convention of the Association for Behavior Analysis, San Francisco, CA.

Babbitt, R. L., Hoch, T. A., Sestero, D. G., & Cataldo, M. F. (1991, May). *Organizational and service evaluation of a pediatric behavioral feeding program.* Poster presented at the Convention of the Association for Behavior Analysis, Atlanta, GA.

Baer, D. M., Wolf, M. M., & Risley, T. R. (1968). Some current dimensions of applied behavior analysis. *Journal of Applied Behavior Analysis, 1,* 91–97.

Bernal, M. E. (1972). Behavioral treatment of a child's eating problem. *Journal of Behavior Therapy and Experimental Psychiatry, 3,* 43–50.

Blackman, J. A., & Nelson, C. L. A. (1985). Reinstating oral feedings in children fed by gastrostomy tube. *Clinical Pediatrics, 24,* 434–438.

Blackman, J. A., & Nelson, C. L. A. (1987). Rapid introduction of oral feedings to tube-fed patients. *Developmental and Behavioral Pediatrics, 8,* 63–67.

Brown, J. E., Davis, E., & Flemming, P. L. (1979). Nutritional assessment of children with handicapping conditions. *Mental Retardation, 17,* 129–131.

Budd, K. S., McGraw, T. E., Farbisz, R., Murphy, T. B., Hawkins, D., Heilman, N., & Werle, M. (1992). Psychosocial concomitants of children's feeding disorders. *Journal of Pediatric Psychology, 17,* 81–94.

Christophersen, E. R., & Hall, C. L. (1978). Eating patterns and associated problems encountered in normal children. *Issues in Comprehensive Pediatric Nursing, 3,* 1–16.

Clauser, B., &. Scibak, J. W. (1990). Direct and generalized effects of food satiation in reducing rumination. *Research in Developmental Disabilities, 11,* 23–36.

Cooper, J. O., Heron, T. E., & Heward, W. L. (1987). *Applied behavior analysis.* Columbus, OH: Merrill.

Cupoli, J. M., Hallock, J. A., & Barnes, L. A. (1980). Failure to thrive. *Current Problems in Pediatrics, 10,* 1–43.

Dahl, M., & Sundelin, C. (1986). Early feeding problems in an affluent society. *Acta Paediatrica Scandinavica, 75,* 370–379.

Duker, P. C. (1981). Treatment of food refusal by the overcorrective functional movement training method. *Journal of Behavior Therapy and Experimental Psychiatry, 12,* 337–340.

Finney, J. W. (1986). Preventing common feeding problems in infants and young children. *Pediatric Clinics of North America, 33,* 775–788.

Fisher, W. P., Piazza, C., Bowman, L., Owens, J. C., Hagopian, L., & Slevin, I. (1992). A comparison of two approaches for identifying reinforcers for persons with severe and profound disabilities. *Journal of Applied Behavior Analysis, 25,* 491–498.

Forsyth, B. W., Leventhal, J. M., & McCarthy, P. J. (1985). Mothers' perceptions of feeding and crying behaviors. *American Journal of Diseases of Children, 139,* 269–272.

Foxx, R. M., Snyder, M. S., & Schroeder, F. (1979). A food satiation and oral hygiene punishment program to suppress chronic rumination by retarded persons. *Journal of Autism and Developmental Disorders, 9*, 399–413.

Geertsma, M. A., Hyams, J. S., Pelletier, J. M., & Reiter, S. (1985). Feeding resistance after parenteral hyperalimentation. *American Journal of Diseases of Children, 139*, 255–256.

Greer, R. D., Dorow, L., Williams, G., McCorkle, N., & Asnes, R. (1991). Peer-mediated procedures to induce swallowing and food acceptance in young children. *Journal of Applied Behavior Analysis, 24*, 783–790.

Gross, A. M., & Drabman, R. S. (Eds.). (1990). *Handbook of clinical behavioral pediatrics.* New York: Plenum Press.

Hatcher, R. P. (1979). Treatment of food refusal in a two-year-old child. *Journal of Behavior Therapy and Experimental Psychiatry, 10*, 363–367.

Haynes, S. N., & O'Brian, W. H. (1990). Functional analysis in behavior therapy. *Clinical Psychology Review, 10*, 649–668.

Hoch, T. A., Babbitt, R. L., Hackbert, L., & Stanton-Brugman, J. (1992, May). *Assessing self-feeders' food preferences to assist in treatment of food selectivity and refusal.* Poster presented at the Convention for the Association for Behavior Analysis, San Francisco, CA.

Hoch, T. A., Babbitt, R. L., Krell, D. M., & Hackbert, L. (in press). Contingency contacting: Combining positive reinforcement and escape extinction procedures to treat persistent food refusal. *Behavior Modification.*

Hyman, S. L., Porter, C. A., Page, T. J., Iwata, B. A., Kissel, R., & Batshaw, M. L. (1987). Behavior management of feeding disturbances in urea cycle and organic acid disorders. *Journal of Pediatrics, 111*, 558–562.

Illingworth, R. S. (1969). Sucking and swallowing difficulties in infancy: Diagnostic problem of dysphagia. *Archives of Disease in Childhood, 44*, 655–665.

Illingworth, R. S., & Lister, J. (1964). The critical or sensitive period, with special reference to certain feeding problems in infants and children. *Journal of Pediatrics, 65*, 839–848.

Iwata, B. A., Riordan, M. M., Wohl, M. K., & Finney, J. W. (1982). Pediatric feeding disorders: Behavioral analysis and treatment. In P. J. Accardo (Ed.), *Failure to thrive in infancy and early childhood* (pp. 297–329). Baltimore: University Park Press.

Johnston, J. M., & Pennypacker, H. S. (1980). *Strategies and tactics of human behavior research.* Hillsdale, NJ: Lawrence Erlbaum.

Jones, T. W. (1982). Treatment of behavior-related eating problems in retarded students: A review of the literature. In J. H. Hollis & C. E. Meyers (Eds.), *Life threatening behavior: Analysis and intervention* (pp. 3–26). Washington, DC: American Association on Mental Deficiency.

Kazdin, A. E. (1982). *Single case research design: Methods for clinical and applied settings.* New York: Oxford University Press.

Koepke, J. M., & Thyer, B. A. (1985). Behavioral treatment of failure-to-thrive in a two-year-old. *Child Welfare, 64*, 511–516.

Krasnegor, N. A., Cataldo, M. F., & Arasteh, J. D. (Eds.). (1986). *Child health behavior: A behavioral pediatric approach.* New York: John Wiley.

Lamm, N., &. Greer, R. D. (1988). Induction and maintenance of swallowing responces in infants with dysphagia. *Journal of Applied Behavior Analysis, 21*, 143–156.

Linscheid, T. R. (1978). Disturbances of eating and feeding. In P. R. Magreb (Ed.), *Psychological management of pediatric problems: Early life conditions and chronic diseases* (Vol. 1, pp. 191–218). Baltimore: University Park Press.

Luiselli, J. K. (1989). Behavioral assessment and treatment of pediatric feeding disorders in developmental disabilities. In M. Hersen, R. M. Eisler, & P. M. Miller (Eds.), *Progress in behavior modification* (Vol. 24, pp. 91–131). Newbury Park, CA: Sage.

Luiselli, J. K., & Gleason, D. J. (1987). Combining sensory reinforcement and texture-fading procedures to overcome chronic food refusal. *Journal of Behavior Therapy and Experimental Psychiatry, 18*, 149–155.

O'Brien, F., Bugle, C., & Azrin, N. H. (1972). Training and maintaining a retarded child's proper eating. *Journal of Applied Behavior Analysis, 5*, 67–72.

Pace, G. M., Ivancic, M. T., Edwards, G. L., Iwata, B. A., & Page, T. J. (1985). Assessment of stimulus preference and reinforcer value with profoundly retarded individuals. *Journal of Applied Behavior Analysis, 18*, 249–255.

Palmer, S., & Horn, S. (1978). Feeding problems in children. In S. Palmer & S. Ekvall (Eds.), *Pediatric nutrition in developmental disorders* (pp. 107–129). Springfield, IL: Charles C. Thomas.

Palmer, S., Thompson, R. J., Jr., & Linscheid, T. R. (1975). Applied behavior analysis in the treatment of childhood feeding problems. *Developmental Medicine and Child Neurology, 17*, 333–339.

Parsons, M. B., & Reid, D. H. (1990). Assessing food preferences among persons with profound mental retardation: Providing opportunities to make choices. *Journal of Applied Behavior Analysis, 23*, 183–195.

Perske, R., Clifton, A., McClean, B. M., & Stein, J. I. (Eds.) (1977). *Mealtimes for severely and profoundly handicapped persons: New concepts and attitudes.* Baltimore: University Park Press.

Riley, A. W., Parrish, J. M., & Cataldo, M. F. (1989). Training parents to meet the needs of children with medical or physical handicaps. In C. E. Schaefer & J. M. Briesmeister (Eds.), *Handbook of parent training: Parents as cotherapists for children's behavior problems* (pp. 305–336). New York: John Wiley.

Riordan, M. M., Iwata, B. A., Wohl, M. K., & Finney, J. W. (1980). Behavioral treatment of food refusal and selectivity in developmentally disabled children. *Applied Research in Mental Retardation, 1*, 95–112.

Riordan, M. M., Iwata, B. A., Finney, J. W., Wohl, M. K., & Stanley, A. E. (1984). Behavioral assessment and treatment of chronic food refusal in handicapped children. *Journal of Applied Behavior Analysis, 17*, 596–610.

Routh, D. K. (Ed.). (1988). *Handbook of pediatric psychology.* New York: The Guilford Press.

Singer, L. T., Nofer, J. A., Benson-Szekeley, L. J., & Brooks, L. J. (1991). Behavioral assessment and management of food refusal in children with cystic fibrosis. *Developmental and Behavioral Pediatrics, 12*, 115–120.

Starin, S. P., & Fuqua, R. W. (1987). Rumination and vomiting in the developmentally disabled: A critical review of the behavioral, medical, and psychiatric treatment research. *Research in Developmental Disabilities, 8*, 575–604.

Thompson, R. J., & Palmer, S. (1974). Treatment of feeding problems — A behavioral approach. *Journal of Nutrition Education, 6*, 63–66.

Tuchman, D. N. (1988). Dysfunctional swallowing in the pediatric patient: Clinical considerations. *Dysphagia, 2*, 203–208.

Vogel, S. (1986). Oral motor and feeding problems in the tube fed infant: Suggested treatment strategies for the occupational therapist. In F. S. Cromwell (Ed.), *Occupational therapy for people with eating dysfunctions.* New York: Haworth Press.

Warren, L. R., & Fox, C. A. (1987). The use of videofluoroscopy in the evaluation and treatment of children with swallowing disorders. In C. Pehoski (Ed.), *Problems with eating: Interventions for children and adults with developmental disabilities* (pp. 9–14). Rockville, MD: The American Occupational Therapy Association.

Ylvisaker, M., & Weinstein, M. (1989). Recovery of oral feeding after pediatric head injury. *Journal of Head Trauma Rehabilitation, 4*, 51–63.

Diagnosis and Management of Pediatric Feeding and Swallowing Disorders: Role of the Speech-Language Pathologist

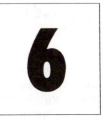

6

CHAPTER

Maureen A. Lefton-Greif, Ph.D., CCC-SP

The role of the speech-language pathologist (SLP) in the evaluation and management of dysphagia[1] is widely recognized. According to the 1985 American Speech Language and Hearing Association (ASHA) Omnibus Survey, 35% of the SLP respondents were delivering dysphagia treatment to both "communicatively disordered and noncommunicatively disordered clients" (ASHA, 1987). By 1988, 42% of the SLPs surveyed were regularly involved in servicing patients with dysphagia (Shewan, 1988). SLPs report that 11% of their caseloads are comprised of patients exhibiting dysphagia (Slater, 1992).

Evaluating Children with Feeding and Swallowing Disorders: General Concepts

Media images such as the happy well-fed Gerber™ baby have evoked warm yet simplistic feelings about the feeding and nurturing process. Safe, efficient, and enjoyable feeding is dependent on a complex series of neuromuscular processes which ensure the rapid and appropriately timed movements of the oral cavity, pharynx, larynx, and esophagus (Logemann, 1988a, 1988b). Eating and swallowing behaviors are modified by the child's cognitive, fine, and gross motor abilities (Christensen, 1989). Furthermore, the infant or child's early feeding circumstance is "distinctively linked with their mother or other care person" (Bosma, 1990, p. 79).

"Dysphagia . . . is a symptom of disease that may be affecting any part of the swallowing tract from the mouth to the stomach" (Donner, 1986, p. 1) and may present as respiratory compromise, growth failure, and/or negative behavior at mealtimes. These symptoms may then be attributed to or correlated with a local anatomic and/or neuromuscular basis (Alexander, 1983; Kramer, 1985; Logan & Bosma, 1967)

---

[1] "Dysphagia is a swallowing disorder characterized by difficulty in oral preparation for the swallow or in moving material from the mouth to the stomach. Subsumed in this definition are problems in positioning food in the mouth and in the oral manipulation preceding the swallow including suckling, sucking, and mastication." (ASHA, 1987, p. 57)

and occasionally to behavioral adaptations to the home environment or the feeding and swallowing situation (DiScipio, Kaslon, & Rubin, 1978; Kenny, 1990; Palmer & Horn, 1978). Environmental factors including "parental stress, depression, or family instability" may predispose some children to feeding disorders (Singer, 1990, p. 61). Additionally, systemic difficulties (e.g., cardiorespiratory diseases) may interfere with the child's ability to coordinate feeding and swallowing maneuvers (Imhoff & Wigginton, 1991).

Feeding and swallowing patterns are considered abnormal when they interfere with airway protection, nutrition or hydration adequacy, and/or the enjoyment of the feeding situation for either the child, or parent and/or caregiver[2] (Harris, 1986). The goal of a feeding and swallowing assessment is to develop a management protocol which enables safe and efficient feeding that is enjoyable for both the child and the caregivers.

Assessment of feeding safety requires the identification of factors that predispose the youngster to airway compromise as well as conditions that lead to elimination of airway contamination during oral intake. The ability to meet nutrition and hydration goals is dependent on oral-pharyngeal efficiency (rate of intake per unit of time) without compromise of airway safety. These goals are often met through a team approach including input from a nutritionist in conjunction with the initiation of therapies to increase oral-pharyngeal efficiency. Finally, the most subjective management goal is the facilitation of an enjoyable interaction between the child and caregiver.

Differences Between Pediatric and Adult Evaluations

Normal and disordered swallowing mechanisms in the adult have been extensively

discussed (Groher, 1984, 1992; Logemann, 1983). However, there are limitations associated with the application of the adult model to the pediatric population. As stated by Bosma (1990), "The clinical approach to these (feeding) impairments in early pediatric age is notably different from that to dysphagia which is acquired in the neurologically mature adult" (p. 79). Feeding and swallowing function are dynamic processes under constant change mediated by the differential growth and development of the structures comprising the upper aerodigestive tract. The growth rate is dramatic enough to have substantial effects on infant vocalization. Bosma (1975) stated,

> The gestures of prelinguistic sounds and of early speech are accomplished by structures at their current moment of development in histology, in form and dimension, and in spatial arrangement within this region. A month later, speech is accomplished by a different anatomy. (p. 469)

Likewise, the infant's feeding and swallowing behavior must continually adapt to this changing system. Throughout all stages of growth, the infant's pharynx is responsible for four primary functions including: airway maintenance, food and liquid passage, respiration, and phonation (Bosma, 1963; Buchholz, Bosma, & Donner, 1985). Consequently, identification of children at risk for feeding and swallowing impairment is dependent on assessing a dynamic system which continually accommodates to growth and development while supporting safe and efficient food and liquid delivery.

An Evaluation Perspective

The model of three developmental strategies describing the emerging vocalizations during infancy proposed by Stark,

---

[2] The parent is generally the primary caregiver. Although this role is not limited to the parent, the terms caregiver and parent will be used interchangeably throughout this chapter.

Rose, and Benson (1974), may be applicable to the evaluation of evolving feeding and swallowing patterns in the pediatric client. The first strategy identifies emerging oral motor patterns in relation to developmental milestone acquisition. This method is classically used to describe the acquisition and progression of oral preparatory and oral stage patterns (Alexander, 1983; Lewis, 1982; Morris & Klein, 1987). The second approach is based on the infant's developmental trajectory and is used in developing prognostic indicators and therapeutic intervention plans. The third tactic compares the infant's patterns with those observed in the adult in an attempt to track successive approximations as the child gradually develops into the adult model. The latter strategy is potentially the most potent factor in developing a management approach because the adult model is inherently at greater risk for airway compromise than is the infant's system. In the neonate, the relatively close approximation between the base of the tongue and the laryngeal aditus facilitates airway protection during swallowing. As the pharynx lengthens and develops, this natural protective anatomic arrangement is lost. Consequently, the infant must continually adapt to a changing system that is at increasingly greater risk for airway compromise. At the same time, nutritional demands grow.

Pediatric Populations at Risk for Development of Feeding and Swallowing Disorders

Imhoff and Wigginton (1991) evaluated 300 infants for potential feeding and swallowing problems and observed five major etiologic categories among children displaying signs of pediatric dysphagia. These included: neurologic dysfunction, cardiorespiratory problems, sensory deprivation, structural abnormalities, and primary behavioral problems. Data from a Georgetown University Program for Child Development identified the most common feeding problems as, "prolonged subsistence on pureed foods; difficulty in sucking, swallowing, or chewing; bizarre food habits; multiple food dislikes; delay in self feeding; mealtime tantrums" (Palmer & Horn, 1978, p. 107). At the Johns Hopkins Hospital, the SLP service has developed a list of five basic indicators identifying children at risk for feeding and swallowing disorders (Table 6–1).

Components of a Pediatric Feeding and Swallowing Evaluation

Groher (1984) stated that the goals of the clinical evaluation are to "(1) establish a possible cause of dysphagia; (2) assess the patient's ability to protect the airway; (3) determine the practicality of oral feeding and/or recommend alternative methods for nutritional management; (4) determine the need for additional diagnostic tests or studies; and (5) establish baseline clinical data" (p. 91). To accomplish these goals, pediatric feeding and swallowing evaluation must include four primary components: a careful history, examination of the oral motor mechanism, observation of a

TABLE 6–1. Conditions associated with difficulties with oral intake in children that indicate need for feeding and swallowing evaluations.

I. Documented or suspected airway compromise as evidenced by
   A. Chronic pulmonary problems
   B. Clinical signs associated with aspiration
II. Diagnosis of a failure to thrive (FFT)
III. Suspicion of oromotor dysfunction
IV. Questions about the appropriateness of feeding patterns
V. The presence of a confirmed diagnostic entity which may predispose the child to impairments in deglutition
   A. Upper aero-digestive tract anomalies
   B. Acquired anatomic defects
   C. Systemic problems or syndromes

trial feeding, and specialized imaging studies as clinically indicated (Groher, 1984; Logemann, 1983; Tuchman, 1989). A multidisciplinary evaluation that addresses medical needs, nutritional requirements, and compliance in the home environment is a prerequisite to a successful management plan.

Evaluation and management approaches will differ in the acute and chronic care settings. In the acute care setting, contact may be brief, goals are short-term, patient stability is variable, and progress is associated with improvement of medical status and is expected to be rapid. In the chronic care setting, contact is ongoing, goals are long-term, the patient is generally stable, and progress is viewed from a rehabilitation perspective and expected to be slower and progressive. The characteristics associated with the setting will guide the evaluation process and the ensuing management plans.

Medical History

In the acute care setting, because the medical record frequently provides historic information about birth, the neonatal period, overall development, past medical conditions, and on occasion feeding development, additional history taking can be very focused. The goal is to identify medical, neurological, developmental, and etiological factors that predispose the child to a feeding and swallowing disorder. Likewise, knowledge of medications, syndromes, and systemic problems (e.g., cardiopulmonary, respiratory distress) that increase demands on pharyngeal function and boost nutritional requirements is essential because these factors may affect the ability of the child to swallow competently.

Developmental History

The developmental history should include the identification of the acquisition and emerging sequences of fine and gross motor and speech and language milestones. Developmental screening tools are avail-

able and typically compare the child's development to normative behavior and/or assesses the child's rate of growth (Frankenburg & Dodds, 1967; Illingworth, 1990). Comprehensive developmental assessments are completed in conjunction with other disciplines, such as developmental pediatricians, education specialists, or psychologists. Ultimately, predictions about the child's potential capacity for development are based on compilation of data reflecting processes that either enhance or inhibit the child's growth.

Feeding History

The primary caregiver or the primary "feeder" may be the best informant for providing details of the feeding history. The interviewer needs to discern the caregiver's perception of the feeding and swallowing problem. Open-ended questions, (e.g., asking the parent to describe the feeding problem) may enable the examiner to develop an overview perspective of clinical symptoms and etiologies that are either indicative of feeding and/or swallowing dysfunction or predispose a child to such problems (Table 6–1).

The examiner needs to know the child's current feeding patterns and manner of nutritional intake (Table 6–2). Mealtimes generally should range between 10 and 30 minutes (Singer, 1990). Average meal times of less than 10 minutes may signal a "rushed" pattern of interaction between the child and caregiver. Additionally, children with oral motor difficulties may require more time for safe and enjoyable feeding. Mathisen, Skuse, Wolke and Reilly (1989) found that inner-city children (approximately 1 year of age) with diagnoses of oral-motor dysfunction and nonorganic failure to thrive were fed meals in an average of 8.5 minutes as compared to a control group of infants (matched for age, race, sex, ordinal position, birth weight and gestation, mother's age and years of education, and type of dwelling and crowding index) without nonorganic

TABLE 6-2. Information needed about nutritional patterns and experiences in relation to methods of feeding.

Nutritional Patterns and Experiences	Method of Feeding		
	Tube Only	Oral Only	Oral and Tube
Tube Feeding			
Type of feeding tube _____	+		+
When initiated _____ Why initiated _____ +/− fundoplication [TYPE] _____	+		+
Formula amount per feeding _____ Bolus vs. Continuous _____ Feeding schedule _____ Position during feeding _____	+		+
Proportion of diet via tube _____	+		+
Oral stimulation? Type _____ Amount _____	+	+/−	+
Any adverse response to oral tactile simulation (e.g., touch, food, temperature) _____ Increase in oral secretions? _____	+	+/−	+
Oral Feeding			
Types of foods _____ Types of liquids _____		+	+
Manner of presentation _____		+	+
Meals per day _____ Snacks per day _____ Amount per meal _____ Amount per snack _____		+	+
Duration of meals _____		+	+
Feeding position _____ Primary "feeder" _____		+	+
"Easy" foods _____ "Difficult" foods _____ Foods disliked _____ Foods liked _____		+	+
Self feeding skills _____		+	+

failure to thrive, who were fed in an average of 21.1 minutes, suggesting an inability of the mother to "suitably accommodate to the needs" of her youngster. Conversely, mealtimes that are too long in duration may signal inefficient feeding and can po-

tentially interfere with other quality of life experiences.

The youngster's early feeding history may indicate a predisposition towards a feeding and swallowing problem. Factors to explore include: strength of suck; nasopharyngeal reflux; fatigue with feeding; cyanosis, apnea, or bradycardia associated with oral intake; poor weight gain; length of time in the hospital following birth; oxygen or ventilator dependency; descriptions of the infant's general feeding patterns; any disruption of oral feeding; and any special adaptations or therapeutic interventions used to assist with feeding.

Clinical Evaluation

The examiner observes interaction patterns between the caregiver and the child. Specific notice is made of communication skills, body contact, and the quality of interaction. The child is observed at rest for body posture and positioning needs, the presence of special equipment (ranging from seating devices to oxygen tanks), alertness, temperament, general use of communication (e.g., speech, language, voice, and articulation skills, use of augmentative communication systems), and clinical signs associated with oral or pharyngeal dysfunction (e.g., drooling, coughing, baseline of upper aerodigestive tract sounds).

The child's body tone and posture are screened as support systems underlying digestive, respiratory, and phonatory functions. The examiner identifies patterns of normal and abnormal motor development.

In the acute care setting, the examiner often has the luxury of hospital monitoring equipment. A baseline of respiratory and heart rates and pulse oxygen levels should be established during rest. Changes in any of these physiologic patterns during increases in activity or with feeding may indicate general system intolerance and/or airway compromise during feeding. The child also is monitored for the presence of obvious upper aerodigestive tract noises.

Oral Motor Examination

Patterns of function and the integrity of the structures that facilitate or interfere with the feeding and swallowing process need to be defined. Each structure is evaluated for precision, strength, range of motion, and as appropriate, symmetry of move-

ment. Additionally, adequacy of function specific to the feeding and swallowing process is assessed.

The progression of reflex development is noted. Specific reflexes are normal for different stages of development. Reflexes that persist beyond the normal time period are considered primitive or immature. Rooting which is normal at birth is a primitive or immature response when it is present beyond 4–5 months of age. There are also abnormal reflexes which are not part of the normal developmental repertoire including marked tongue thrust, a tonic bite, and a hypersensitive gag. Immature or abnormal reflexes generally reflect neurogenic problems and can interfere with the development of mature feeding patterns (Alexander, 1983; Lewis, 1982; Morris, 1985; Morris & Klein, 1987).

General Appearance of Craniofacial Region

The head and face are examined for general appearance, appropriateness of size relationships among the structures, symmetry, and overall tone at rest and during activity. Facial expressions should be observed for appropriateness, symmetry, range of movement, and hypo- or hyper-muscular activity during spontaneous movements and volitional tasks. A screening of cranial nerves function is conducted to assess the potential of muscular control and the sensory integrity of the muscles involved in deglutition, speech, and expression (Logemann, 1983; Weiss, 1988). Cranial nerves screened for oral phase function include V, VII, X, and XII (Logemann, 1983). The pharyngeal phase of deglutition is dependent on muscles innervated by cranial nerves IX, X, and XI (Logemann, 1983).

Lips

Lips are assessed for strength and ability to form a seal to prevent excessive food and/or liquid leakage. The effects of inadequate lip closure can range from "incontinence of food" to drooling (Robbins, 1985). Leakage of very small amounts of formula at the beginning of bottle feeding is considered to be grossly within normal limits. Inadequate lip closure during speech can be manifested by difficulty with bilabial sounds (e.g., /m/, /b/, and /p/) and vowels that require lip spreading (e.g., /i/) or lip rounding (e.g., /u/).

Tongue

The tongue is the "primary mobile agent" involved during the oral and pharyngeal stages of deglutition and it is the principle articulator during speech (Robbins, 1985, p. 339). It is examined for its size relative to the oral cavity, strength, symmetry of movement, range of motion, and patterns of abnormal movement (e.g., fasciculations, tongue thrusting). Lingual function is age-dependent.

Sucking patterns are evaluated in the infant and baby who bottle feeds or nurses. Nutritive (Wolff, 1968) and non-nutritive (Bosma, 1986; Wolff, 1968) sucking rates occur at the frequency of approximately one and two sucks per second, respectively. Thus infants can suck up to 30 times per minute, and there "is a 1:1 correlation between suck and swallow in the initial phase of feeding" (Mathew, 1991, p. 517). The burst pattern and rate of sucking are dependent on multiple factors including nipple type (Mathew, 1991) and the child's state of health (Conway, 1989; Mathew, 1991; Singer, 1990). The examiner observes non-nutritive patterns while the infant is sucking on a pacifier and a gloved finger, and focuses on the strength, rate, and duration of the sucking. Any changes in respiratory patterns, heart rate, and oxygen saturation levels are noted. Increased instability or significant effort during non-nutritive tasks generally indicates that an infant is not ready for oral feeding and requires a non-nutritive program which progressively primes the patient for nutritive stimulation.

In the older child, lingual function is assessed for its capacity to form a bolus and transfer it to the posterior portion of the oral cavity during feeding, and to demon-strate movements associated with consonant and vowel productions during speech. Depending on the age and cognitive abilities of the child, lingual movements are assessed during spontaneous activity, imitation, speech, and feeding. The examiner assesses tongue protrusion/retraction, lateralization, elevation, movement patterns in relation to the normal developmental sequence of lingual movements during nutritive and non-nutritive tasks (Morris & Klein, 1987). Oral diadochokinetic testing of rapid consonant-vowel sequences may be used to assess precision and speed of rapid articulatory patterns (Robbins & Klee, 1987).

Palate

The hard palate is examined for the presence of a cleft or submucous cleft, and the relative size, shape, and height of the palatal arch in relation to the entire oral cavity. Children who were intubated early in life frequently exhibit a midline indentation in the hard palate. This midline crevice and/or the presence of a high vaulted palatal arch are sometimes associated with post-swallow food residue particularly in the child with inefficient lingual function. Additionally, the presence of a relatively high palate in a child with impaired lingual function, may interfere with sucking by compromising intra-oral pressure build-up. Arch malformations may hinder the development of normal dentition.

A cleft of the palate is associated with nasopharyngeal regurgitation during feeding. If other components of the oral-pharyngeal mechanism are intact, the child should be able to feed safely. Children with multiple structural dysfunctions are at greater risk for suck, swallow, and breathing coordination difficulties. This is particularly true in the infant under 4 months of age who is still an obligate nasal breather.

The soft palate is assessed for effective length of closure in relation to the posterior pharyngeal wall. Normal palatal movements are upward and posterior during phonation and gagging. These motions should be brisk and symmetrical. Ineffective or sluggish movements tend to be associated with nasopharyngeal reflux during feeding and hypernasality during speech. It is very difficult to visualize soft palate movement in the child under 6 months of age because the tongue is relatively large in relation to the oral cavity and consequently obscures the examiner's line of vision. A bifid uvula may be indicative of a submucous cleft.

Oral Sensation

The assessment of oral sensation depends on the child's age and neurological and cognitive status. The palatal gag is the most frequently assessed reflex. Lack of a palatal gag response does not mean that aspiration is inevitable. The palatal gag response only stimulates movement of the soft palate and not "the total pharyngeal response of a gag reflex" (Logemann, 1983, p. 110). When a palatal gag reflex is absent, other structural functions mediated by the Xth cranial nerve must be examined and a hypothesis formulated about the effects of all the findings on swallowing function. Consequently, laryngeal dysfunction (e.g., dysphonia, a weak cry, stridor) in conjunction with a absent palatal gag reflex may be indicative of neurogenic dysfunction which may put the child at risk for aspiration, and thus needs further assessment.

Hyper- and hyposensitive reactions are potential indicators of dysphagia. A hypersensitive reaction may have evolved in response to "threatening" types of stimulation (Kenny, 1990). Hyperactive responses can include tonic bite, tongue thrusting, and an over-reactive gag. It has been hypothesized that a position of cervical hyperextension, which is frequently observed in children with central nervous system impairment, develops as a compensatory maneuver to "open" the airway (Beecher & Alexander, 1990). This is the same position used to "open" the airway in cardiopulmonary resuscitation (CPR). When the hypotonic child's head is in a position of cervical hyperextension, the tongue with gravity assistance may passively occlude the airway; and a tongue thrust pattern may be a response aimed at reopening the pharyngeal airway. Lack of a swallow response despite substantial accumulation of salivary secretions in the posterior portion of the oral cavity is a hyposensitive response and frequently identifies a patient who has difficulty handling liquids.

Laryngeal Function

The laryngeal mechanism is the primary structure that protects the airway from foreign bodies. Theories and techniques for assessing phonatory function have been extensively discussed in the literature and are beyond the scope of this chapter. (See Aronson, 1985 and Wilson, 1987, for comprehensive accounts of the assessment and management of phonatory disorders.) The evaluation and management of laryngeal problems is discussed in depth in Chapter 8.

An understanding of the adequacy of laryngeal function is partially derived from clinical observations about the appropriateness of loudness, pitch, and vocal quality relative to the patient's age and sex. Deviations in any of these parameters can be indicative of laryngeal dysfunction. Patients exhibiting phonatory problems need to be referred to an otolaryngologist to assess the reason for the problem and to evaluate airway patency.

A "wet" or "gurgly" phonatory quality is the most frequently mentioned dysphonic pattern associated with pharyngeal dysphagia. At baseline, a wet phonatory pattern may represent the inability of a patient to "handle" his own secretions. When associated with feeding, "wetness" is typically thought to be indicative of laryngeal penetration. Unfortunately, 40% of adults with neurogenic impairment are silent aspirators (Linden & Siebens, 1983). Arvedson, Rogers, Buck, Smart, and Msall (1992) retrospectively reviewed videofluoroscopic evaluations of 186 children and observed aspiration in 48 (26%) of the subjects. Silent aspiration occurred in 45 (94%) of the children demonstrating airway contamination. Thus, although aberrant phonatory patterns or coughing may be associated with pharyngeal dysphagia, it is generally accepted that lack of these clinical indicators does not guarantee airway safety.

The examiner should palpate the thyroid cartilage to analyze the extent of laryngeal elevation during swallowing. Normal elevation is brisk, and the thyroid cartilage returns to its resting position at the completion of the swallow. In the infant, the larynx is located relatively high in the neck so that its upward elevation is limited. The extent of laryngeal elevation during the clinical feeding and swallowing assessment is subjective and based on the examiner's previous evaluation experience. When imaging studies (e.g., videofluoroscopy) are clinically warranted, they can track laryngeal movement objectively.

Patients with tracheostomy tubes are at risk for airway contamination during feeding secondary to the tethering of the laryngeal mechanism and neurophysiologic changes in laryngeal function that may adversely affect the closing of the vocal cords (Buckwalter & Sasaki, 1984). The reason for the tracheostomy tube placement may provide predictive information about swallowing competency. Patients for whom the tracheostomy was placed because of pulmonary toileting needs are probably at greatest risk for aspiration. Patients with tracheostomies because of airway obstruction (e.g., subglottic stenosis or vocal fold paralysis) may be more competent in protecting the airway during swallowing.

Patients with tracheostomy tubes frequently are screened for aspiration by being fed foods mixed with blue food coloring. The tracheostomy site is monitored for the appearance of blue-tinged secretions during and after the feeding session. The appearance of blue-tinged secretions indicates the presence, but not etiology, of aspiration. Patients with tracheal secretions demonstrating airway contamination should be considered for videofluoroscopic evaluation of swallowing function.

Speech and Language Evaluation

Speech, language, and cognitive levels are generally screened during a feeding and swallowing evaluation. Depending on the child's primary needs at the time of evaluation (e.g., assessment of aspiration potential versus ability to control drooling), a complete evaluation of these skills may be warranted at this time or deferred until more immediate issues are addressed.

The acquisition of speech and language milestones is viewed from two perspectives. First the rate and sequence of acquisition are observed as clinical indicators of cognitive and communication skills. Levels of communicative competency influence the direction of the feeding and swallowing assessment and intervention. For example, a child who is able to follow simple commands may be able to volitionally cough to enhance airway protection. As noted above, Stark et al.'s (1974) three strategies are used to assess these areas. The best assessments of communication development evolve from serial evaluations conducted at 3-month intervals for the child (under 1 year of age) who is at risk for problems (Rossetti, 1986, 1990).

Articulatory proficiency, voice, and resonance are also evaluated as reflecting motor control and the maturation of the developing oral-pharyngeal mechanism. Comparisons between oral motor patterns used during speech production and those used during feeding may generate therapeutic approaches and prognostic expectations. Specific patterns of oral motor movement may suggest adaptations used to overcome structural and/or functional processes that interfere with the basic functions of the oral pharyngeal mechanism. The child "may employ different oral actions in speech appropriate to his local sensory and motor development as well as to her auditory and visual imitation monitor experience" (Bosma, 1963, p. 103).

It is beyond the scope of this chapter to review speech and language acquisition, normal patterns of oral movement and the concomitant effects on feeding and speech production. Knowledge of these areas is critical to the development of an appropriate evaluation and management plan for each child. Extensive accounts of these areas have appeared in the literature (Alexander, 1983; Lahey, 1988; Lewis, 1982; Morris, 1985; Morris & Klein, 1987; Rossetti, 1986, 1990).

Observation of a Trial Feeding

Although it would be ideal to observe a child in his or her natural feeding situation, it is rarely possible. However, even in the acute care setting, there are variables that can be manipulated to optimize the trial feeding. Observation should coincide with a regularly scheduled mealtime to enhance the feeding incentive. Supportive medical and/or nursing personnel may need to be present for monitoring of medical status, suctioning, or other care needs. The primary caregiver should be present during this portion of the evaluation process so that the child's "natural" feeding circumstance can be duplicated as closely as possible.

Observation of a trial feeding allows the examiner to define normal and abnormal (or primitive) patterns of oral intake; identify optimal stimuli for feeding (e.g., bolus characteristics, including size, textures, and temperatures); identify the patient requiring "priming" or desensitization prior to scheduling a formal videofluoroscopic evaluation; observe the child/caregiver interaction; define special adaptive equipment or positioning needs for a dedicated imaging evaluation; develop strategies for tailoring imaging studies to the needs of the specific child (e.g., if fatigue is a potential component contributing to increased airway compromise, then a videofluoroscopic evaluation should be planned which taxes the system while minimizing radiation exposure); and plan for special needs and/or strategies during feeding (e.g., assuring the availability of suctioning equipment and/or stroking the tongue of the child who begins a suck-swallow sequence in response to lingual stimulation) (Beecher, 1988; Beecher & Alexander, 1990; Logemann, 1990).

If possible, the parent should feed the child using foods, utensils, special adaptations (e.g., thickening formula or cutting a large hole in the nipple), and positioning equipment used at home. The child is monitored for clinical signs associated with aspiration including: cough, choke, and/or gag episodes; changes respiratory rate or function patterns; changes in vocal quality or upper aerodigestive tract noises; episodes of oxygen desaturation; and episodes of apnea or bradycardia.

Another clinical tool is placement of a stethoscope over the thyroid cartilage to listen to swallow and breath sounds. This technique, cervical auscultation, sometimes aids in the identification of swallowing difficulties by amplifying sounds that are generally inaudible to the unassisted ear (Bosma, 1986; Logan & Bosma, 1967). The following sounds can be monitored: the presence or absence of a swallow, the number of sucks produced prior to the initiation of a swallow, increases in upper aerodigestive tract noises, and the presence of inaudible but spontaneous vocalizations (e.g., patients with athetoid cerebral palsy). In addition, a gross estimate of bolus size and a rough estimate of the duration of time between oral presentation and the elicitation of a swallow can be made.

Indications for Specialized Studies

In the acute care setting, the child's stability is a factor in the consideration of proceeding with specialized studies. Sometimes a child is too medically fragile to risk an episode of aspiration and the determination of when to proceed with specialized studies is made in consultation with other team members. Factors to consider in deciding to proceed with specialized evaluations include the child's current medical status and the prognosis for a change in disposition, risks associated with the specific procedure, the risks associated with "optimal" feeding methods during the interim between the referral and the planned specialized study, the scheduling constraints, caregiver needs, scheduling of other procedures, and the time interval between the specialized evaluation and the potential of changing the current feeding regime.

Videofluoroscopic Feeding and Swallowing Evaluation

In the acute care setting, the two most frequent reasons for referral are to assess the risk of aspiration as a potential contributor to respiratory distress and to determine whether a feeding and swallowing impairment can explain poor weight gain. These questions generally require a videofluoroscopic evaluation of swallowing function (see Chapter 10). Ideally, the formal feeding and swallowing assessment should be scheduled as close in time as possible to the anticipated resumption of oral feeding.

It is not always possible to follow an ideal clinical and videofluoroscopic assessment protocol. When a child is too medically fragile to risk any aspiration and there are contraindications for tube feeding, the child's "first" feeding experience might unfortunately be barium. The pros and cons of barium as a first meal must be carefully considered because both the patient and examiner are put into an "experimental" situation. A management approach needs to be developed which balances the "minimal" amount of nutritive presentations necessary to "prime" the child for a formal swallow assessment while keeping the child healthy. Some children can be "primed"

by being presented with approximately 1 ounce of their "best" consistency daily and participating in an aggressive non-nutritive intervention program. Again this decision must be made in conjunction with the child's primary physician.

Oral and pharyngeal stage competency need to be assessed along different continuums. Oral stage function is synonymous with efficiency to maintain nutrition and to provide a pleasurable experience; it also prepares the pharynx for the bolus delivery. Pharyngeal phase function is viewed from the perspective of safety and minimizing risks of airway contamination (see Table 6–3).

Oral and pharyngeal stage performance may be influenced by multiple external factors including rate and manner of food presentation, type of consistency, and positioning. Internal factors that can affect oral and/or pharyngeal performance include the child's general health, respiratory stability, cognitive status, underlying etiologic processes, previous feeding experiences, and the disposition (e.g., alertness, ability to cooperate, and crying), and fatigue or performance over time. All intervening variables need to be noted to assess the reliability and validity of this examination.

Management of Pediatric Feeding and Swallowing Problems

The primary foci of a feeding and swallowing management program are:

1. reduction or elimination of factors that potentially contribute to airway compromise,

2. maintenance of adequate nutrition and hydration intake, and

3. facilitation of a positive interaction between the parent and the child.

Frequently a trial period of implementing recommendations is initiated prior to

TABLE 6–3. Summary of videofluoroscopic findings for oral and pharyngeal stage function in relation to variables manipulated during the evaluation.

Oral Stage Function	*	*	*	*
Within normal limits				
Minimal deviation: Probably no effect on oral intake.				
Mild deviations: Possible effect on oral intake; Should be functional with minimal intervention; Good prognosis for adequate PO intake.				
Moderate deviation: Difficulty with sustaining adequate PO intake; Requires ongoing compensatory measures; Fair prognosis; may need supplemental nutrition/hydration support.				
Marked deviation: Adequate intake unlikely even with maximum support; Presentations for therapeutic trials and/or pleasure; Limited prognosis; requires supplemental nutrition/hydration support.				
Profound deviation: Oral intake inadequate; Poor prognosis; requires alternate nutrition/hydration route.				
Pharyngeal Stage Function				
Within normal limits				
Minimal deviation: Slight variation without suspected/documented risk of airway compromise; PO intake should be WNL.				
Mild deviations: Slight risk of aspiration 2° to other factors (e.g., alertness, integrity of other structures; positioning, rate of PO intake); PO intake possibly affected.				
Moderate deviation: At risk for airway compromise with good response to compensatory measures (diet, t_x maneuvers); Able to protect airway; PO intake probably affected (rate, bolus size/consistency); Requires ongoing compensatory measures; Fair prognosis; may need supplemental nutrition/hydration support.				
Marked deviation: Risk/documented airway compromise controlled only with maximum supervision; PO intake is affected; PO presentations for therapeutic trials and/or pleasure under professional supervision; Limited prognosis; requires supplemental nutrition/hydration support.				
Profound deviation: Demonstrated inability to protect airway; Elimination of consistency from PO diet; Poor prognosis; requires alternate nutrition/hydration route.				

* Variables manipulated during the study may include factors such as: bolus characteristics (texture, amount, temperature), manner of presentation (bottle, spoon, cup), special adaptations (positioning, and specific modifications of feeding devices).

adopting a more permanent management plan. This is the case, for example, when nasogastric feedings are used for a temporary period of time prior to the placement of a more permanent gastrostomy tube. Treatment strategies are continually evaluated

and modified according to the patient's needs. As Linden-Castelli (1991) noted,

One skill (that the SLP must possess) is that of formulation; that is, one should be able to take an array of existing and acquired data and to generate a hypothesis regarding what treatment strategy to employ and why. The clinician should also have the skills of 'online' reasoning and observation and be able to modify a planned treatment strategy. (p. 255)

The management plan is a comprehensive decision which is based partially on the child's overall prognosis, the etiology of the feeding and swallowing impairment, the home environment, local care facilities, and past medical history. Risks of aspiration may be managed more aggressively in the child with documented respiratory compromise than with the child who has no history of pneumonia, wheezing, and/or reactive airway disease. Likewise the child with progressive neurologic disease may decompensate over time and potentially requires an increasingly aggressive management plan. A management plan for children is designed in conjunction with the child's parents and pediatrician and frequently is based on judgments related to quality of life issues.

Recommendations can range from eliminating specific consistencies from an oral diet to complete reliance on nonoral methods of feeding. The ideal treatment for swallowing dysfunction probably includes activities which encourage swallowing because: (a) complications associated with deprivation of oral stimulation (e.g., hypersensitivity or defensive types of behavior) are minimized (Morris, 1985; Morris & Klein, 1987); (b) muscles are used in unique ways during feeding and their magnitude of activity appears to be task dependent (Perman et al., 1989) suggesting that swallowing may be the best exercise for pharyngeal dysphagia; and (c) "real" foods and drinks may evoke pleasurable responses that cannot be simulated outside of the true feeding situation (Linden-Castelli, 1991).

It may be necessary to re-investigate swallowing function by videofluoroscopy. This is particularly true for the child who aspirates silently. Evaluations should be repeated when it is expected that the results will change the child's feeding and swallowing management plan by either upgrading or increasing oral intake. Conversely, the child with a progressive problem or whose problems associated with oral intake persist might need to be re-evaluated to develop a more aggressive management plan. Although videofluoroscopy is currently the "gold-standard" for evaluation of swallowing function, it is not without the risks associated with repeated radiation exposure.

Principles of Therapy

Therapeutic interventions described for the pediatric population generally are directed at improving the efficiency of oral stage function by increasing the strength, coordination, and the range of motion of the oral structures; decreasing the potential development of hypersensitive responses to oral tactile stimulation; adjusting body position to increase overall stability, and/or use of gravity to direct food to the stronger structures; and encouraging activities to simulate actions that are consistent with improved oral and/or pharyngeal function. Descriptive accounts suggest the improvement of oral stage efficiency with treatment (Alexander, 1983; Lewis, 1982; Morris, 1985; Morris & Klein, 1987); however, objective data that support a causative relationship between therapeutic exercises and improved pharyngeal stage function have not been reported. Because pharyngeal muscle activity differs during deglutition versus nondeglutition tasks (Perman et al., 1989), the most desirable management strategies encourage swallowing. Compensatory maneuvers enable the patient to adapt to or counterbalance a variety of pharyngeal dysfunctions (Beecher, 1988; Beecher & Alexander, 1990; Linden-Castelli, 1991; Logemann, 1983, 1986). These maneuvers need to be verified by an imaging study which demonstrates safe swallow function.

Therapeutic interventions used with adults are classified as either "direct" or "indirect" (Logemann, 1983). Direct therapy strategies use foods and/or liquids and are aimed at reinforcing appropriate deglutition skills with or without the use of specified compensation strategies. Initially, direct therapy interventions are conducted in the presence of the SLP to ensure the safe and appropriate use of the techniques. Once a predetermined level of competency is achieved, the supervisory role may be transferred to the family and/or other team members.

In the pediatric population the terms "direct" and "indirect" therapies are analogous to "nutritive" and "non-nutritive" stimulation, respectively. The use of a pacifier is a form of non-nutritive stimulation for the infant. The goals of non-nutritive stimulation are designed to provide exercises that facilitate the strength, range of motion, and precision of movement among the structures comprising the oral-pharyngeal mechanism; simulate patterns needed for patterns such as bolus formation and transfer; provide oral sensory input for the child; and normalize oral stage interactions for the parent-child dyad.

The SLP uses "speech-like" gestures to facilitate oral motor patterns that are characteristic of skills required for both articulatory proficiency and deglutition (Morris, 1985; Morris & Klein, 1987; Robbins, 1985). Sounds that require movements similar to those needed for oral stage efficiency are sometimes helpful in facilitating the desired movement patterns. The examiner observes the child and notes the appearance of oral motor sequences that approximate the desired repertoire. Sometimes the child who bunches her tongue during spoon presentations will demonstrate a flattened tongue body during neutral vowel productions. For this child, the most efficient therapeutic approach might be encouraging speech sound production to reinforce desirable tongue configurations during oral intake. See Morris (1985) for a comprehensive description of oral motor patterns used during speech and nonspeech oral motor activities, as well as accounts of dys-

function and the potential concomitant speech and nonspeech difficulties.

Nutritive stimulation uses foods and liquids in a systematic manner to promote appropriate deglutition. For example, placing very small pieces of graham cracker on the molar table can encourage the lateralization of the tongue as a precursor for chewing. The literature has extensive accounts of evaluation and therapeutic interventions for non-nutritive and nutritive stimulation techniques (see Alexander, 1983; Lewis, 1982; Morris, 1985; Morris & Klein, 1987).

Feeding Suggestions

Feeding suggestions for the pediatric patient may include best food consistencies (see Table 6–3), amounts per feeding, delivery mode (e.g., special spoons, straw, specific nipples), optimal positioning, and any special techniques tailored to the particular child's needs (Griggs, Jones, & Lee, 1989). Such techniques may include positioning for gastroesophageal reflux precautions, use of suctioning, cervical auscultation during bottle feeding, and monitoring of oxygen saturation levels during oral intake. Sometimes recommendations specify feeding schedules such that the "best" consistencies are used to maximize safety and caloric intake at mealtimes and more difficult consistencies are offered as snacks or under therapeutic supervision.

Recommendations that "improve, enhance, foster, or assist function" and require little or no active patient participation are referred to as "facilitation" strategies in the adult literature (Linden-Castelli, 1991, p. 256). Techniques for positioning the child, suggestions for changes in nipples or feeding devices, and presentations of specific textures are examples of facilitation techniques. Forms of non-nutritive and/or nutritive stimulation might be considered faciliatory maneuvers. An example is deep pressure applied midline to the tongue body to facilitate tongue "cupping" for bolus formation. Conversely, "compensations" are strategies that require the patient to actively participate to "remedy, equalize, or restore function" (Linden-Castelli, 1991, p. 257). The child who can imitate a cough following a swallow sequence is engaging in a compensatory technique. In general, facilitation techniques are generally used with the pediatric patient. Of course, active participation is required of the caregiver in complying with any of these recommendations.

Further Management Considerations

CPR training is recommended for caregivers of all children with dysphagia. Additionally, families need to be educated about symptoms suggestive of aspiration and given emergency backup instructions should problems arise.

Plans for Follow-Up and/or Reevaluation

Future evaluation and/or therapeutic intervention plans need to be discussed and decided on in conjunction with primary referral source and whenever possible with the family and other team members involved in the child's management. Family participation is crucial to the development of an accurate assessment and management plan. The family is aware of the pragmatic realities in the home environment and their compliance ultimately will determine the success of the management plan. They can assist by identifying the child's strengths and weaknesses in the hospital situation. The serious consequences of aspiration-related events necessitate identifying decompensations or patterns consistent with potential difficulties in controlled situation and in the "safe" environment.

The pediatric patient should not be subjected to further radiation exposure unless the results of such a study will signifi-

cantly alter the feeding management protocol or promote a definitive diagnosis of the child's underlying problem. Children who exhibit behavioral feeding problems and/or oral stage difficulties without concomitant symptoms suggestive of deviant pharyngeal stage function and those with extreme hypersensitivity may not be appropriate candidates for a videofluoroscopic evaluation of feeding and swallowing function. When pharyngeal stage dysfunction is suspected in these children, the child may need to be "primed" prior to conducting a videofluoroscopic assessment.

Counseling

Development of a successful management plan depends on establishing a rapport with the referral source and the child's parents. Some caregivers will have experienced multiple difficulties and disappointments stemming from the child's recurrent and/or chronic medical needs. These parents may be confused, upset, angry, and/or scared about a feeding and swallowing evaluation which might identify a "new" problem. Educating and counseling the caregiver are integral components of the evaluation and management process. The feeding specialist should explain feeding and swallowing function to the parent in terms that are part of the parent's language repertoire. Parents should be encouraged to be active participants in the evaluation and management decision-making process so that the recommendations made are workable in the home and compliance is enhanced.

Conclusion

In the past, some children with feeding and swallowing problems were not identified and developed sequelae associated with respiratory or growth compromise. Others were fortunate enough to tolerate difficulties without major disruptions to their health or growth. Children with severe feeding and swallowing impairments were destined to rely solely on tube feedings for their nutrition and hydration requirements. Currently, a greater number of options are available to children with feeding and swallowing problems. As more sophisticated evaluation and management techniques become increasingly available, these children will be enabled to increase their capacity for safe, efficient, and enjoyable oral intake.

References

Alexander, R. P. (1983). Developing prespeech and feeding abilities in children. In S. J. Shanks (Ed.), *Nursing and the management of pediatric communication disorders* (pp. 165–222). San Diego, CA: College-Hill Press.

American Speech-Language-Hearing Association (1987). Ad Hoc Committee on Dysphagia (1986). Ad Hoc Committee on Dysphagia report, *ASHA, 29,* 57–58.

Aronson, A. E. (1985). *Clinical voice disorders* (2nd ed.). New York: Thieme.

Arvedson, J. C., Rogers, B. T., Buck, G., Smart, P., & Msall, M. (1992, November). *Pediatric dysphagia: 186 videofluoro swallow studies.* Paper presented at the American Speech-Language-Hearing Association Convention, San Antonio, TX.

Beecher, R. B. (1988, February). *Videofluoroscopic swallow studies with the pediatric patient: What, who, when, why, how, what do.* Paper presented at the meeting of the Illinois Speech-Language Hearing Association, Chicago, IL.

Beecher, R. B., & Alexander, R. (1990, March). *Pediatric oral-pharyngeal motility (videoswallow) studies: Their use, analysis and application.* Workshop at Children's National Medical Center, Washington, DC.

Bosma, J. F. (1963). Maturation of oral and pharyngeal functions. *American Journal of Orthodontics, 49*(163), 94–104.

Bosma, J. F. (1975). Anatomic and physiological development of the speech apparatus. In D. B. Tower (Ed.), *Human communication and its disorders* (Vol. 3, pp. 469–483). New York: Raven.

Bosma, J. F. (1986). Development of feeding. *Clinical Nutrition, 5,* 210–218.

Bosma, J. F. (1990). Evaluation and therapy of impairments of suckle and transitional feeding. *Journal of Neurologic Rehabilitation, 4*(2), 79–84.

Buchholz, D. W., Bosma, J. F., & Donner, M. W. (1985). Adaptation, compensation, and decompensation of the pharyngeal swallow. *Gastrointestinal Radiology, 10,* 235–239.

Buckwalter, J. A., & Sasaki, C. T. (1984). Effect of tracheotomy on laryngeal function. *Otolaryngologic Clinics of North America, 17*(1), 41–48.

Christensen, J. R. (1989). Developmental approach to pediatric neurogenic dysphagia. *Dysphagia, 3,* 131–134.

Conway, A. E. (1989). Young infant's feeding patterns when sick and well. *Maternal-Child Nursing Journal, 18,* 255–350.

DiScipio W. J., Kaslon, K., & Ruben, R. J. (1978). Traumatically acquired conditioned dysphagia in children. *Annals of Otolaryngology, 87,* 509–514.

Donner, M. W. (1986). Editorial. *Dysphagia, 1,* 1–2.

Feinberg, M. J., & Ekberg, O. (1991). Videofluoroscopy in elderly patients with aspiration: Importance of evaluating both oral and pharyngeal stages of deglutition. *American Journal of Radiology, 165,* 293–296.

Frankenburg, W. K., & Dodds, J. B. (1967). The Denver Developmental Screening Test. *Journal of Pediatrics, 71,* 181–191.

Griggs, C. A., Jones, P. M., & Lee, R. E. (1989). Videofluoroscopic investigation of feeding disorders of children with multiple handicaps. *Developmental Medicine and Child Neurology, 31,* 303–308.

Groher, M. E. (Ed.). (1984). *Dysphagia diagnosis and management.* Stoneham, MA: Butterworth.

Groher, M. E. (Ed.). (1992). *Dysphagia diagnosis and management* (2nd ed.). Stoneham, MA: Butterworth-Heinemann.

Harris, M. B. (1986). Oral-motor management of the high-risk neonate. *Physical and Occupational Therapy, 6,* 231–253.

Illingworth, R. S. (1990). *Basic developmental screening: 0–4 years* (5th ed.). Oxford: Blackwell Scientific Publications.

Imhoff, S. M., & Wigginton, V. M. (1991). Identifying feeding and swallowing problems in young infants. *Clinics in Communication Disorders, 1,* 56–67.

Kramer, S. (1985). Special swallowing problems in children. *Gastrointestinal Radiology, 10,* 241–250.

Kenny, D. J. (1990, March). *Integration of mastication, tongue, teeth, jaw.* Paper presented at the Third Symposium on Dysphagia, Baltimore, MD.

Lahey, M. (1988). *Language disorders and language development*. New York: Macmillan.

Lewis, J. A. (1982). Oral motor assessment and treatment of feeding difficulties. In P. J. Accardo (Ed.), *Failure to thrive in infancy and early childhood* (pp. 265–295). Baltimore, MD: University Park Press.

Linden-Castelli, P. (1991). Treatment strategies for adult neurogenic dysphagia. *Seminars in Speech and Language, 12,* 255–260.

Linden, P., & Siebens, A. A. (1983). Dysphagia: Predicting laryngeal penetration. *Archives of Physical Medicine and Rehabilitation, 64,* 281–284.

Logan, W. J., & Bosma, J. F. (1967). Oral and pharyngeal dysphagia in infancy. *Pediatric Clinics of North America, 14,* 47–61.

Logemann, J. A. (1983). *Evaluation and treatment of swallowing disorders*. San Diego, CA: College-Hill Press.

Logemann, J. A. (1986). *Manual for the videofluorographic study of swallowing*. San Diego, CA: College-Hill Press.

Logemann, J. A. (1988a). Dysphagia in movement disorders. In J. Jankovic & E. Tolosa (Eds.), *Advances in neurology: Vol. 49. Facial dyskinesias*. New York: Raven.

Logemann, J. A. (1988b). Swallowing physiology and pathophysiology. *Otolaryngologic Clinics of North America, 21*(4), 613–623.

Logemann, J. A. (1990, March). *Nutrition and swallowing disorder interaction*. Paper presented at the Third Symposium on Dysphagia, Baltimore, MD.

Mathew, O. P. (1991). The science of bottle feeding. *The Journal of Pediatrics, 119,* 511–519.

Mathisen, B., Skuse, D., Wolke, D., & Reilly, S. (1989). Oral-motor dysfunction and failure to thrive among inner-city infants. *Developmental Medicine and Child Neurology, 31,* 293–302.

Morris, S. E. (1985). Developmental implications for the management of feeding problems in neurologically impaired infants. *Seminars in Speech and Language, 6,* 293–315.

Morris, S. E., & Klein, M. D. (1987). *Pre-feeding skills*. Tucson, AZ: Therapy Skill Builders.

Palmer, S., & Horn, S. (1978). Feeding problems in children. In S. Palmer & S. Ekvall (Eds.), *Pediatric nutrition in developmental disorders* (pp. 107–129). Springfield, IL: Charles C. Thomas.

Perman, A. L., Luschei, E. S., & Du Mond, C. E.

(1989). Electrical activity from the superior pharyngeal constrictor during reflexive and nonreflexive tasks. *Journal of Speech and Hearing Research, 32,* 749–754.

Robbins, J. (1985). Swallowing and speech production in the neurologically impaired adult. *Seminars in Speech and Language, 6,* 337–348.

Robbins, J., & Klee, T. (1987). Clinical assessment of oropharyngeal motor development in young children. *Journal of Speech and Hearing Research, 52,* 271–278.

Rossetti, L. M. (1986). *High-risk infants: Identification, assessment, and intervention*. Boston: College-Hill Press.

Rossetti, L. M. (1990). *Infant-toddler assessment: An interdisciplinary approach*. Boston: College-Hill Press.

Sheppard, J. J., & Mysak, E. D. (1984). Ontogeny of infantile oral reflexes and emerging chewing. *Child Development, 55,* 831–834.

Sherman, J. M. (1988). The respiratory system. In R. Kaye, F. A. Oski, & L. A. Barness (Eds.), *Core textbook of pediatrics* (pp. 205–214). New York: Lippincott.

Shewan, C. M. (1988). 1988 omnibus survey: Adaptation and progress in times of change. *ASHA, 30*(8), 27–30.

Singer, L. (1990). When a sick child won't — or can't — eat. *Contemporary Pediatrics, 7*(12), 60–76.

Slater, S. C. (1992). 1992 omnibus survey: Portrait of the professions. *ASHA, 34,* 61–65.

Stark, R. E., Rose, S. N., & Benson, P. J. (1974). Classification of infant vocalizations. *British Journal of Disorders of Communication, 13,* 41–47.

Stroh, K., Robinson, T., & Stroh, G. (1986). A therapeutic feeding programme: I. Theory and practice. *Developmental Medicine and Child Neurology, 28,* 3–10.

Tuchman, D. N. (1989). Cough, choke, sputter: The evaluation of the child with dysfunctional swallowing. *Dysphagia, 3,* 111–116.

Weiss, M. H. (1988). Dysphagia in infants. In Y. P. Krespi & A. Blitzer (Eds.), *Otolaryngologic Clinics of North America, 21*(4), 727–736.

Wilson, D. K. (1987). *Voice problems of children* (3rd ed.). Baltimore, MD: Williams & Wilkins.

Wolff, P. H. (1968). The serial organization of sucking in the young infant. *Pediatrics, 42,* 943–956.

The Role of Occupational Therapy in Diagnosis and Management

7

CHAPTER

Linda Miller Schuberth, M.A., OTR/L

Occupational therapy is based on the principle that purposeful activity or "occupation" can be used therapeutically to facilitate the performance of daily life skills in persons with disabilities (American Occupational Therapy Association, 1986). The profession places major emphasis on independent eating and self-feeding by working not only with oral motor skills such as sucking, chewing, and swallowing, but also upper extremity function for manipulation of appropriate utensils. Because of this background, the occupational therapist plays an important role in the multidisciplinary team approach to feeding and swallowing disorders. Specific occupational therapy responsibilities include assessing and treating oral motor and swallowing dysfunction, assisting in the modified barium swallow study, making recommendations regarding positioning and adaptive equipment, and serving as a liaison with caregivers to ensure that recommendations are carried out. There may be areas of overlap with other specialties, particularly the speech-language pathologist. Traditionally, the occupational therapist has focused more on self-feeding skills, whereas the province of the speech therapist has been oral motor dysfunction and its effects on sound production and articulation.

As both disciplines broaden their scopes, members of either specialty may develop expertise in the area of feeding and swallowing, and be the team member to carry the more general title of "feeding therapist." This chapter discusses assessment and management for children with neurological impairment due either to congenital problems, such as cerebral palsy, or acquired causes, such as severe head trauma or neurodegenerative disease.

Oral Motor Dysfunction

Eating and swallowing are highly integrated sensorimotor functions. Coordination of the lips, tongue, jaw, cheeks, and soft palate is necessary to manipulate the food bolus while reflexive control of the pharynx protects the airway. The sequence of normal oral motor development and its relationship to acquisition of eating skills and speech production are discussed in Chapter 2. Oral motor dysfunction in children most often occurs as a result of neurological impairment which leads to abnormal muscle tone, persistent oral reflexes, and sensory-perceptual deficits. Although not discussed in this chapter, other conditions such as craniofacial anomalies, gastrointestinal disorders, and chronic pulmonary disease may also be associated with oral motor dysfunction.

Postural Tone Abnormalities

Abnormalities of postural muscle tone are important and often overlooked contributors to oral motor dysfunction. Swallowing requires not only intact oral motor function but also the support and stability provided by general postural muscle tone. Normal muscle tone and strength in the hips, pelvis, trunk, and shoulder girdle allow upright posture, alignment of the head and neck, and a stable base to anchor oral and pharyngeal musculature. In addition, the development of righting and equilibrium reactions requires integration of primitive postural reflexes such as the symmetrical and asymmetrical tonic neck and tonic labyrinthine.

Muscle tone abnormalities generally are classified as increased, decreased, or fluctuating. Children with hypertonia are often dominated by mass patterns of flexion or extension that not only interfere with postural alignment, but also affect rib cage expansion and esophageal motility (Morris, 1989). They often exhibit a tendency for upper lip retraction, tonic bite, jaw thrusting, and limited jaw movements, all of which hinder graded oral motor control. Hypotonic children often have difficulty maintaining an upright posture, have slow and poorly coordinated movements, and may exhibit poor lip closure and limited tongue mobility. Children with fluctuating muscle tone have slow, irregular, and oscillating involuntary movements that limit stability. Muscle tone abnormalities have been associated with drooling, uncoordinated breathing, decreased oral exploration, and difficulty initiating, grading, or sustaining oral motor patterns (Ottenbacher, Bundy, & Short, 1983).

Abnormal Oral Motor Patterns

Protective oral reflexes such as suck/swallow and rooting are necessary for the nutritional intake of the newborn infant. During normal development, they are integrated into the highly coordinated patterns of oral movements necessary for mature swallowing (Morris & Klein, 1987). In conditions such as cerebral palsy, early damage to the motor cortex may interrupt the integration process. The pathological persistence of these reflexes beyond 6 months of age interferes with normal oral motor development and, in combination with other postural tone abnormalities, may result in the following problems:

1. Prolonged suckling

2. Exaggerated tongue thrust

3. Open mouth posture

4. Tonic bite

5. Jaw thrust

6. Jaw clenching

7. Jaw or tongue retraction

8. Lip pursing

Oral Tactile Sensitivity

A growing number of children with oral motor and swallowing disorders appear to have either increased or decreased awareness of sensory stimuli in and around the mouth and pharynx. Often this is generalized to the rest of the body. Oral tactile hypersensitivity is commonly seen in children who have been tube fed for prolonged periods. This is characterized by an aversion to being touched around the face and mouth which results in food refusal. A hyperactive gag reflex is usually present and may contribute to difficulty advancing to higher texture foods. Decreased oral awareness may result in drooling, poor chewing, retained food in the mouth, and a depressed gag reflex. Pharyngeal hyposensitivity may result in lack of awareness of residual food pooled in structures around the airway. This not only makes aspiration or penetration more likely, but also reduces the cough response once the food enters the airway. The following scenarios are typical of children with sensitivity abnormalities:

The infant who has never developed a strong suck and requires an enteral feeding tube to maintain his or her nutritional requirements.

The child with abnormal muscle tone and posture who missed normal oral sensory experiences such as hand- and foot-to-mouth play or mouthing of toys.

The older child with failure to thrive or aspiration who later is fed by an alternate method, usually a gastrostomy tube.

The child who has had oral surgery and may interpret touch around the mouth as a negative experience.

Assessment

As a member of the multidisciplinary team, the occupational therapist evaluates the sensorimotor aspects of feeding and swallowing function. This includes food presentation, bolus manipulation, and pharyngeal swallow function. An organized approach to assessment includes a careful feeding history obtained from the primary caregiver, a hands-on clinical evaluation of both general postural muscle tone and specific oral motor function, and videofluoroscopy when indicated.

General information that should be obtained prior to the assessment includes medical diagnosis, reports of previous gastrointestinal or related procedures, past and current medications, developmental level, and overall medical and nutritional status.

Feeding History

The feeding history is best obtained by interviewing the primary caregiver. It should include:

1. a discussion of the caregiver's major concerns about the child's feeding,

2. a developmental feeding history,

3. a description of the current feeding method, and

4. specific questions related to swallowing dysfunction.

The developmental areas include overall postural tone and general movement capabilities as well as the emergency and quality of specific oral motor skills such as sucking, transition to solid foods, spoon feeding and cup drinking, use of utensils, and general behavior at mealtime. Details of the current feeding method should include food textures and preferences, average amount consumed, length of time required to complete a meal, quality of oral motor skills, special feeding practices, and any problems encountered when the child is fed by someone other than the primary caregiver. Finally, questions about signs and symptoms of specific problems such as aspiration and gastroesophageal reflux/esophagitis must always be included.

Clinical Examination

The occupational therapist performs a "hands-on" comprehensive clinical examination designed to evaluate general development, oral motor function, and feeding. The examination focuses on specific oral motor function as well as a variety of related factors which influence the feeding process.

General Developmental Evaluation

The initial observation and handling of the patient provide information about overall muscle tone and general developmental status including motor and cognitive capabilities. The neuromotor evaluation focuses on the effects of abnormal muscle tone and primitive reflexes on the child's posture and movement transitions.

Oral Motor Inspection

The oral motor inspection begins with observation and inspection of the musculature of the cheeks, lips, and jaw, looking for asymmetry and for tone or sensory abnormalities. It then proceeds intraorally to the gums, dentition, hard palate, and tongue, and, lastly, to the soft palate, pharynx, and oral motor reflexes. Movement of the soft palate and pharyngeal wall can be assessed during phonation and during stimulation of the gag reflex with tongue blade pressure, usually on the back third of the tongue. Hypo- or hyperresponsiveness of the gag reflex is gauged by how far back on the tongue it is elicited. Laryngeal elevation, identified by observation and palpation, is used to determine if swallowing is occurring. Objective sensory testing is difficult in neurologically impaired children, especially those with low cognitive function. Hypersensitivity is measured by the degree of aversion to oral tactile tests.

Feeding Evaluation

The feeding evaluation provides an opportunity to assess oral motor function by observing the swallowing process during a typical meal when fed by the primary caregiver, the self-feeding child, and the occupational therapist. Four areas are important:

1. *Posture and positioning.* Posture is strongly influenced by general muscle tone. Positioning is determined by how the caregiver holds the child, by independent sitting, or by the use of adaptive seating devices. Assessment focuses on the presence of abnormal muscle tone and maintenance of adequate body alignment.

2. *Caregiver/child interaction.* The feeding process requires both physical and so-

cial interaction between the caregiver and child. The essential elements are the quality of the nurturing relationship and, specifically, how problem behaviors such as tantrums and food refusal are handled.

3. *Food presentation.* The method and rate of food delivery to the mouth strongly influence the quality of swallowing. Utensils used, food texture, bolus size, rate of feeding, and the effect of oral tactile hypersensitivity should be assessed.

4. *Oral motor function.* Observation of the quality and coordination of oral motor movement during feeding and swallowing is essential. The evaluation includes: (a) identification of abnormal oral-motor patterns, (b) assessment of feeding efficiency as determined by the rate of eating and the amount of food loss, (c) detection of signs of aspiration and/or gastroesophageal reflux, and (d) detection of nasopharyngeal reflux.

Cervical Auscultation

Some clinicians use cervical auscultation during swallowing to identify patients who aspirate. Aspiration is thought to occur during swallows that sound less sharp or have a bubbly quality when compared to normal (Hamlet, Nelson, & Patterson, 1990). The usefulness of this technique is limited by its subjectivity and by the lack of research validating the physiologic source of the sounds. It may, however, provide additional information when videofluoroscopy is not possible.

Formal Assessment Tools

Many oral motor/feeding assessment tools are available that allow a structured approach to the clinical examination. They include:

1. *Pre-Speech Assessment Scale* (Morris, 1982). Designed for use with neurologically impaired children from birth to age 2, this tool is based on the presumption that development of feeding patterns is one of the critical components of speech production. It examines 27 prespeech performance

areas and takes between 2½ to 3 hours to administer. Although considerable time is required to develop familiarity with this test, it nevertheless provides an excellent resource in defining terminology and reviewing normal oral motor development.

2. *Behavioral Assessment Scale of Oral Functions in Feeding* (Stratton, 1982). Developed for use with multiply handicapped adolescents or adults, this scale provides a quick assessment of nine areas of oral motor function grading with a 6-point scale in each area. It is intended to be used in conjunction with an assessment of overall muscle tone and postural patterns.

3. *Oral-Motor/Feeding Rating Scale* (Jeim, 1990). This evaluation has five sections organized on one concise form and is useful for children 1 year of age through adulthood. The main section examines eight feeding patterns and rates three specific oral motor movements in each. Other sections evaluate related areas of feeding function. It is designed to be administered at feeding time and usually requires 20 minutes to 1 hour, depending on additional information from the primary feeder.

4. *Multidisciplinary Feeding Profile (MFP)* (Kenny et al., 1989). The MFP is the first statistically based protocol for the quantitative assessment of severely disabled children. It is comprehensive in nature, can be completed in 30–40 minutes, and is designed to be administered by clinicians from several disciplines.

5. *Vulpe Assessment Battery* (Vulpe, 1969). This battery provides a comprehensive assessment of the child's overall development from birth to 5 years. The section on eating contains 47 items including oral reflexes, eating behaviors, motor functions, self-feeding, use of utensils, and social behaviors during mealtime.

Videofluoroscopy

The modified barium swallow study is the radiographic procedure of choice for assessing the oral and pharyngeal anatomy and the physiology of the stages of swallowing. It is particularly useful for identifying children who either aspirate or are at high risk for aspiration, and also serves as a basis for the development of treatment programs (Fox, 1990). The occupational therapist's role is twofold: (1) to determine the necessity of this procedure based on the results of the clinical evaluation and (2) to take part in performance of the study, including positioning and feeding the child. The initial clinical evaluation determines positioning, bolus characteristics, rate and sequence of presentation, and environmental factors that could potentially affect the outcome. Positioning should simulate the child's normal eating position, but adequate support must also be provided to maximize good postural alignment and optimize safe swallowing.

Texture presentation is extremely important and should be based on the child's developmental age and clinical evaluation. During the study, several food textures may be used to simulate different food groups. Solid or thickened food textures simulating a preferred food (cookie coated with Esophatrast®) are less likely to be aspirated and should be offered first. Some clinicians advocate initially using thin barium to best define the cause and amount of aspiration (Logemann, 1983). However, thin barium may result in residual contrast in the laryngeal vestibule or airway, which may interfere with accurate assessment of subsequent swallows of thicker textures. In addition, in children where fatigue during the meal is a factor in compromising airway protection, saving the more difficult thick texture until later in the study is more likely to demonstrate aspiration/penetration. Thin barium can be offered by cup, bottle, or syringe. The therapist should never force feed, and when using a syringe, exercise caution not to squirt the contrast into the pharynx. Placing it on the tongue allows assessment of the oral phase of bolus formation and decreases the risk of aspiration.

Children who demonstrate food refusal, tantruming, and crying may become more agitated during the procedure, making completion of the study difficult or resulting in aspiration that may not reflect the child's usual swallowing status. In spite of these difficulties, it may be critical to view at least a few swallows before designing and implementing feeding programs in children with medical illnesses or clinical signs related to aspiration. If severe aversive behaviors are present at the initial evaluation, a program of oral stimulation may be beneficial before attempting videofluoroscopy. On the other hand, in difficult children without clear signs of aspiration, videofluoroscopy may not be warranted. Instead, cervical auscultation combined with a thorough history and clinical evaluation may provide enough information to begin a program to increase oral intake. If clinical signs of aspiration develop during treatment, reevaluation may be necessary.

Management/Therapy

For most children, the goal of management is to optimize feeding and swallowing skills so that they can eat as independently and efficiently as possible. For children who are unable to eat, treatment focuses on enhancement of prefeeding oral motor skills. To design and implement a comprehensive oral motor/feeding program, the occupational therapist interacts with parents, other members of the multidisciplinary team, and community-based resources. Specific treatment objectives are based not only on the results of the oral motor assessment, but also on the child's cognitive level, general behavior, social/environmental factors, and general health. The components of a program include positioning, specific oral motor therapy, determination of appropriate food quantity and texture, and use of adaptive equipment. The best outcomes are achieved when clinical problems are identified early, appropriate management programs are implemented promptly, and families or caregivers are included in the decision-making process.

It is helpful to think of the oral motor therapeutic process in terms of non-nutritive and nutritive goals. Readiness for feeding is an important determinant of the direction of therapy. In children who are unsafe oral eaters, daily non-nutritive oral stimulation is used to reduce hypersensitivity, facilitate management of secretions, establish or retrain the swallowing mechanism, maintain coordination of breathing and swallowing, and develop oral movements for sound play and communication. Objectives for a nutritive oral motor program include increasing oral intake, advancing food textures, transition to appropriate use of utensils, and improvement of self-feeding.

The oral motor intervention techniques employed by occupational, physical, and speech therapists are based on a number of theories. Neurodevelopmental treatment (NDT) established by Karl and Berta Bobath utilized handling and positioning to inhibit patterns of abnormal reflex activity and facilitate patterns of normal movement (Bobath, 1977). Based on Rood's neurophysiological theory, Stockmeyer (1967) has advocated facilitation of sensory receptors to enhance motor strength and control. A multisensory approach using controlled application of sensory stimuli to activate, inhibit, or facilitate desired motor responses has been described by Farber (1982). Morris (Morris & Klein, 1987) has developed a commonly used comprehensive resource that includes prefeeding development, assessment, and specifics of oral motor treatment and self-feeding. General procedures, such as proper body positioning, oral sensory preparation, and presentation of therapeutic activities and food to promote normal oral motor patterns and coordination of sucking, swallowing, and breathing, are outlined.

Positioning

Individuals who need oral motor intervention often have associated neuromotor deficits that result in difficulty maintaining a stable sitting position. The initial therapeutic objective is the establishment of proper positioning which decreases the influence of abnormal muscle tone, promotes swallowing, and minimizes the risk of aspiration. The upright sitting position is most efficient because the forces of gravity assist peristalsis and muscle function of the esophagus (Inglefinger, 1973). The feet, knees, and pelvis are supported at 90° flexion, with the head and trunk in midline and slight head and neck flexion. Pelvic stabilization is a critical requirement for optimal postural seating (Harryman & Warren, 1992). Specialized seating systems may be necessary to provide proper alignment and stability (Figures 7–1, 7–2). Occasionally, an upright position may not be the best. Some children with poor head control are more stable in a reclined position. Others with poor lip closure and tongue thrusting lose large amounts of food when upright, but retain more when reclined. In spite of these advantages, the reclining position may adversely affect food manipulation in the oral phase and result in poor protection of the airway, increasing the risk of aspiration or penetration.

Oral Motor Techniques

Treatment sessions consist of a series of oral motor techniques followed by a functional activity. The choice of specific oral motor techniques is based on the results of the clinical examination and videofluoroscopy. Techniques can be grouped into six categories: general sensory stimulation, intraoral stimulation, jaw control, sensorimotor techniques, food placement, and thermal stimulation.

General Sensory Stimulation

Graded use of a toothette, NUK® toothbrush, soft toys, or vibrators increases sensory awareness and encourages oral exploration. In children with generalized tactile defensiveness, sustained deep pressure can be incorporated into a handling or play session. In addition, rhythm and purpose will

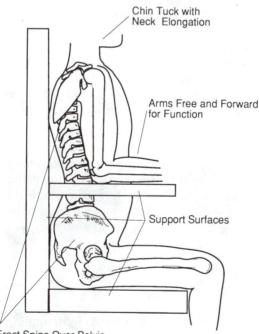

Chin Tuck with Neck Elongation

Arms Free and Forward for Function

Support Surfaces

Erect Spine Over Pelvis Perpendicular to Support Surface

FIGURE 7–1. Components of normal seating.

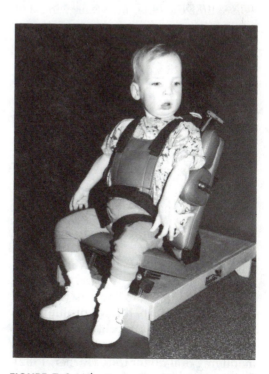

FIGURE 7–2. Adaptive seating system.

help increase the child's tolerance to touch (DeGangi, Craft, & Castellan, 1991). Therapy begins with less sensitive areas of the body, such as the back, front of the lower legs, back of forearms, and dorsum of hands and feet, and progresses to more sensitive areas, including the mouth, neck, palms, and soles.

Intraoral Stimulation

Intraoral stimulation decreases oral tactile hypersensitivity by the sequential application of pressure to specific oral structures. Initially, firm pressure is applied to the upper outer gum by stroking in an anterior to posterior direction beginning in the midline (Mueller, 1972). The rate and range of stroking is guided by the response of the child. Stimulation is then provided to the lower gums, hard palate, and, lastly, to the tongue. Because this generally increases saliva flow, the child should be allowed to swallow as necessary. Pressure applied to the tongue is particularly useful in decreasing a hyperactive gag reflex, beginning on the tongue tip and extending backward to just in front of the gag trigger point (Wolfe & Glass, 1992).

Jaw Control

Jaw control uses manual support and guidance to facilitate active lip closure, graded jaw movements, and swallowing. Usually, the therapist sits to the child's side using his or her nondominant arm to provide head and neck support. The therapist's middle finger is placed under the child's chin at the base of musculature, the index finger just below the lower lip, and the thumb tucked into the palm or resting on the cheek (Figure 7–3). Alternatively, if the child's positioning is stable, jaw control can be provided while sitting face to face.

Sensorimotor Techniques

Swallowing can be improved through a variety of specific muscle inhibition and facilitation techniques that work primarily by modifying oral motor tone (Farber, 1982). In the hypertonic child, deep pressure applied with a cloth bib around the mouth and shaking of the cheeks and lips with the therapist's middle and index fingers can enhance elongation of the facial musculature. When muscles are hypotonic, tapping, vibration, quick stretch, and stretch pressure may improve the function and increase tone. In either case, specific therapy to the tongue is important. Lateral or diagonal shaking of the tongue encourages graded movement and muscle elongation, whereas firm tapping in the middle of the tongue promotes cupping and a midline resting position (Alexander, 1992).

Food Placement

Placement of food between the opposing surfaces of the teeth helps to improve tongue lateralization, a prerequisite for effective chewing. Small pieces of food such as fruit wrapped in gauze, cookies, crackers, or cereal can be positioned laterally in the mouth to provide a source of stimulation.

Thermal Stimulation

Thermal stimulation uses cold touch to increase the sensory readiness of the swallowing mechanism (Lazzara, Lazarus, & Logemann, 1986; Logemann, 1986). A small long-handled mirror is chilled and applied to the anterior faucial arches to stimulate swallowing. Because this technique may be difficult in infants and small children, chilled

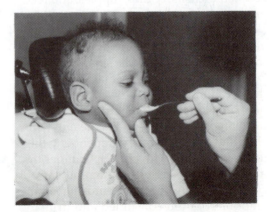

FIGURE 7–3. Manual jaw control.

foods can also be used to trigger the swallow reflex (Wolf & Glass, 1992). The clinical efficacy of this technique remains controversial.

Bolus Modification

Bolus modification is the technique of altering food texture and/or size of the food bolus offered (Wolf & Glass, 1992). Patients with dysphagia have more difficulty handling liquids than solids (Linden & Siebens, 1982). Bolus modification is particularly useful for those who aspirate. Thickening the food increases bolus cohesiveness and slows transit time, allowing better food manipulation and decreasing the risk of aspiration. A general guideline for thickening is one tablespoon of rice cereal to two ounces of liquid. In addition, presenting a single or smaller bolus results in improved oral and pharyngeal phase control and better coordination of breathing and swallowing.

Adaptive Equipment

Neurologically impaired children may have difficulty not only with swallowing, but also with the upper extremity function required to deliver the food to the mouth. The occupational therapist deals with both parts of this process and is uniquely skilled in the areas of food delivery and self-feeding. In addition to upper extremity neuromuscular therapy, there are a variety of specially adapted utensils, bottles, nipples, and feeders available to assist in food delivery (Morris & Klein, 1987). Examples include universal cuffs with wrist support that position the utensil and adds wrist stability (Figure 7–4); scoop dishes that contain the food so that it can more easily be "scooped" onto a utensil (Figure 7–5); electric feeders that mechanically deliver food to the mouth for children who are totally dependent (Figure 7–6); spoons with built-up handles that help with poor grip strength; and cut-out cups that allow both monitoring of the amount of liquid consumed and drinking without head hyperextension.

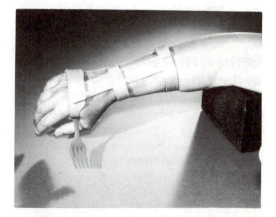

FIGURE 7–4. Universal cuff with wrist support. (Photo provided by Fred Sammons, Inc. © 1992 BISSELL Healthcare Company.)

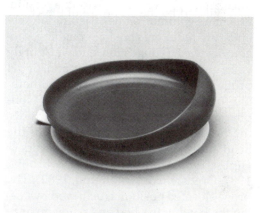

FIGURE 7–5. Scoop dish. (Photo provided by Fred Sammons, Inc. © 1992 BISSELL Healthcare Company.)

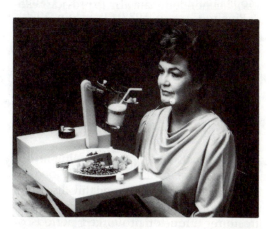

FIGURE 7–6. Electric feeder. (Photo provided by Fred Sammons, Inc. © 1992 BISSELL Healthcare Company.)

Specific Clinical Problems

Gastroesophageal Reflux/Aspiration

Gastroesophageal reflux and aspiration secondary either to reflux or to pharyngeal dysfunction are often seen in children with neurological impairments. Because the occupational therapist performs feeding assessments and provides feeding therapy, she or he is in a unique position to detect clinical signs of these problems. Vomiting either during or between meals is the most obvious indicator of reflux. Esophagitis secondary to reflux may cause pain and produce arching, sweating, or food aversion. The more common signs of aspiration secondary to reflux are choking, coughing, gagging, increased congestion, and wet/gurgly voice quality. Videofluoroscopy and/or pH probe is often recommended by the therapist to confirm these clinical findings. Nonpharmacologic therapy for reflux includes the prone position with elevation of the head and thickened feedings (Meyers & Herbst, 1982; Orenstein, Magill, & Brooks, 1987; Orenstein & Whitington, 1982). The prone elevated position is achieved by raising the head of the bed and using an antireflux harness. Recent studies have questioned the efficacy of these commonly used techniques in the treatment of gastroesophageal reflux (Bailey, Andres, Danek, & Pineiro-Carrero, 1987; Orenstein, 1990). Aspiration secondary to pharyngeal dysfunction is treated by use of a combination of oral motor techniques, bolus modification, and tube feeding, when indicated.

Prolonged Tube Feeding

Occupational therapists are seeing an increasing number of children with medical as well as neurodevelopmental disorders who have been fed by nasogastric or gastrostomy tubes for prolonged periods of time. Many have difficulty making the transition to oral feedings due to poor coordination of breathing and swallowing or the presence of oral tactile hypersensitivity resulting from the lack of normal swallowing stimulation. Because oral contact is difficult, initial therapy consists of sensorimotor techniques designed to develop prefeeding skills (Morris, 1977). Readiness for oral feeding is determined on the basis of overall medical status, clinical examination, and/or videofluoroscopy. Nutritional and cardiorespiratory status must be stable. The clinical examination must demonstrate head and neck control and enough oral motor function to handle secretions. Videofluoroscopy is usually performed to assess the risk of aspiration and the effectiveness of treatment techniques.

When judged medically appropriate, tastes of food may be introduced. Some children are resistant to advancing from purees to higher textures because they have missed critical oral motor developmental periods (Illingworth & Lister, 1964). Intervention is aimed at providing graded oral tactile stimulation and gradually introducing textured food on a continuum from pureed to chunky to crunchy to harder chewing foods (Wolf & Glass, 1992). Often these transitions from tube feeding to higher textures are lengthy. Goals must be realistic, and caregivers must be encouraged to follow through.

Head Injury

Transient or prolonged dysphagia is a common sequela of head injury in children and adolescents. In the case of severe head injury, there is often damage to cranial nerves or the brainstem which affects the sensorimotor control mechanisms necessary to maintain a safe swallow. In addition, many head injured patients remain in coma for prolonged periods of time and, because of their dependence on tube feeding, are deprived of swallowing stimulation. There has been considerable recent interest in this problem because it has been shown that head injured patients with dysphagia require rehabilitative hospital stays more than twice as long as those without dysphagia (Field & Weiss, 1989). In most cases, the central therapeutic problem is the safe transition from tube to oral feedings in a patient emerging from coma. Both the timing of the initial feeding and the progression of food texture are critical elements. The medical history and the bedside clinical evaluation are the most important indicators of feeding readiness. Most patients must be able to follow simple commands and demonstrate volitional oral motor responses (Rancho Level III) (Malkus & Stenderup, 1974). Videofluoroscopy may also be warranted in some cases. Figure 7–7 outlines a typical evaluation protocol (Brockmeyer-Stubbs, personal communication).

Excessive Drooling

Drooling is a frequent problem in children with sensorimotor impairments. It may be related to decreased head control; poor jaw, tongue, and lip movement; or delay in the pharyngeal phase of swallowing. To move efficiently for swallowing, the jaw and tongue need support from the shoulder girdle and neck muscles (Morris & Klein, 1987). Therapy aimed at improving head and trunk control will often result in better spontaneous swallowing. Techniques such as jaw control, pressure on the tongue, and elongation of the perioral musculature facilitate swallowing and, when used in conjunction with proper positioning, optimize the child's ability to swallow.

Poor Suck/Swallow in Infants

In the normal infant, sucking and swallowing occur in a coordinated, rhythmic pattern (Wolf & Glass, 1992). At the start of a feeding, sucking is aggressive, averaging 1 suck per second with a 1:1 ratio of sucking to swallowing. As the feeding progresses and slows, the ratio declines to 2 to 3 sucks

per swallow. Infants with neurological impairments or structural anomalies often have difficulty establishing this normal sucking pattern. Abnormal postural tone, oral tactile hypersensitivity, poor lip closure, and tongue retraction may all be contributing factors. A disorganized and inefficient pattern of sucking, swallowing, and breathing results in either fatigue, which prevents adequate nutritional intake, or pharyngeal incoordination, which may lead to aspiration. Initial therapy consists of positioning to assure proper body alignment. In addition to using specific sensorimotor techniques to improve oral motor function, the therapist establishes the pace and rhythm of feeding by periodically interrupting the sucking cycle. Special adaptive equipment, including nipples and bottles designed to improve flow and reduce fatigue, may also be helpful.

Inadequate Self-Feeding Skills

In addition to specific oral motor problems, the occupational therapist also deals with a variety of associated feeding difficulties. Neurologically impaired children often have sensorimotor problems affecting the trunk and upper extremities. Inability to grasp and poor hand-to-mouth coordination interfere with independent feeding. Therapy includes adequate positioning and the use of a variety of adaptive utensils and equipment designed to promote independence in self-feeding.

Behavioral Problems

Many children with feeding disorders also have behavioral difficulties either as a primary or secondary problem, especially in the case of food refusal or food selectivity (Blackman & Nelson, 1985, 1987). When a joint effort with behavioral psychology is necessary, the occupational therapist initially evaluates oral motor function to assure the safety of swallowing and also rec-

OCCUPATIONAL THERAPY
HEAD TRAUMA ORAL MOTOR/FEEDING EVALUATION

PATIENT NAME _____ DATE _____ TIME _____ a.m./p.m.

MEDICATIONS _____

NUTRITIONAL STATUS AT TIME OF EVAL. :   NPO _____ G–TUBE _____ NG TUBE _____

RANCHO LEVEL: _____

DATE OF INJURY: _____ ETIOLOGY _____

POSITIONING: _____

CHECK ( ) all responses that apply to the patient

ORAL TONE: Hypertonic _____ Athetoid _____ WNLs _____ Asymmetry _____

GAG RESPONSE: Hyperactive _____ Hypoactive _____

LIP CLOSURE AT REST: Open mouth _____ Retracted upper lip _____ Closed mouth _____

TRACHEOSTOMY TUBE PRESENT: Yes _____ No _____

GURGLY WET VOCAL QUALITY/CONGESTION AT START OF EVALUATION: Yes _____ No _____

SENSATION TO TOUCH IN PERIORAL/INTRAORAL REGION: Hypersensitive ____ Hyposensitive ____

   Asymmetrical _____ Right _____ Left _____ WNLs _____

COUGHING: Unable _____ Volitional _____ Productive _____ Unproductive/Weak ____

EVIDENCE OF OROPHARYNGEAL STRUCTURAL ABNORMALITY (e.g. scarring, lacerations, or malocclusions)

         Yes _____ No _____ Comments _____

EVIDENCE OF ABNORMAL REFLEXES: Yes _____ No _____ Comments _____

TONGUE MOBILITY: Pt. demonstates full ROM in anterior/posterior direction   Yes _____ No _____

               Pt. demonstates full lateralization to right side   Yes _____ No _____

               Pt. demonstates full lateralization to left side   Yes _____ No _____

               Pt. demon. ability to elavate tongue to top of upper lip   Yes _____ No _____

               Pt. can cup tongue in response to oral stimulation   Yes _____ No _____

BEHAVIOR: Oriented _____ Lethargic _____ Impulsive _____ Food Refusal _____ Motivated _____

RECOMMENDATIONS AT CONCLUSION OF CLINICAL EVALUATION

_____ NPO: RATIONALE _____

                       _____

                       _____

_____ PO: Puree _____ Ground _____ Chopped Fine _____ Regular _____

         Thickened Liquids _____ Thin Liquids _____

_____ Use of OM treatment techniques: Jaw control _____ Lip closure _____ Thermal _____

                                Tongue depression _____ Multiple swallows _____

                                Head positioning _____ Bolus modification _____

VIDEOFLUOROSCOPY PLANS: (positioning, texture sequence, adaptive feeding utensils, and additional comments)

_____

_____

OUTCOME OF VIDEOFLUOROSCOPY: (penetration, aspiration, oral motor vs. pharynx, pooling, etc) _____

_____

Rater's Initials _____

             Revised : K. Brockmeyer–Stubbs, OTR/L 4/93

                      L. Miller Schuberth, MA, OTR/L 4/93

FIGURE 7–7. Head trauma oral-motor/feeding evaluation.

RATER'S GUIDE TO HEAD TRAUMA
ORAL–MOTOR FEEDING EVALUATION

Clinical Observations	Food Presentations	1	2	3	4	5	6	7	8	9	10	11	12
Lip Closure	No active lip closure												
	Partial lip closure												
	Full closure on utensils/finger food												
Tongue Mobility	Incomplete lateralization												
	Incomplete cupping tongue @ bolus/spoon												
	Functional mobility												
Chewing Pattern	Linear – sucking pattern												
	Vertical – munching pattern												
	Rotary – mature pattern												
Oral Transit Time	1 to 3 seconds												
	4 to 10 seconds												
	More than 10 seconds												
Congestion	Present												
	Absent												
Cheek Tone	Pocketing of food present												
	Chewing on one side only												
Other Clinical Signs	Coughing												
	Gagging												
	Vomiting												
	Marked change in respiration												

Intake: _____ solids oz.
_____ liquid oz.

TIME STARTED: _____ TIME ENDED: _____
Meal Items: (list)

Revised : K. Brockmeyer–Stubbs, OTR/L 4/93
L. Miller Schuberth, MA, OTR/L 4/93

FIGURE 7–7. Continued.

ommends appropriate food textures. During the course of behavior intervention, oral motor therapy, and/or reevaluation may be required.

References

Alexander, R. (1992, July). *Neurodevelopmental treatment course in pediatrics.* Presented at Neurodevelopmental Treatment Association, Baltimore, MD.

American Occupational Therapy Association. (1986). Uniform terminology system for reporting occupational therapy services. In *Reference manual of the official documents of the American Occupational Therapy Association, Inc.* (Vol. 9, pp. 12–18). Rockville, MD: Author.

Baily, D. J., Andres, J. M., Danek, G. D., & Pineiro-Carrero, V. M. (1987). *The Journal of Pediatrics, 110,* 187–189.

Blackman, J. A., & Nelson, C. L. A. (1987). Rapid introduction of oral feeding to tube-fed patients. *Journal of Developmental and Behavioral Pediatrics, 8,* 63–66.

Bobath, B. (1977). The neurodevelopmental approach to treatment. In P. H. Pearson & C. E. Williams (Eds.), *Physical therapy services in the developmental disabilities* (pp. 114–185). Springfield, IL: Charles C. Thomas.

DeGangi, G., Craft, P., & Castellan, J. (1991). Treatment of sensory, emotional, and attentional problems in regulatory disordered infants. *Infants and Young Children, 3,* 9–19.

Farber, S. D. (1982). *Neurorehabilitation: A multisensory approach.* Philadelphia: W. B. Saunders.

Field, L. H., & Weiss, C. J. (1989). Dysphagia with head injury. *Brain Injury, 3,* 19–26.

Fox, C. A. (1990). Implementing the modified barium swallow evaluation in children who have multiple disabilities. *Infants and Young Children, 3,* 67–77.

Hamlet, S. L., Nelson, R. J., & Patterson, R. L. (1990). Interpreting the sounds of swallowing: Fluid flow through the cricopharyngeus. *Annals of Otology, Rhinology, and Laryngology, 99,* 749–752.

Harryman, S. E., & Warren, L. R. (1992). Positioning and power mobility. In G. Church & S. Glennen (Eds.), *The handbook of assistive technology* (pp. 55–92). San Diego, CA: Singular Publishing Group.

Illingworth, R. S., & Lister, M. B. (1964). The critical or sensitive period, with special reference to certain feeding problems in infants and children. *The Journal of Pediatrics, 65,* 839–848.

Inglefinger, F. (1973). How to swallow, and belch and cope with heartburn. *Nutrition Today, 8,* 4–13.

Jeim, J. M. (1990). *Oral-Motor/Feeding Rating Scale.* Tucson, AZ: Therapy Skill Builders.

Kenny, D. J., Koheil, R. M., Greenberg, J., Reid, D., Milner, M., Moran, R., & Judd, P. L. (1989). Development of a multidisciplinary feeding profile for children who are dependent feeders. *Dysphagia, 4,* 16–28.

Lazzara, G. D. L., Lazarus, C., & Logemann, J. A. (1986). Impact of thermal stimulation on the triggering of the swallowing reflex. *Dysphagia, 1,* 73–77.

Linden, P., & Siebens, A. A. (1983). Dysphagia: Predicting laryngeal penetration. *Archives of Physical Medicine and Rehabilitation, 64,* 281–283.

Logemann, J. A. (1983). *Evaluation and treatment of swallowing disorders.* San Diego: College-Hill Press.

Logemann, J. A. (1986). Treatment for aspiration related to dysphagia: An overview. *Dysphagia, 1,* 34–38.

Malkus, D., & Stenderup, K. (1974). *Levels of Cognitive Functioning.* Downey, CA: Rancho Los Amigos Hospital.

Meyers, W. F., & Herbst, J. J. (1982). Effectiveness of positioning therapy for gastroesophageal reflux. *Pediatrics, 69,* 768–772.

Morris, S. E. (1977). *Program guidelines for children with feeding problems.* Madison, WI: Childcraft Education Corporation.

Morris, S. E. (1982). *Pre-Speech Assessment Scale: A rating scale for the measurement of prespeech behaviors from birth through two years.* Clifton, NJ: J. A. Preston.

Morris, S. E. (1989). Development of oral-motor skills in the neurologically impaired child receiving non-oral feedings. *Dysphagia, 3,* 135–154.

Morris, S. E., & Klein, M. D. (1987). *Pre-feeding skills.* Tucson, AZ: Therapy Skill Builders.

Mueller, H. (1972). Facilitating feeding and prespeech. In P. H. Pearson & C. E. Williams (Eds.), *Physical therapy services in the developmental disabilities* (pp. 283–310). Springfield, IL: Charles C. Thomas.

Orenstein, S. R. (1990). Prone positioning in infant gastroesophageal reflux: Is elevation of the head worth the trouble? *The Journal of Pediatrics, 117,* 184–187.

Orenstein, S. R., Magill, H. L., & Brooks, P. (1987). Thickening of infant feedings for therapy of gastroesophageal reflux. *The Journal of Pediatrics, 110,* 181–186.

Orenstein, S. R., & Whitington, P. F. (1983). Positioning for prevention of infant gastroesophageal reflux. *The Journal of Pediatrics, 103,* 534–537.

Ottenbacher, K., Bundy, A., & Short, M. A. (1983). The development and treatment of oral motor dysfunction: A review of clinical research. *Physical and Occupational Therapy in Pediatrics, 3,* 1–13.

Stockmeyer, S. A. (1967). An interpretation of the approach of Rood to neuromuscular dysfunction. *American Journal of Physical Medicine, 46,* 400–455.

Stratton, M. (1981). Behavioral assessment scale of oral functions in feeding. *American Journal of Occupational Therapy, 35,* 719–721.

Vulpe, S. (1969). *Vulpe Assessment Battery for the Atypical Child.* Toronto: National Institute on Mental Retardation.

Wolf, L. S., & Glass, R. P. (1992). *Feeding and swallowing disorders in infancy: Assessment and management.* Tucson, AZ: Therapy Skill Builders.

Surgical Approach to Diagnosis and Management: Otolaryngology

CHAPTER

David Eric Tunkel, M.D.

Swallowing and respiratory functions are intimately related in children. Dysphagia may be the presenting symptom of an upper airway abnormality, and respiratory distress from an upper aerodigestive tract lesion may preclude an infant from achieving a normal feeding pattern. The role of the otolaryngologist in the evaluation and treatment of the young child with swallowing and feeding dysfunction centers on the complex relationship between airway protection during swallowing and airway patency for ventilation.

The otolaryngologist can directly visualize the larynx and pharynx in a dynamic manner to assess functional disorders, and in a static sense to diagnose anatomic lesions. Fiberoptic endoscopic techniques to visualize the laryngopharynx in awake children can assess dynamic issues, and operative laryngoscopy/bronchoscopy in anesthetized children can evaluate fixed anatomic lesions. Surgical intervention is directed at the various disease states and anatomic lesions in an individualized manner to optimize respiration and swallowing.

Evaluation

Evaluation of the young child with swallowing disorder involves a full head and neck examination to look for obstructive nasal or pharyngeal lesions, abnormal neuromotor function, or stigmata of craniofacial syndromes which may be associated with feeding disorders.

The retrodisplaced tongue, small mandible, and wide U-shaped cleft of the secondary palate collectively known as the Pierre-Robin sequence is easily noted on examination. Children with this syndrome often require special positioning and feeding maneuvers to promote effective swallowing and to avoid upper airway obstruction at the level of the tongue base (Figure 8–1). Macroglossia is seen in trisomy 21 and with abdominal wall defects in Beckwith-Wiedemann syndrome.

Nasal patency is assessed by passing catheters or by direct visualization with fiberoptic telescopes. Posterior choanal atresia (Figure 8–2) in neonates is often recognized when cyanosis occurs with initial attempts at feeding, due to an inability to

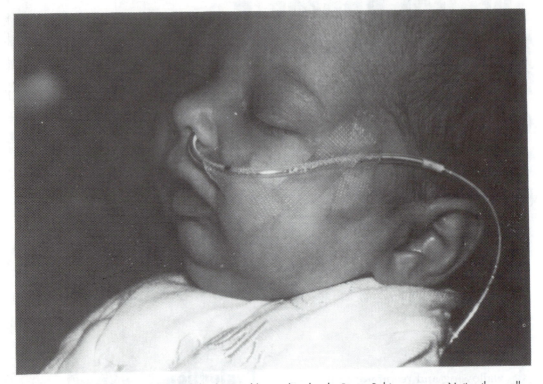

FIGURE 8–1. Three-week-old child with feeding problems related to the Pierre-Robin sequence. Notice the small recessed mandible.

breathe nasally while feeding orally. Surgical repair can allow nasal airflow and uneventful oral feeding. Nasal masses can be inflammatory, congenital, or neoplastic, and obstructed nasal airflow can adversely affect feeding in neonates due to "obligate" nasal breathing during suckling.

Examination of the oral cavity and oropharynx includes a thorough evaluation of lip structure and the competence or oral closure, tongue size and mobility, integrity and movement of the soft palate, and size of the tonsils. The presence of a gag reflex with pharyngeal stimulation is often elicited.

Endoscopic Evaluation of the Larynx and Hypopharynx

The use of fiberoptic and rigid telescopes allows a thorough examination of the upper aerodigestive tract in both a dynamic manner in the awake child and a static manner in the anesthetized child.

Laryngeal examination in cooperative older children can be performed with the standard mirror technique of indirect laryngoscopy. The majority of young children and all infants require the use of flexible fiberoptic endoscopes to perform hypopharyngeal and laryngeal examination. This method allows the examiner to assess the airway and pharynx from the nasal vestibule to the glottis with a full assessment of laryngopharyngeal movement and anatomy during respiration and even swallowing (Tunkel & Zalzal, 1992).

This study is usually performed with an awake child held in a sitting, upright position (Figure 8–3). Topical anesthesia is applied to the nose using tetracaine or lidocaine solutions. Videorecording devices are useful for documenting lesions

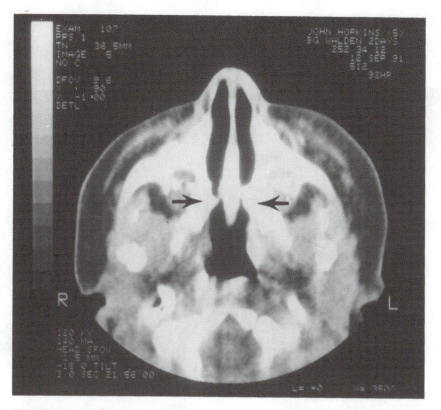

FIGURE 8–2. Axial computerized tomogram of a 2-day-old child with bilateral choanal atresia which presented as cyanosis during feeding. Arrows point to bony atresia plate in the posterior nasal cavity.

and reviewing findings with parents and colleagues.

The fiberoptic endoscope is passed through each side of the nose to assess nasal and choanal patency, and the nasopharynx is inspected for mass lesions and adenoid size. Velopharyngeal closure can be studied in a child old enough to speak during the examination. Closure of the nasopharyngeal inlet can be directly observed, and deficiencies of palate or pharyngeal wall motion leading to hypernasal speech or nasal regurgitation of foods can be documented.

The pharynx is then inspected from a superior view from the nasopharynx, viewing the supraglottic larynx, the tongue base, and the hypopharynx. Excessive secretions in the vallecula and the pyriform sinuses may be observed in children with impaired pharyngeal muscle function. By observing the supraglottic structures during breathing, a dynamic assessment of epiglottic, aryepiglottic fold, and arytenoid motion is obtained. Laryngomalacia, the most common cause of stridor in the neonate, is best diagnosed with this examination.

The true vocal cords are observed for mass lesions, and vocal cord mobility is assessed during respiration and crying or speech to evaluate for vocal cord paralysis or paresis. Erythema of the arytenoids and posterior glottis can be suggestive of laryngeal inflammation from gastroesophageal reflux.

The subglottic larynx and the trachea cannot be evaluated safely during the awake fiberoptic examination due to the

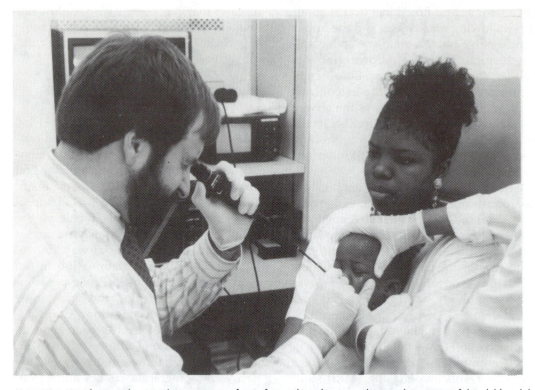

FIGURE 8–3. Fiberoptic laryngeal examination of an infant with stridor. Note the upright position of the child and the video display equipment in the background.

risk of laryngospasm and respiratory compromise. These areas are best evaluated with radiographic studies or with operative laryngoscopy/bronchoscopy with airway control under general anesthesia or local anesthesia with sedation.

The most definitive anatomic evaluation of the upper aerodigestive tract is obtained with direct endoscopic evaluation under general anesthesia in the operating room. The Hopkins rod telescopic system and the operating microscope are aids in defining subtle hypopharyngeal or laryngeal lesions. Direct inspection, palpation, and biopsy of lesions can be performed intraoperatively. The location and anatomy of laryngeal clefts and tracheoesophageal fistula, often suggested by barium studies, are best confirmed using these procedures (Benjamin, 1981). Operative endoscopy also affords the ability to treat some hypopharyngeal and laryngeal

lesions with the use of standard microlaryngeal excision techniques or excision with the carbon dioxide laser.

Esophagoscopy using the rigid open tube or the flexible esophagoscope can be performed at the same anesthetic when indicated in the evaluation of the child with dysphagia. Fiberoptic bronchoscopy can be performed in the operating suite in a sedated child with local anesthesia, using fiberoptic scopes with diameters less than 3 millimeters (mm). Tracheomalacia and vascular compression of the trachea by anomalous great vessels can be observed in this manner.

Ancillary Radiographic Studies

The use of videofluoroscopy and the modified barium swallow is discussed in Chapter 9. Certainly this study provides excellent anatomic and functional details about the swallowing mechanism and the upper aerodigestive tract. A child with concomitant respiratory and swallowing abnormalities should have airway fluoroscopy performed at the same time as contrast swallow study. Fluoroscopy of the airway can detect tracheomalacia, focal tracheal compression from aberrant intrathoracic vessels, subglottic stenosis, and other airway lesions.

Roentgenograms of the neck in the anteroposterior and lateral planes can help assess adenoid and tonsillar size, epiglottic size and shape, retropharyngeal profile, and subglottic diameter. In the setting of acute swallowing disorders, they are most useful to rule out an inflammatory process or a foreign body, as will be detailed later in this chapter. The neck films should be taken with higher kilovoltage settings to emphasize soft tissue detail (Zalzal, 1989).

Computerized tomographic (CT) and magnetic resonance imaging (MRI) studies of the upper aerodigestive tract are obtained only in selected cases during the evaluation of a child with feeding disorder. These studies can define the anatomy of cervical or thoracic masses that may compress the airway or esophagus and cause feeding problems (i.e, hemangioma or lymphangioma). MRI is useful for studying the various vascular anomalies that can compress the trachea and esophagus in the thorax, defining the anatomy of abnormalities usually detected initially by contrast esophagography or bronchoscopy.

Specific Disorders

The following section discusses the presentation, diagnosis, and treatment of some of the more common conditions seen by otolaryngologists when evaluating young children with feeding problems. This is by no means an exhaustive listing of the various anatomic and functional disorders of the upper aerodigestive tract. The emphasis is placed on specific laryngotracheal diseases that may present with feeding difficulties, although respiratory symptoms may coexist or even predominate the clinical picture.

Laryngomalacia

Laryngomalacia is the most common congenital anomaly affecting the larynx, comprising over 60% of all neonatal laryngeal problems (Holinger, 1980). Coarse inspiratory stridor occurs when flaccid supraglottic laryngeal structures, including the epiglottis, aryepiglottic folds, and arytenoids, prolapse into the airway lumen. Fiberoptic laryngeal examination in the awake child is diagnostic. Prone positioning can alleviate stridor, and agitation or feeding can worsen the stridor. Concomitant airway pathology has been demonstrated in up to one fifth of infants with laryngomalacia; thus, full airway evaluation with radiographic studies and/or endoscopy is advised (Gonzales, Reilly, & Bluestone, 1987).

Most children with laryngomalacia do well with conservative treatment. A small subset of children develop increased stridor during feeds, and adequate oral nutrition cannot be accomplished due to increased respiratory efforts. Failure to thrive, obstructive apnea, and cyanosis are indications for surgical intervention, with the former being the most frequent indication for surgery to relieve laryngomalacia. Holinger and Konior (1989) noted feeding difficulties in over three-quarters of patients that required surgery for laryngomalacia.

Tracheotomy will relieve airway obstruction in children with severe laryngomalacia. However, the current initial surgical approach is that of "epiglottoplasty," or trimming of redundant supraglottic structures using operative endoscopic techniques to reduce the amount of obstructive tissue prolapse on inspiration (Figure 8–4) (Zalzal, Anon, & Cotton, 1987). This procedure often stabilizes the airway to allow feeding without airway compromise, and

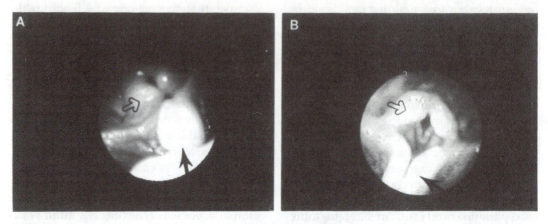

FIGURE 8–4. Fiberoptic images of a 3-month-old infant with failure to thrive from severe laryngomalacia. **A.** Severe collapse of supraglottic structures during inspiration. Note folding of epiglottis (*black arrow*) and collapse of arytenoid mucosa (*open arrow*), blocking visualization of vocal cords. **B.** One week after epiglottoplasty. Note reduction of epiglottic folding and arytenoid collapse, with easy visualization of vocal cords during inspiration.

tracheotomy is avoided. Objective improvement of airway obstruction after epiglottoplasty for laryngomalacia was documented by Marcus, Crockett, and Davidson-Ward (1990) with pre- and postoperative polysomnography.

Vocal Cord Paralysis

True vocal cord paralysis is the second most common cause of stridor in neonates, and both unilateral and bilateral vocal cord motion abnormalities can be seen in children. Bilateral vocal cord paralysis is the most common cause of severe upper airway obstruction presenting at birth. Vocal cord paralysis can be congenital or acquired, and diagnosis is best made by fiberoptic examination of the larynx in an awake child during phonation and respiration.

An abnormal cry, with hoarseness or a weak breathy character, should alert the clinician to the possibility of vocal cord paralysis. Vocal cord paralysis has been associated with birth trauma, forceps delivery, chest and neck surgery, and intracranial and intrathoracic congenital abnormalities (Grundfast & Harley, 1989). The

abductor function of the larynx allows lateral movement of the vocal cords which opens the glottis during inspiration. It is this function that is usually impaired by vocal cord paralysis and, with bilateral paralysis, causes severe airway obstruction at the level of the vocal cords. The inability of the paralyzed vocal cords to fully adduct, or close, against each other, leads to hoarseness or weak cry and often to aspiration of liquid foods.

The etiology of vocal cord paralysis and the presence of other neuromotor abnormalities can dictate the degree of associated swallowing problems. Vocal cord paralysis due to central nervous system disorders at the level of the brainstem may be accompanied by other lower cranial nerve deficits, further complicating swallowing efforts. The internal branch of the superior laryngeal nerve, the sensory nerve to the supraglottic larynx, leaves the vagus nerve (cranial nerve X) high in the neck. The recurrent laryngeal nerve, which provides motor innervation to all intrinsic laryngeal muscles except the cricothyroid muscle and sensory innervation to the infraglottic larynx, leaves the vagus nerve in the chest. Thus, vocal cord paralysis of central etiology, or from "high vagal" lesions, is associated with swallowing difficulties from glottic incompetence and laryngeal sensory deficits.

Unilateral vocal cord paralysis in neonates can be associated with congenital anomalies within the chest and neck. It is also seen after intrathoracic or cervical procedures for congenital heart disease or tracheoesophageal anomalies, presumably due to injury to the recurrent laryngeal nerve in the neck or chest (Robertson & Birch, 1976). A child with a unilateral vocal cord paralysis rarely requires tracheotomy for airway obstruction, although stridor may be a significant symptom in the small infant. Feeding issues usually predominate, with aspiration occurring because of incompetent laryngeal closure at the glottic level. Compensation usually occurs, with the normal mobile vocal cord attaining the motion necessary for glottic closure. Thickening of feeds and positioning with the mobile cord dependent during feeds are useful maneuvers until such compensation is evident.

In older children with persistent voice disorder (hoarseness or breathiness) or persistent aspiration from vocal cord paralysis, vocal cord medialization procedures have been performed to shift the immobile vocal cord to a more medial position to allow closure against the opposite mobile vocal cord. These procedures involve endoscopic injection of materials (gelfoam = temporary, teflon = permanent) into the paraglottic space, or open laryngeal surgery to insert various spaces into the space between the thyroid cartilage and its inner perichondrium (Koufman, 1986; Lewy, 1986).

Bilateral vocal cord paralysis usually presents with airway obstruction, and tracheotomy is required for persistent paralysis with airway compromise. Aspiration may occur from incomplete glottic closure, but the respiratory issues are paramount. Bilateral vocal cord paralysis is associated with central nervous system anomalies such as the Arnold-Chiari malformation, and a full neurologic workup with radiographic imaging to rule out intracranial pathology is indicated in children with this disorder.

Tracheotomy is performed in young children with bilateral vocal cord paralysis to secure the airway. When bilateral vocal cord paralysis is seen in children with increased intracranial pressure, endotracheal intubation is preferable to tracheotomy, because vagus nerve function and vocal cord motion may improve when the intracranial process is relieved. The child with a ventriculoperitoneal shunt who presents with stridor and vocal cord paralysis needs to have the shunt function evaluated.

Electromyography can be performed under general anesthesia with electrodes placed endoscopically into the posterior cricoarytenoid muscle (the vocal cord *abductor*), to measure reinnervation potentials to prognosticate the return of vocal cord abductor function (Koch, Milmoe, & Grundfast, 1987).

Definitive procedures to improve the laryngeal airway in neonates and young children with bilateral vocal cord paralysis are usually performed only after vocal cord motion has not returned after 6 to 12 months of observation (Narcy, Contecin, & Viala, 1990). These procedures involve open or endoscopic approaches to remove or lateralize the vocal cord or the arytenoid cartilage to increase the airway size between the two immobile vocal cords. Arytenoidectomy can be performed endoscopically with the carbon dioxide laser. Transverse cordotomy, detachment of the vocal cord from its insertion onto the arytenoid, can improve the airway (Dennis & Kashima, 1989). Open approaches to remove the arytenoid or to lateralize the arytenoid and vocal cord with sutures, can be performed through lateral pharyngotomy or anterior laryngofissure approaches (Narcy et al., 1989).

Nerve-muscle pedicle reinnervation is a procedure pioneered by Tucker, who implanted innervated omohyoid tissue into the posterior cricoarytenoid muscle. Return of abductor vocal cord function has been observed after this procedure (Tucker, 1986). Tucker was able to remove the tracheotomies in 9 of 18 patients with bilateral vocal cord paralysis after reinnervation.

Any procedure that opens the fixed glottic aperture to improve the airway increases the risk of breathy voice and even aspiration. Current trends in surgery for vocal cord paralysis involve study of phrenic nerve to laryngeal nerve reinnervation procedures, as well as refinement of the nerve-muscle procedure for more reliable return of vocal cord motion (Crumley, 1982, 1983). The reliability of reinnervation procedures to allow successful decannulation is not universally accepted, and additional study is needed. Hopefully, future advances in the treatment of children with bilateral vocal cord paralysis may avoid the voice problems associated with the more reliable arytenoidectomy or lateralization procedures.

Laryngeal Clefts

Congenital laryngeal clefts are rare anomalies that occur because of incomplete closure of the tracheoesophageal septum and/or cricoid cartilage in the sixth week of fetal life. Neonates with laryngeal clefts present with cough, cyanosis, or respiratory distress with feeding attempts. Aspiration pneumonia may be a recurrent problem, and stridor or weak cry can be observed.

Posterior laryngeal clefts may be part of a much larger defect involving the tracheoesophageal common "party" wall, and separate tracheoesophageal fistulas may be present. Esophageal atresia, gastroesophageal reflux, and other congenital anomalies may be associated. When confined to the larynx, these posterior defects may involve only the interarytenoid muscles, with or without a mucosal defect, or may extend partially or totally through the

cricoid cartilage posteriorly. Several classification systems have been devised, with Benjamin and Inglis (1989) proposing a four-grade system (Figure 8–5).

The defect in posterior laryngeal clefts allows food, especially liquids, to spill through the posterior glottis into the airway. Diagnosis is usually suggested on contrast swallow study with videofluoroscopy. Confirmation of diagnosis is sometimes difficult, especially in the "minor" supraglottic or type 1 clefts. Fiberoptic laryngoscopy in the awake state may not show a cleft, because redundant arytenoid mucosa may occlude the cleft during this examination. Operative direct laryngoscopy under general anesthesia allows manual distraction of the arytenoids to visualize the cleft (Figure 8–6). Radiographic and endoscopic studies in the child with a laryngeal cleft must be aimed at ruling out any other associated tracheal or esophageal anomalies that may be contributing to dysphagia or aspiration.

Type 1 laryngeal clefts are often managed conservatively, with thickened feeds and positioning. When aspiration continues to be a problem, small clefts can be repaired endoscopically with microlaryngeal suture techniques, avoiding the need for tracheotomy (Koltai, Morgan, & Evans, 1991). More extensive laryngeal clefts require open surgical repair through an anterior laryngofissure, with tracheotomy placement for airway protection in the perioperative period (Myer, Cotton, Holmes, & Jackson, 1990).

Subglottic Stenosis

Subglottic stenosis is a congenital or acquired narrowing of the subglottic airway. Presentation usually consists of some combination of biphasic stridor, low pitched cough, or recurrent croup like illness. In the neonatal intensive care unit, subglottic stenosis usually presents as repeated extubation failure.

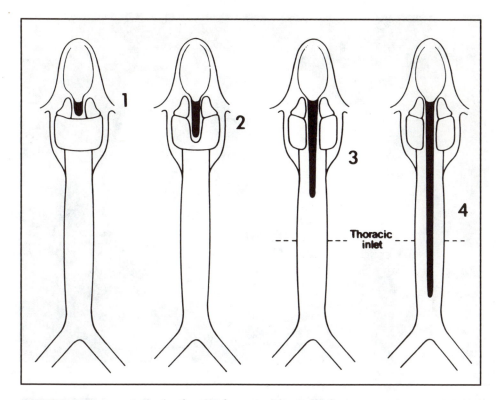

FIGURE 8–5. Benjamin/Inglis classification of posterior laryngeal clefts: 1 = supraglottic interarytenoid clefts; 2 = partial cricoid defects; 3 = complete cricoid defects +/− cervical tracheal involvement; 4 = laryngotracheoesophageal clefts into the thorax. (From Benjamin, B., & Inglis, A. [1989]. Minor congenital laryngeal clefts: Diagnosis and classification. *Annals of Otology, 98,* 417–420, reprinted with permission.)

Congenital subglottic stenosis is thought to be secondary to abnormal formation of the cricoid cartilage and the associated soft tissues. More commonly, subglottic stenosis is seen as an acquired lesion secondary to laryngeal injury from intubation or trauma. The diagnosis can be made by neck radiographs or airway fluoroscopy, and confirmed by laryngoscopy and bronchoscopy (Figure 8–7). Subglottic stenosis itself does not cause dysfunctional swallowing; however, these children often have feeding irregularities from increased respiratory effort or from the tracheotomy that may be required to relieve airway obstruction.

Management of children with subglottic stenosis is dictated by the severity of the clinical presentation and the degree of narrowing at endoscopy. In general, acquired lesions are more severe than congenital stenoses and more often require tracheotomy and subsequent laryngeal reconstruction for airway management (Tunkel & Zalzal, 1992). An alternative to tracheotomy in neonates with subglottic stenosis who have failed extubation is the anterior cricoid split, which involves an anterior midline division of the lower thyroid cartilage, the cricoid cartilage, and the first two or three tracheal rings and stenting with an endotracheal tube to expand the subglottic diameter (Cotton & Seid, 1980). More severe subglottic obstruction requires early tracheotomy, followed by open laryngotracheal reconstruction using a variety of cartilage grafting and stenting techniques to allow decannulation (Zalzal, 1988).

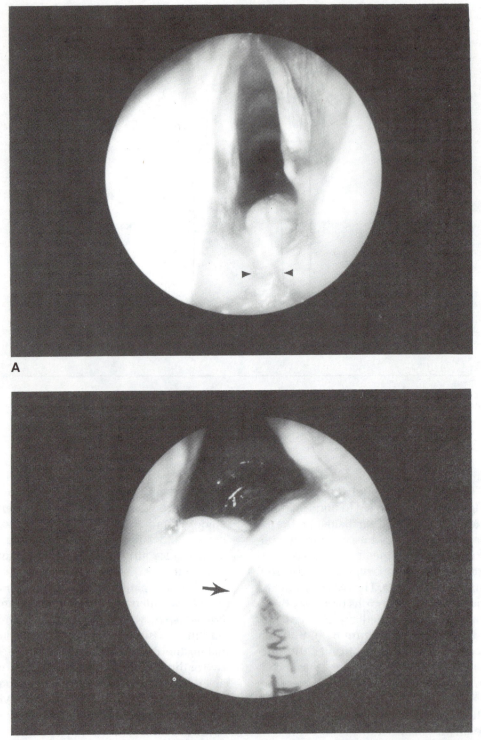

A

B

FIGURE 8–6. Operative endoscopic photographs of a type 1 laryngeal cleft. **A.** Arrows point to defect in interarytenoid area. **B.** Same patient after orotracheal intubation. Note endotracheal tube has fallen through cleft posteriorly (*arrow*). (Photographs courtesy of Dr. Bernard Marsh.)

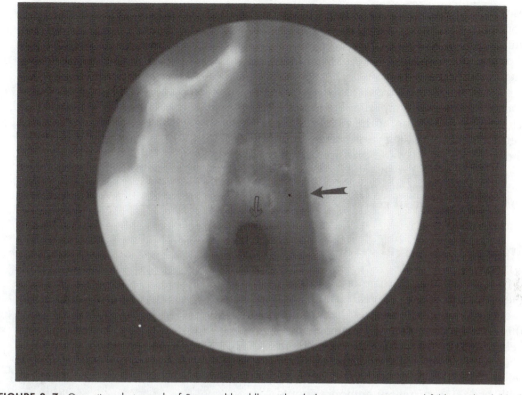

FIGURE 8–7. Operative photograph of 3-year-old toddler with subglottic stenosis. True vocal fold noted with black arrow, stenotic airway lumen with open arrow. (Photograph courtesy of Dr. Bernard Marsh.)

Vascular Rings

A variety of vascular malformations of the great vessels in the chest cause respiratory and feeding symptoms in young children. In general, even when these anomalies compress the esophagus, respiratory symptoms overshadow feeding problems. Biphasic or expiratory low-pitched stridor occurs from tracheal compression, and recurrent pneumonia may occur from aspiration and/or faulty pulmonary secretion clearance from bronchial or partial tracheal obstruction.

The compressive vascular rings may consist of full rings of great vessels, such as seen with the double aortic arch, or a partial ring of a vessel with a fibrous or ligamentous vessel remnant completing the ring, as seen in the right aortic arch with

ligamentum arteriosus (Sachs & Lee, 1989). The most common vascular anomaly is an abnormal innominate artery compressing the anterior trachea, causing stridor and pneumonia when obstruction is high grade.

"Dysphagia lusoria" is a term used to describe swallowing difficulties from an aberrant intrathoracic vessel. The most common cause of dysphagia lusoria is from esophageal compression by an aberrant course of the right subclavian artery.

Diagnosis of vascular rings is suggested by the presence of a right sided aortic arch or a double aortic arch on chest radiographs. Pulsatile tracheobronchial compression can be seen with fiberoptic or rigid bronchoscopy performed for evaluation of stridor. Compression of the esophageal barium column on contrast barium esophagography is highly suggestive of an aberrant great vessel (Figure 8–8). Vascular anatomy can be defined by echocardiography or MRI, precluding the need for angiography in many cases.

Surgery is contemplated when the above respiratory symptoms are severe. This involves division of the ring, or suspension of the offending vessels away from the trachea. Vascular compression of the trachea may cause a segmental tracheomalacia with symptoms that persist even after corrective vascular surgery.

Tracheoesophageal Fistula

A full discussion of the diagnosis and treatment of tracheoesophageal fistula and esophageal atresia is beyond the scope of this chapter. The isolated tracheoesophageal fistula, or "H-type," may be subtle in presentation and accounts for only 4% of these anomalies (Adkins, 1990). Coughing with feeds, or recurrent pneumonia, should provoke an evaluation for such an abnormality. Contrast videofluoroscopy may demonstrate the fistula, and confirmation can be obtained with rigid bronchoscopy and esophagoscopy (Benjamin, 1991). Tracheal examination for a fistulous opening posteriorly is more fruitful than esophageal endoscopy when looking for an H-type fistula.

Aerodigestive anomalies associated with tracheoesophageal fistula include laryngeal clefts, tracheal stenosis, esophageal atresia or stenosis, and tracheomalacia. Vocal cord motion impairment after repair of these tracheoesophageal anomalies may be more common than clinically evident (Robertson & Birch, 1976).

Cricopharyngeal Achalasia

Incomplete relaxation of the cricopharyngeus muscle during swallowing has been described in neonates (Shapiro & Healy, 1988). Regurgitation of feeds and aspira-

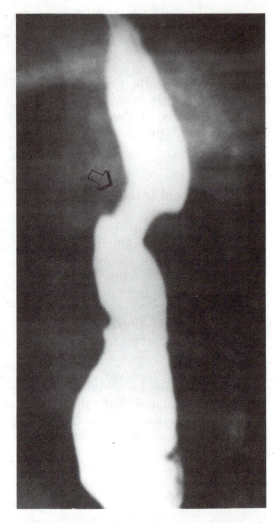

FIGURE 8–8. Barium esophagram of a stridulous 5-week-old infant demonstrating the indentation of the esophagus by a vascular ring (*arrow*).

tion are seen early in life. In one series, 11 of 15 patients had associated central nervous system diseases, including cerebral palsy, meningomyelocele, Arnold-Chiari malformation, and seizures (Reichert, Bluestone, Stool, Sieber, & Sieber, 1977). Diagnosis is usually made by videofluoroscopy. Prognosis is variable, with spontaneous recovery seen most frequently in those children without central neuromuscular disorders.

Treatment of cricopharyngeal achalasia has included enteral feedings, dilatation, and cricopharyngeal myotomy. Surgical indications for myotomy in this group of young patients remain undefined. Cricopharyngeal myotomy was "only moderately" helpful in the two patients that underwent this procedure in Reichert et al.'s (1977) study, and concomitant gastroesophageal reflux may be aggravated by myotomy.

Velopharyngeal Incompetence (VPI)

Nasal regurgitation of feedings, usually liquids, is often seen in children with more global neuromuscular and swallowing disorders. The more common manifestation of velopharyngeal incompetence, incomplete closure of the nasopharyngeal inlet by the pharyngeal walls and soft palate, is hypernasal voice during certain speech sounds. In severe cases, an incompetent velopharyngeal mechanism allows nasal regurgitation of food.

Structural abnormalities from overt cleft palate and submucous cleft palate can lead to velopharyngeal incompetence. A small subset of patients develop hypernasal speech and—or nasal regurgitation after adenoidectomy with or without tonsillectomy. Most of these postoperative problems resolve without treatment.

Velopharyngeal closure problems can be studied with fiberoptic nasopharyngoscopy to directly observe movement of the soft palate, the lateral pharyngeal walls, and the posterior pharyngeal wall (D'Antonio, Muntz, Marsh, Marty-Grames, & Backensto-Marsh, 1988). The size and location of deficiencies of sphincteric closure can be documented to plan therapy. "Phonation studies" using videofluoroscopy of intranasal and oral contrast during speech and swallow can also assess velopharyngeal function.

Most patients with VPI have therapy directed to improve hypernasal speech. Speech therapy and obturators play a role, but surgery is the mainstay of treatment of severe cases. Cleft palate closure, place-

ment of pharyngeal flaps, and redirection of pharyngeal or soft palate musculature all play a role in surgical treatment of VPI (Crockett, 1990).

Head and Neck Masses

Neoplasms affecting the head and neck can affect the swallowing mechanisms by direct compressive or obstructive mass effect as well as by causing cranial nerve dysfunction.

Hemangiomas can occur in the subglottis, causing stridor and airway symptoms, as well as occur in the pharyngeal walls or postcricoid hypopharynx, causing feeding problems. Reduction in size of these lesions is expected in the first three years of life when confined to the larynx. More extensive head and neck hemangiomas may cause persistent symptoms, although some reduction in size is expected in the first seven years of life. Laryngeal hemangiomas can be treated with observation, systemic steroids, endoscopic laser excision, or early tracheotomy depending on the severity of symptoms (Shikhani, Marsh, Jones, & Holliday, 1986).

Cystic hygromas, or lymphangiomas, can expand during upper respiratory infections and cause compressive airway and feeding symptoms. Surgery is the mainstay of treatment. Recurrences are common because of lack of clear distinction between normal and infiltrated tissues, and the desire to avoid radical surgery for a histologically "benign" lesion.

Rhabdomyosarcoma is the most common pediatric soft tissue malignancy. Lower cranial nerve deficits from skull base involvement may lead to dysphagia with cough, hoarseness, and even aspiration. Treatment of these tumors involve multimodality oncologic therapy, and supportive feeding assistance directed at specific swallowing difficulties.

A variety of non-neoplastic pharyngeal masses can lead to dysphagia and foreign body sensation, depending on location and size. Lingual thyroid tissue and vallecular cysts (Figure 8–9) can cause globus symptoms because of the mass effect at the tongue base. Lingual thyroid can respond to hormone suppression therapy, while cysts can be removed or marsupialized endoscopically.

Dysphagia of Acute Onset

Swallowing difficulties of rapid onset in children that present to the otolaryngologist usually are due to acute infectious laryngeal or pharyngeal disorders and ingested foreign bodies. These patients require prompt evaluation as acute airway compromise may accompany or follow the initial symptoms of dysphagia.

Swallowed foreign bodies are most typically found in the 9-month to 3-year-old age group. A history of foreign body ingestion, aspiration, coughing, or "mouthing" of objects may be present, but the absence of such a history should not lessen clinical suspicion. Radiographs of the chest and neck may diagnose a radiopaque foreign body (Figure 8–10). A normal X-ray study does not rule out the presence of a small or radiolucent object in the upper aerodigestive tract, and operative laryngoscopy, esophagoscopy, and bronchoscopy may be necessary to diagnose foreign body ingestion and to remove the offending object. Foreign body aspiration into the tracheobronchial tree should always be considered, but in these cases dysphagia is replaced by wheezing, asymmetric breath sounds, or stridor.

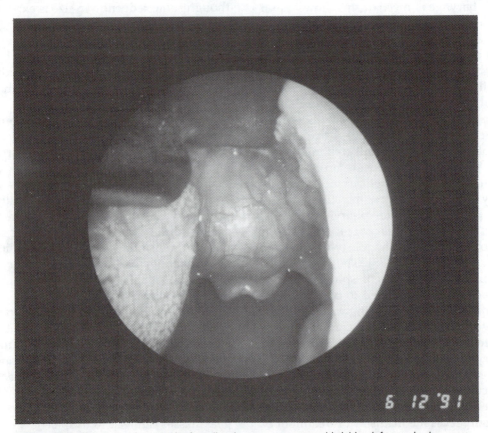

FIGURE 8–9. Operative photograph of a vallecular cyst in a 6-year-old child with foreign body sensation when swallowing. Note posterior displacement of the tip of the epiglottis.

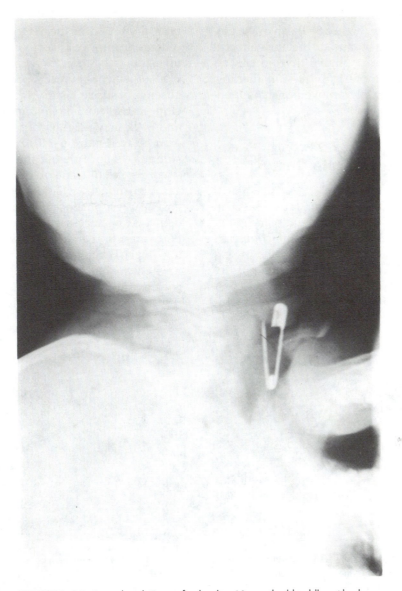

FIGURE 8–10. Lateral neck X-ray of a drooling 18-month-old toddler with a hypopharyngeal open safety pin.

Tonsillitis and peritonsillar abscess are common causes of acute dysphagia and odynophagia in children. Antimicrobial treatment of tonsillitis is directed against group A beta-hemolytic streptococcus, although viral etiologies are common. Peritonsillar abscess usually requires a drainage procedure along with antibiotic treatment, and drainage has been performed by needle aspiration, incision, or ton-

sillectomy (Ophir, Bawnik, Poria, Porat, & Marshak, 1988).

Epiglottitis should be considered in the young child with acute dysphagia, stridor, and toxicity. This condition, more correctly termed acute bacterial supraglottitis, occurs primarily in the 3- to 6-year-old age group and presents with rapidly progressive sore throat, drooling, and respiratory compromise. A diagnostic lateral neck

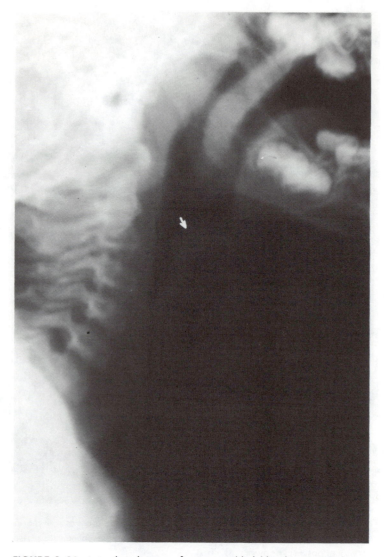

FIGURE 8–11. Lateral neck X-ray of a 3-year-old child with acute epiglottitis. Note the thickened "thumbprint" epiglottis (*arrow*).

radiograph shows a thickened epiglottis and obliteration of the vallecula (Figure 8–11). Airway control is the preeminent issue, and prompt intubation is the standard of care to prevent airway obstruction. Antimicrobial treatment is directed against *Hemophilus influenza B* (Tunkel & Zalzal, 1992).

Acute dysphagia, abnormal neck posture, and toxicity can be seen in children with retropharyngeal abscesses. Diagnosis of retropharyngeal abscess is suggested by pharyngeal examination and a widened retropharyngeal soft tissue space on lateral neck X-ray. This diagnosis is confirmed by fluoroscopic examination or by contrast computerized tomography of the neck (Figure 8–12). Treatment consists of surgical drainage by a transoral or transcervical approach and systemic antibiotics (Elliott, Bernard, Briggs, & McDonald, 1992; Guarisco & Grundfast, 1988).

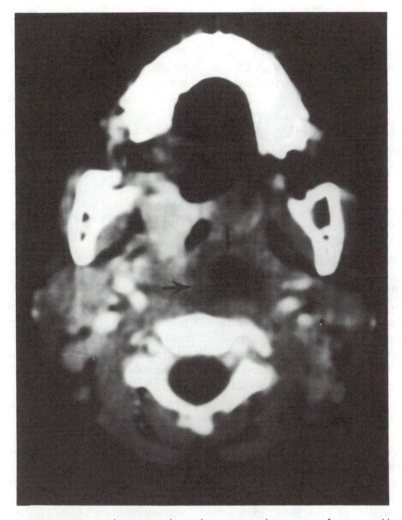

FIGURE 8–12. Axial contrast-enhanced computerized tomogram of a 4-year-old with fever, neck stiffness, and dysphagia. Note lucent area representing a large retropharyngeal abscess (*arrows*).

Surgery for Aspiration

A variety of surgical techniques have been devised for intractable aspiration. These are usually directed at the specific anatomic or functional problems that are compromising the laryngeal protective mechanisms. Intractable aspiration from central nervous lesions can be treated with laryngeal closure or diversion procedures or even laryngectomy, all of which necessitate a tracheostoma for breathing (Blitzer, Krespi, Oppenheimer, & Levin, 1988).

These procedures were developed for adults with severe brainstem or head and neck disorders, and are rarely used in the pediatric age group.

Aspiration secondary to vocal cord paralysis is often treated with the previously described medialization procedures to close the glottic aperture during swallow. Augmentation of an immobile vocal cord by endoscopic Teflon injection, or medialization by an external laryngoplasty approach, has been used in children with aspiration due to unilateral vocal cord paralysis. Tracheotomy, even with a cuffed tube in place, does not prevent aspiration, as will be described later. Pulmonary toilet can be improved with tracheotomy for suctioning children with severe aspiration.

Swallowing Function in Children After Tracheostomy

The swallowing function of pediatric patients with long-term tracheostomy for airway management has not been systematically studied. Certainly the indication for tracheotomy is often predictive of the degree of dysphagia that is seen in these children. Children with upper airway obstruction from pharyngeal hypotonia as seen in severe cerebral palsy often require tracheotomy. It can be expected that children with central nervous disease affecting the pharyngeal musculature will have long-term feeding problems even after tracheotomy alleviates respiratory problems. The child who undergoes a tracheotomy for isolated congenital subglottic stenosis usually swallows well with the tracheotomy in place, because no concomitant pharyngoesophageal or neuromuscular issues exist.

The placement of a tracheotomy tube fixes the laryngotracheal complex to the anterior neck skin, limiting the elevation of this complex during swallow. This elevation allows for closure of the supraglottic larynx during deglutition by elevation under the tongue base, and is a physiologic means of preventing aspiration (Stool & Eavey, 1990). The adductor reflex function of the vocal cords, closure of the glottis with superior laryngeal nerve stimulation, is blunted after tracheotomy (Buckwalter & Sasaki, 1984). Thus tracheotomy appears to diminish the efficacy of airway protection during swallowing at two levels: by limiting supraglottic sphincteric action and elevation by "tethering" the larynx and by blunting the normal response of vocal cord closure to sensory input from the hypopharynx and supraglottis.

It is reasonable to suspect that aspiration may be common due to the aforementioned factors. This can be studied radiographically with contrast pharyngoesophagography or, more simply, by dyeing feeds and observing the color of tracheal secretions. Indeed, Cameron, Reynolds, and Zuidema (1973) detected aspiration in over two thirds of adult patients after tracheotomy by placing blue dye on the tongues of 61 patients.

Treatment of Sialorrhea

Sialorrhea, or drooling, is a problem that coexists with disordered oromotor function in children with cerebral palsy. Problem drooling is almost always due to impaired clearance of saliva from the mouth and pharynx, rather than from increased saliva production. Various combinations of poor tongue coordination, delay of the bolus in the mouth and pharynx, pharyngeal dyscoordination, and upper esophageal sphincter spasticity can be seen in the drooling child with neuromuscular disease (Ekedahl, Mansson, & Sandberg, 1974). Sialorrhea causes problems in the daily care of multiply handicapped children, with impaired oral intake, increased oral and perioral infections, and need for frequent clothing changes.

Saliva is produced by both major and minor salivary glands. The major salivary glands (parotid, submandibular, and sublingual glands) produce 90% of saliva volume during the resting state (Myer, 1989). Salivary secretion is controlled by the parasympathetic nervous system. Parotid gland parasympathetic innervation originates in the inferior salivary nucleus, travels with the glossopharyngeal nerve to the otic ganglion via the auriculotemporal nerve (Figure 8–13). Submandibular gland parasympathetics originate in the superior salivary nucleus, travel with the facial nerve to the submandibular ganglion via the chorda tympani nerve. Management of sialorrhea has been directed at the major salivary glands themselves and their innervation.

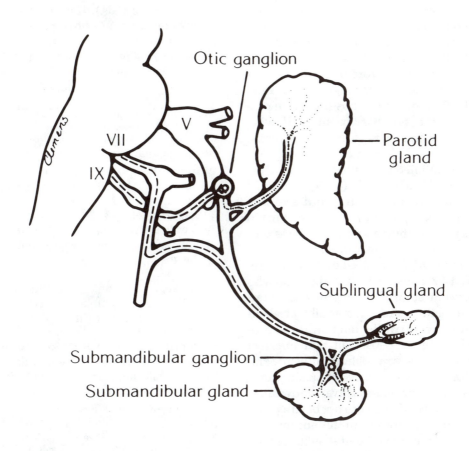

FIGURE 8-13. Parasympathetic innervation of the major salivary glands. (From Myer, C. M. [1989]. Sialorrhea. *Pediatric Clinics of North America, 36,* 1495–1500, reprinted with permission.)

The evaluation of the drooling child involves an extensive evaluation of the swallowing mechanism to assess oromotor tone, pharyngeal function, and salivary clearance changes with positioning. A full head and neck examination is performed looking for oral and pharyngeal abnormalities or obstructive lesions. With the assistance of speech-language pathologists and occupational therapists, the effects of concentration, positioning, emotional states, and so on are correlated with sialorrhea.

The primary treatment of sialorrhea in children with neuromuscular impairment has been physical therapy. Behavioral techniques to improve oromotor tone and pharyngeal function, as well as appropriate positioning, have been effective in improving salivary clearance in some children. Medical treatment with anticholinergic drugs has been associated with side effects such as constipation, urinary retention, blurred vision, and behavioral changes (Tunkel & Furin, 1991). Radiotherapy for sialorrhea has had variable responses, and the potential for future malignant transformation exists.

The surgical treatment of sialorrhea has included various combinations of salivary gland removal, duct ligation, duct rerouting, and interruption of parasympathetic input. Bilateral chorda tympani nerve section and tympanic neurectomy is performed with a surgical approach through the middle ear, but this has been associated with late failure with recurrent drooling from presumed reinnervation of interrupted parasympathetics.

Crysdale and White (1989) advocate bilaterally rerouting of the submandibular gland duct orifices from their native position under the ventral tongue in the anterior floor of mouth to a position more posterior in the oropharynx, thus allowing salivary clearance without tongue assistance and oral closure competence. This can be combined with sublingual gland excision. Wilkie and Brody (1977) combined bilateral submandibular gland excision with posterior rerouting of the parotid ducts from the buccal mucosa into the tonsillar fossa.

Shott, Myer, and Cotton (1989) reviewed 52 patients with sialorrhea who underwent surgical treatment and determined that bilateral submandibular gland excision and parotid duct ligation provided the most consistent and effective control of drooling. Although this operation has the theoretical risk of causing xerostomia by eliminating salivary flow from four major glands, this has not been a problem in Shott's series or in this author's experience. Transient parotid swelling is seen in most patients after parotid duct ligation, but this resolves shortly after surgery.

The surgical approach to the treatment of sialorrhea has provided effective cessation of drooling to improve the daily care of neuromuscularly impaired children. Meticulous dental care is required postoperatively to avoid dental caries associated with decreased salivary flow. The drooling child deserves a multidisciplinary evaluation aimed at analysis of oromotor factors which impede salivary clearance, and surgery should be considered for those children with problem drooling that does not respond to behavioral and physical therapy.

References

Adkins, J. C. (1990). Congenital malformations of the esophagus. In C. D. Bluestone &

S. E. Stool (Eds.), *Pediatric Otolaryngology* (2nd ed., pp. 973–984). Philadelphia: W. B. Saunders.

Benjamin, B. (1981). Endoscopy in esophageal atresia and tracheoesophageal fistula. *Annals of Otology, Rhinology, and Laryngology, 90,* 376–382.

Benjamin, B., & Inglis, A. (1989). Minor congenital laryngeal clefts: Diagnosis and classification. *Annals of Otology, Rhinology, and Laryngology, 98,* 417–420.

Blitzer, A., Krespi, Y. P., Oppenheimer, R. W., & Levine, T. M. (1988). Surgical management of aspiration, *Otolaryngologic Clinics of North America, 21,* 743–750.

Buckwalter, J. A., & Sasaki, C. T. (1984). Effect of tracheotomy on laryngeal function. *Otolaryngologic Clinics of North America, 17,* 41–48.

Cameron, J. L., Reynolds, J., & Zuidema, G. D. (1973). Aspiration in patients with tracheotomies. *Surgery, Gynecology, and Obstetrics, 136,* 68–70.

Cotton, R. T., & Seid, A. B. (1980). Management of the extubation problem in the premature child; anterior cricoid split as an alternative to tracheotomy. *Annals of Otology, Rhinology, and Laryngology, 89,* 508–511.

Crockett, D. M. (1990). Velopharyngeal incompetence. In G. B. Healy (Ed.), *Common problems in pediatric otolaryngology* (pp. 275–288). Chicago: Year Book Medical Publishers.

Crumley, R. L. (1982). Experiments in laryngeal reinnervation. *Laryngoscope, 92,* 1–27.

Crumley, R. L. (1983). Phrenic nerve graft for bilateral vocal cord paralysis. *Laryngoscope, 93,* 425–428.

Crysdale, W. S., & White, A. (1989). Submandibular duct relocation for drooling: A ten year experience with 194 patients. *Otolaryngology/Head and Neck Surgery, 101,* 87–92.

D'Antonio, L., Muntz, H. R., Marsh, J. L., Marty-Grames, L., & Backensto-Marsh, R. (1988). Practical application of flexible fiberoptic nasopharyngoscopy for evaluating nasopharyngeal function. *Plastic and Reconstructive Surgery, 82,* 611–618.

Dennis, D. P., & Kashima, H. (1989). Carbon dioxide laser posterior cordectomy for treatment of bilateral vocal cord paralysis. *Annals of Otology, Rhinology, and Laryngology, 98,* 930–934.

Ekedahl, C., Mansson, I., & Sandberg, N.

(1974). Swallowing dysfunction in the brain-damaged with drooling. *Acta Otolaryngologica, 78,* 141–149.

Elliott, C. A., Bernard, P. A., Briggs, V. A., & McDonald, P. (1992). Posterolateral cervicotomy in retropharyngeal abscesses. *Laryngoscope, 102,* 585–587.

Gonzales, C., Reilly, J. S., & Bluestone, C. D. (1987). Synchronous airway lesions in infancy. *Annals of Otology, Rhinology, and Laryngology, 96,* 77–80.

Grundfast, K. M., & Harley, E. (1989). Vocal cord paralysis. *Otolaryngologic Clinics of North America, 22,* 569–597.

Guarisco, J. L., & Grundfast, K. M. (1988). A technique for insertion and removal of an intraoral drain following treatment of a retropharyngeal abscess. *Laryngoscope, 98,* 242–243.

Holinger, L. D. (1980). Etiology of stridor in the neonate, infant, and child. *Annals of Otology, Rhinology, and Laryngology, 89,* 397–400.

Holinger, L. D., & Konior, R. J. (1989) Surgical management of severe laryngomalacia. *Laryngoscope, 99,* 136–142.

Koch, B. M., Milmoe, G., & Grundfast, K. M. (1987). Vocal cord paralysis in children studied by monopolar electromyography. *Pediatric Neurology, 3,* 288–293.

Koltai, P. J., Morgan, D., & Evans, J. N. G. (1991). Endoscopic repair of supraglottic laryngeal clefts. *Archives of Otolaryngology/Head and Neck Surgery, 117,* 273–278.

Koufman, J. A. (1986). Laryngoplasty for vocal cord medialization: An alternative to teflon. *Laryngoscope, 96,* 726–731.

Lewy, R. B. (1976). Experience with vocal cord injection. *Annals of Otology, Rhinology, and Laryngology, 85,* 440–450.

Marcus, C. L., Crockett, D. M., & Davidson-Ward, S. L. (1990). Evaluation of epiglottoplasty as treatment of severe laryngomalacia. *Journal of Pediatrics, 117,* 706–710.

Myer, C. M. (1989). Sialorrhea. *Pediatric Clinics of North America, 36,* 1495–1500.

Myer, C. M., Cotton, R. T., Holmes, D. K., Jackson, R. K. (1990). Laryngeal and laryngotracheoesophageal clefts: Role of early surgical repair. *Annals of Otology, Rhinology, and Laryngology, 99,* 98–104.

Narcy, P., Contecin, P., & Viala, P. (1990). Surgical treatment for laryngeal paralysis in infants and children. *Annals of Otology, Rhinology, and Laryngology, 99,* 124–128.

Ophir, D., Bawnik, J., Poria, Y., Porat, M., & Marshak, G. (1988). Peritonsillar abscess: A prospective evaluation of outpatient management by needle aspiration. *Archives of Otolaryngology/Head and Neck Surgery, 114,* 661–663.

Reichert, T. S., Bluestone, C. D., Stool, S. E., Sieber, W. K., & Sieber, A. M. (1977). Congenital cricopharyngeal achalasia. *Annals of Otology, 86,* 603–610.

Robertson, J. R., & Birch, H. G. (1976). Laryngeal problems following infant esophageal surgery. *Laryngoscope, 86,* 965–970.

Sachs, F., & Lee, K. J. (1987). The chest. In K. J. Lee (Ed.), *Essential otolaryngology* (4th ed., pp. 794–795). New York: Medical Examination Publishing Company.

Shapiro, J., & Healy, G. B. (1988). Dysphagia in infants. *Otolaryngologic Clinics of North America, 21,* 737–741.

Shikhani, A. H., Marsh, B. R., Jones, M. M., & Holliday, M. J. (1986). Infantile subglottic hemangiomas: An update. *Annals of Otology, Rhinology, and Laryngology, 95,* 336–347.

Shott, S. R., Myer, C. M., & Cotton, R. T. (1989). Surgical management of sialorrhea. *Otolaryngology/Head and Neck Surgery, 101,* 47–50.

Stool, S. E., & Eavey, R. D. (1990). Tracheotomy. In C. D. Bluestone & S. E. Stool (Eds.), *Pediatric otolaryngology* (2nd ed., pp. 1226–1243). Philadelphia: W. B. Saunders.

Tucker, H. M. (1986). Vocal cord paralysis in small children: Principles in management. *Annals of Otology, Rhinology, and Laryngology, 95,* 618–621.

Tunkel, D. E., & Furin, M. J. (1991). Salivary cysts following parotid duct translocation for sialorrhea. *Otolaryngology/Head and Neck Surgery, 105,* 127–129.

Tunkel, D. E., & Zalzal, G. H. (1992). Stridor in infants and children: Ambulatory evaluation and operative diagnosis. *Clinical Pediatrics, 31,* 48–55.

Wilkie, T. F., & Brody, G. S. (1977). The surgical management of drooling: A ten year review. *Plastic and Reconstructive Surgery, 59,* 791–798.

Zalzal, G. H. (1988). Rib cartilage grafts for the treatment of posterior glottic and subglottic stenosis in children. *Annals of Otology, Rhinology, and Laryngology, 97,* 506–511.

Zalzal, G. H. (1989). Stridor and airway compromise. *Pediatric Clinics of North America, 36,* 1389–1402.

Zalzal, G. H., Anon, J. B., & Cotton, R. T. (1987).

Epiglottoplasty for the treatment of laryngomalacia. *Annals of Otology, Rhinology, and Laryngology, 96,* 72–76.

Nutritional Approach to Diagnosis and Management of Pediatric Feeding and Swallowing Disorders

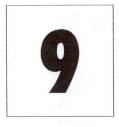

CHAPTER

Kathryn M. Camp, M.S., R.D.
Mary C. Kalscheur, M.S., R.D./L.D.

Infants and children are experts at regulating calorie intake to meet their specific needs for body growth and development (Birch & Deysher, 1986), provided the feeding process is not subject to either external or internal interference (Satter, 1990). Multiple factors can have an impact on normal development so that the acquisition of feeding skills does not proceed in a normal, coordinated manner, and the intrinsic ability to regulate nutrient intake may become disrupted.

Children with feeding and swallowing disorders are at varying degrees of risk for inadequate dietary intake depending, in part, on the extent to which other problems affect their ability to obtain adequate nutrition. Abnormalities in deglutition and feeding may preclude oral feeding or severely reduce the quantity a child can consume orally. These patients are at risk for the development of deficiencies in calories and nutrients, including water and fiber. A large percentage of children with feeding and swallowing disorders have developmental disabilities or chronic illnesses, including neurological, structural,

mechanical, and sensory abnormalities that further exacerbate an already risky situation. Thommessen, Heiberg, Kase, Lansen, and Riis (1991a) and Thommesson, Riis, Kase, Larson, and Heiberg, et al. (1991b) studied 221 developmentally disabled children and found that children with feeding problems, specifically oral-motor dysfunction or those requiring assisted feeding, had a significantly lower energy and nutrient intake and abnormal growth parameters when compared to disabled children without oral motor dysfunction or assisted feeding. Krick and VanDuyn (1984) demonstrated that children with cerebral palsy and oral motor impairment have depressed weight and height for age and depressed weight for height when compared to children with cerebral palsy with no oral motor impairment.

Medical and developmental conditions that can lead to disordered feeding and swallowing with significant implications for nutritional status include:

1. Structural abnormalities of the oral cavity such as cleft lip and palate (Farnan, 1988).

2. Structural abnormalities of the central nervous system such as the Arnold Chiari malformation sometimes seen in children with spina bifida (Putnam et al., 1992).

3. Gastrointestinal disorders such as gastroesophageal reflux (Catto-Smith, Machida, Butzner, Gall, & Scott, 1991), delayed gastric emptying, frequent vomiting, esophagitis, and rumination (Rogers, Stratton, Victor, Kennedy, & Andres, 1992).

4. Prematurity during which time the immature central nervous system is unprepared for sucking. This clinical setting is compounded by the trappings of the technologically dependent premature infant such as ventilator support, nasogastric tube feeding, and repeated medical procedures that may have a negative impact on the acquisition of feeding skills.

5. Chromosomal abnormalities such as Down syndrome, which predisposes infants to low muscle tone and cardiac defects which may lead to fatigue and poor suck (Hull, 1993), and Rett syndrome where progressive neurological deterioration occurs leading to problems with chewing and swallowing (Van Acker, 1991).

6. Static encephalopathy such as cerebral palsy characterized by poor head control and difficulties with sucking, swallowing, and the development of chewing skills (Moffat, 1984).

7. Pulmonary and cardiac problems such as bronchopulmonary dysplasia and congenital heart defects which lead to easy fatigue, poor oxygen saturation, and discomfort on feeding, factors that affect the infant's ability to acquire feeding skills in a normal progression.

Recently, Veldee and Peth (1992) suggested that inability to obtain adequate nutrition may negatively affect swallowing function. They very eloquently argued that, because malnutrition is known to interfere with the function of a variety of muscles with accompanying biochemical alterations within the muscle cells, it may cause or worsen dysphagia. To date, research has not been undertaken to specifically evaluate the impact of malnutrition on the swallowing mechanism. However, clinical experience suggests that identification of children at risk for malnutrition combined with an aggressive approach to repletion in those identified with sub-optimal nutritional status would be prudent.

Feeding and swallowing disorders in the pediatric population require an interdisciplinary approach to assessment and management with carryover beyond the clinic setting due to the complexity of issues and the likelihood that multifactorial sequelae will be encountered. A comprehensive transdisciplinary intervention model, Project SPOON (Tluczek & Sondel, 1991), was developed at the University of Wisconsin Children's Hospital and provides guidelines for intervention that function across all environments and promotes collaboration and coordination of services across multiple disciplines. Additionally, Wodarski (1990a) has described an interdisciplinary nutritional assessment and intervention protocol for children with developmental disabilities with applicability to feeding and swallowing disorders.

Role of the Nutritionist

The nutritionist's role in the assessment and treatment of the pediatric patient with a feeding or swallowing disorder includes assessing nutritional status and providing recommendations for intervention. When working with children with disordered feeding and swallowing, the nutritionist interacts with other team members in a variety of ways. The nutritionist works with the occupational therapist, physical therapist, and speech-language pathologist on issues related to feeding and may be involved in a multidisciplinary feeding assessment. The nutritionist communicates with the physician regarding special nutrient requirements, such as fluid and electrolyte needs, setting energy and protein levels, and aids in the interpretation and significance of biochemical data and other medical issues that affect nutritional status. Coordination with social work and/or nursing personnel is imperative in situations where a family is unable to purchase specialized products or requires additional support in the home to carry out nutritional recommendations. Behavioral issues may affect the child's ability to obtain adequate nourishment, and communication with a psychologist and/or behavior therapist to optimize intake is necessary.

Many children with feeding and swallowing disorders have recognized developmental disabilities. The Individuals with Disabilities Education Act (IDEA) (PL-101-476, 1990, and subsequently amended by PL-102-199, 1991) which expanded PL-94-142 (Education of All Handicapped Children Act of 1975) mandates nutrition services as part of the interdisciplinary program provided for children from birth to 3 years of age who are identified as having developmental disabilities. Providing nutrition services to children with developmental disabilities has long-term benefits including prevention of growth retardation or further disability, improvement of health status, and decrease in medical costs (American Dietetic Association, 1992).

Patient Evaluation

History

A comprehensive history is obtained from chart review and from interviews with the child's parents, caregivers, and perhaps the child. History may include but is not limited to the following areas:

Medical Issues: particularly those related to feeding and swallowing disorders such as history of gastrointestinal and pulmonary problems, frequent fractures, pica (ingestion of non-food items), allergies, recent weight changes, use of prescription and over-the-counter medications, vitamin/mineral or nutritional supplements, previous growth information or measurements, and previous diagnostic swallowing studies;

Early Feeding Experiences: such as oral and nonoral intake and interruptions in feeding due to illness or medical procedures;

Current Appetite and Intake: food preferences, avoidance, and allergies; chewing/swallowing problems, drooling, dentition status, dry mouth, excess saliva, fluid intake, solid intake, texture preference/avoidance;

Eating Patterns: number of meals/snacks, length of time required to complete a meal, fed by others, self-fed, location where meals are eaten, ethnicity of diet, and dietary modification;

Psychosocial Data: occupation, educational level, economic status, religion, living/cooking arrangements, cognitive level, mental status; and

Other Information: age, sex, level of physical activity, and perceived dietary or nutritional problems.

Dietary Assessment

When collecting dietary data, the goal is to estimate the dietary intake to provide specific recommendations so that intake can be improved. The reliability of the information will vary depending on the availability of assessment time, trained personnel, and resources such as diet analysis programs. Obtaining dietary information and translating it into useful information requires use of a validated tool for data collection (e.g., 24-hour recall, food record, food frequency, or combination), translation of recorded information into numerical values for calories and nutrients, comparison of intake to a recognized standard, identification of deviations from standards, and specific recommendations to alter and improve the diet. Techniques used to assess intake in the pediatric population are applicable to the population of children with feeding and swallowing disorders. However, potential difficulties exist when estimating amounts of food and liquid lost during feeding in the child with oral motor dysfunction, assisted feeding, or frequent emesis.

Methods

Twenty-four Hour Recall

A 24-hour recall is a minimal level of dietary assessment in which a nutritionist trained in interviewing techniques asks the child's parents or caregivers to recall the child's exact food intake during the previous 24-hour period. The 24-hour recall does not require extensive work on the part of the parent or caregiver and is the method most commonly used to assess the current intake of children (Eck, Klesges, & Hanson, 1989). It is not considered appropriate for assessing usual food or nutrient intakes in individuals (Gibson, 1990), and its reliability in estimating usual intake in children is questionable (Baranowski, Sprague, Baranowski, & Harrison, 1991; Stein, Shea, Bosch, Contento, & Zybert, 1991.). Greater reliability is attained when multiple recalls are obtained (Treiber et al., 1990), when both parents observe and recall the child's intake together (Eck, Klesges, & Hanson, 1989), or if the parent or primary caregiver acts as informant (Klesges, Klesges, Brown, & Frank, 1987). Children with feeding and swallowing disorders may have multiple caregivers and/or may consume a significant amount of their daily intake outside the home in school and reha-

bilitation settings. On the other hand, parental reporting of food intake may be very accurate in children whose diet is limited due to textural concerns or feeding by gastrostomy tube.

Food Records

Food records require that a parent or caregiver carefully record, at the time of consumption, all foods and beverages eaten for a specified number of days. Details regarding brand names, methods of preparation, portion sizes in household measures or by weight, composite dish ingredients, and so forth, must be recorded. Because food records do not rely on a person's memory, potentially they are more accurate in estimating a child's nutrient intake than dietary recall. Additionally, foods consumed can be recorded for any number of days, thus theoretically providing a better picture of long-term intake. More days are better than fewer days in providing estimates of usual intake for an individual (Guthrie & Crocetti, 1985; Potosky, Block, & Hartman, 1990; St. Jeor, Guthrie, & Jones, 1983). The days chosen to record intake should include weekend days proportionally to account for day-of-the-week effects (Gibson, 1990). However, Larkin, Metzner, and Guire (1991) recently found that random selection of days is preferable when food records are being used to assess the nutrient intake of individuals.

The food record form can be constructed so that information regarding meal timing, meal and snack structure, and food and texture refusal can be obtained in addition to nutrient intake. These data can be invaluable when interpreting dietary data, assessing contributors to inadequate intake, and designing intervention strategies in a neurologically impaired or otherwise handicapped child. They also help the nutritionist identify specific foods and textures that are consistently refused and specific times when appetite is greatest. It is also helpful to record the time and place of consumption because this aids in determining whether a child is fed too often, thus maintaining a depressed appetite, or not often enough. This information will also help to determine whether a child receiving feeding via a gastrostomy is optimally positioned in a feeding environment.

Vitamin and mineral supplements and medications should also be recorded to confirm appropriate supplementation practices and verify that medications are being given as prescribed.

Food Frequencies

Food frequency questionnaires are useful in obtaining descriptive information about food consumption patterns, but they generally do not provide quantitative data on nutrient intake (Gibson, 1990). They may be helpful in combination with a food record for obtaining a more complete picture of usual intake, but they do not substitute for the quantitative information obtained either through a 24-hour recall or a food record.

Evaluating Dietary Information

One method of evaluating dietary data is to determine the nutrient composition of each food in the child's diet record either by hand tabulation or using one of the many computer software programs available. Totals are then compared to the Recommended Dietary Allowances (RDA). Several publications provide nutrient values (Adams, 1988; Gebhardt & Matthews, 1981; Pennington, 1989). Information regarding computer diet analysis systems can be found in articles by Byrd-Bredbenner (1988) and Nieman, Butterworth, Nieman, Lee, and Lee (1992).

In using the RDA as a standard, the practitioner must be aware of its limitations. The RDA is most appropriate for assessing the diets of population groups, not individuals. In addition, the RDA provides guidelines for average amounts to be consumed over time and was designed with a "safety factor" which may exceed the actual requirements of most individuals. Requirements for the RDAs are based on healthy persons, and therefore may not be applicable to individuals with special health and nutritional needs; values may over- or underestimate actual requirements. Often two thirds, or 70 to 75% of the RDA are deemed an appropriate standard of comparison (Cazjka-Narins, 1992a). If intake values are lower than the RDA, nutrient deficiency cannot be assumed but risk of deficiency is possible (National Research Council, 1989).

Biochemical Assessment

Use of biochemical methods to evaluate nutritional status provides a measurable parameter of nutritional status. In cases of malnutrition, biochemical abnormalities often precede actual physical signs or symptoms of malnutrition. Laboratory studies may also be useful in early detection of marginal nutrient deficiencies. However, certain caveats regarding laboratory tests of nutritional status should be kept in mind. First, there is no specific quantifiable value of a biochemical test that clearly distinguishes a deficiency state from a nondeficient one (Krause & Mahan, 1984). Accordingly, standards are usually given as ranges and are somewhat arbitrary. Also the sex and age of the person may affect the level of a nutrient in the body. As a result, multiple ranges of "normal" are given for some nutrients. Levels of nutrients or their metabolites are quite variable and may reflect only recent rather than usual nutrient intake. Results also may be affected by time of day the sample is collected, method of collection, and storage and processing of the sample (Baer, 1976). A biochemical value should be evaluated based on the normal range as stated by the laboratory performing the analysis (Krause & Mahan, 1984).

References such as Grant and DeHoog (1991), Krause and Mahan (1984), and others provide specific information on routine biochemical parameters. Detailed discussion of all the laboratory tests related to nutrition is beyond the scope of this chapter. For a listing of biochemical tests that may be used for evaluation of various nutrients see Czajka-Narins (1992a).

Several tests are especially important to consider for children with developmental disabilities, including:

1. *Major indices of protein status* (serum albumin, transferrin, retinol-binding protein, prealbumin).

2. *Major indices of hematologic status* (hematocrit, hemoglobin, red blood cell indices, and total lymphocyte count) where it is important to be aware that some hemoglobinopathies such as thalassemia minor give CBC results similar to iron deficiency anemia but do not respond to iron therapy. Use of serum ferritin and MCV allows for differentiation in patients with iron deficiency and beta-thalassemia trait. Serum ferritin is diagnostic for iron deficiency anemia because it is not low in any other condition (Wallach, 1986); and levels may be low before anemia or other changes occur.

3. *Vitamin D status* where metabolites must be measured directly because calcium, phosphorus, and alkaline phosphatase may not be useful as indicators of vitamin D deficiency (Lee, Lyne, Kleerekoper, & Logan, 1989). Serum 25-hydroxycholecalciferol (25-OHD) levels can be performed to determine mineral metabolism abnormalities. Elevated levels of parathormone (PTH) are suggestive of possible rickets or osteomalacia due to hypocalcemia. When serum calcium falls below a certain level, PTH increases to promote the transfer of calcium into the blood from the bone and to increase re-

absorption of calcium from the kidney (Czajka-Narins, 1992b).

4. *Zinc status*, particularly if pica is documented or suspected. Danford, Smith, and Huber (1982) found that malabsorption of zinc and iron may be associated with some types of pica. Testing blood lead levels is indicated if the child has a history of pica as lead toxicity has been documented in these children (Kalisz, Ekvall, & Palmer, 1978).

Drug-Nutrient Interactions

Children with feeding and swallowing difficulties frequently receive long-term drug therapy involving medications administered for control of seizures, gastrointestinal disorders, and behavioral problems. It is important to assess drug use, dose, and multiple drug regimens for the possibility of drug-nutrient interactions (Blyler & Lucas, 1987).

There are two categories of interactions between drugs and nutrients. First, drugs may affect the body's intake, absorption, metabolism, and requirements for nutrients. Food intake may be altered through changes in appetite, changes in taste and smell, decreased saliva secretion, gastric irritation, and nausea and vomiting. Second, nutrients in foods or beverages may affect the absorption, metabolism, action, and excretion of the drugs (Mahan & Arlin, 1992). Many excellent references are available dealing with the topic of interactions between drugs and nutrients including books by Roe (1985, 1989), Chapter 21 in Krause and Mahan's (1984) diet therapy book, Appendix 18 in ADA's *Manual of Clinical Dietetics* (1988), and the most current editions of the *Powers and Moore's Food Medication Interactions* (Allen, 1991), the *Nursing Drug Handbook* (Springhouse Corporation, 1989), and the *Physician's Desk Reference* (Medical Economics Data, 1993). In the following section, nutrition-related interactions are presented for the most frequently used categories of drugs in children with feeding and swallowing problems.

Anticonvulsants

Children on anticonvulsant medications are at risk for vitamin D deficiency which may lead to rickets or osteomalacia (Holmes, 1987; Tolman et al., 1975), osteopenia (Lee et al., 1989), and increased tendency to fracture (Hahn, 1976; Holmes, l987; Lee et al., 1989), particularly when therapy is longer than 6 months and in children receiving more than one anticonvulsant medication (Hahn & Avioli, 1984; Pipes & Glass, 1989).

Studies that have looked at possible mechanisms for increased risk of vitamin D deficiency and changes in bone metabolism have demonstrated a decrease in bone mass and serum 25-hydroxycholecalciferol levels (Hahn, 1976). Other factors known to increase the risk of vitamin D deficiency and bone abnormalities, such as inactivity and reduced exposure to sunlight, must also be taken into consideration in children receiving anticonvulsant therapy. Nonambulatory patients on anticonvulsants showed greater radiological evidence of osteopenia compared to ambulatory patients (Hahn & Avioli, 1984). In institutionalized children on anti-seizure medication with infrequent exposure to sunlight, vitamin D production was decreased which in turn increased the risk of bone complications (Lifshitz & Maclaren, 1973). Gough et al. (1986) looked at a variety of factors that affect anticonvulsant osteomalacia including ultra-violet (UV) radiation exposure, diet, and mobility and found that although these factors influenced vitamin D metabolism, anticonvulsants had a more severe effect on bone mineral metabolism. Therefore, in children receiving anticonvulsant therapy, efforts must be made to minimize risk factors that affect vitamin D status and bone metabolism.

Chronic intake of anticonvulsants may lead to deficiencies in other nutrients as well (Roe, 1986). Goggin et al. (1987) found significantly reduced red cell folate levels in adults using phenytoin and carbamazepine alone and in those using more than one anticonvulsant. Evidence of folic acid deficiency was found in 20% of subjects between the ages of 2 and 34 years receiving phenytoin, phenobarbital, carbamazepine, or valproic acid either singly or in combination (Cole et al., 1985). It is important to note that, if folate supplementation is given, vitamin B-12 levels may decrease because increased hematopoiesis increases B-12 requirement (Krause & Mahan, 1984). Therefore, serum vitamin B-12 levels should be measured if a vitamin B-12 deficiency is suspected. In addition, the effectiveness of some anticonvulsants may be decreased by supplements of folic acid, thereby increasing seizure frequency (Pipes & Glass, 1989), hence careful monitoring of serum drug levels is important.

Anticonvulsant therapy may also increase serum iron levels and decrease serum ferritin, total iron binding capacity, and protoporphyrin/heme ratio (Taylor, Kozlowski, Baer, Blyler, & Trahms, 1982). Clinical evidence of cardiac beriberi and subclinical ascorbic acid deficiency has been reported in a child receiving three anticonvulsants (Klein, Florey, Goller, Larese, & VanMeter, 1977).

Biotin may also be compromised in long-term therapy with anticonvulsant drugs. The effects of carbamazepine and primidone in the human intestine were found to be competitive inhibitors of biotin transport (Said, Redha, & Hylander, 1989). Symptoms of biotin deficiency include neurologic disorders, growth retardation, and skin abnormalities.

Use of valproic acid has been associated with secondary carnitine deficiency in children, particularly when valproate is used in conjunction with other anticonvulsant medications (Opala et al., 1991). Carnitine deficiency is also associated with inborn errors of metabolism, dietary deficiency from total parenteral nutrition, soy-based infant formulas, malabsorption, decreased body stores from extreme prematurity or intrauterine growth retardation, and increased urinary losses as in the Fanconi syndrome (Rebouche, 1992). Dietary carnitine helps to maintain tissue stores (Breningstall, 1990). Meat and dairy products are the major source of carnitine in the diet (Broquist, 1988). In children with a feeding or swallowing disorder intake of carnitine-rich foods may be limited due to defined diets and/or textural concerns.

Wodarski (1990b) found that elevated levels of serum cholesterol may be correlated with anticonvulsant use. Forty institutionalized children and adolescents with various developmental disabilities were studied. In eight of the subjects who had an average serum cholesterol higher than 200 mg/dL, high density lipoprotein (HDL) and very low density lipoprotein (VLDL) were the major contributors to the increased total cholesterol, suggesting no increased risk for coronary heart disease.

Sodium and fluid balance may be affected by carbamazepine. Hyponatremia has been reported to occur during carbamazepine use alone (Lahr, 1985; Yassa et al., 1987) or in conjunction with other anticonvulsants, neuroleptics, or diuretics (Kastner, Friedman, & Pond, 1992). The mechanism is unclear but it appears that carbamazepine interferes with function of antidiuretic hormone causing the body to retain fluid. Close monitoring of fluid and electrolyte status is needed in these situations.

Medications Used for Gastrointestinal Disorders

Antacids, which may be used in patients with conditions such as gastroesophageal reflux, cause an increase in gastric pH which may result in decreased absorption of calcium, iron, magnesium and zinc (D'Arcy & McElnay, 1985). An acidic gastric environment is needed for iron to be changed from the ferric to the more easily absorbable ferrous form. Antacids may also bind other minerals preventing their absorption (Murray & Healy, 1991).

Antacids taken in conjunction with drugs may delay absorption due to increased stomach pH which adversely affects dissolution of some drugs (McElnay, Uprichard, & Collier, 1982). Drug absorption may be decreased because the mineral component of the antacid may bind with the drug and form a nonabsorbable complex. In addition, Hurwitz, Robinson, Vats, Whittier, and Herrin (1976) found that the aluminum ion present in many antacids causes a delay in gastric emptying.

Valli, Schalthess, Asper, Escher, and Hacker (1986) reported the formation of an esophageal plug in three patients receiving enteral tube feedings in which antacid was given at the same time. It was theorized that the aluminum salts precipitated the protein; thus, these authors recommended that antacids be given following a feeding and after the tube has been flushed thoroughly with water.

Metoclopramide hydrochloride (Reglan) is often used to prevent or decrease reflux and regurgitation/rumination. It acts by increasing lower esophageal sphincter tone and stimulating motility of the upper GI tract. One of its side effects that may have an impact on nutritional status is tardive dyskinesia which may in turn result in dysphagia. This can be a serious side effect in a population that tends toward oral motor/feeding difficulties. More information on tardive dyskinesia and dysphagia appears in the section on drugs used for behavior problems.

Ranitidine (Zantac®), an H_2-receptor antagonist, may also be used as treatment for infants and children with gastroesophageal reflux. Ranitidine decreases basal and meal stimulated secretion of gastric acid. Nausea, constipation, and decreased absorption of vitamin B-12 during long-term use has been reported (Powers & Moore, 1988). Absorption of ranitidine is compromised by antacids, and dosages should be separated by at least 1 hour (Springhouse Corporation, 1989).

Medications Used for Behavior Problems

In hyperactive children, amphetamines such as dextroamphetamine (Dexedrine) and methylphenidate (Ritalin) may be used to control impulsive behavior and improve attention. These drugs also act on the central nervous system to depress the appetite (Krause & Mahan, 1984). Long-term use may cause growth retardation in children, possibly secondary to drug-induced suppression of appetite (Mattes & Gittelman, 1983; Safer, Allen, & Barr, 1972). Because excess caffeine intake may impede absorption of neuroleptic drugs, thereby decreasing the drug's effect (Smith & Bidlack, 1984), its frequency in the child's diet, via soda and chocolate primarily, should be monitored.

Tranquilizing and antidepressant drugs such as chlorpromazine and lithium carbonate may result in an increase in body weight due to an increase in appetite, food intake, and fluid retention (Levitsky, 1984). Excretion of lithium carbonate can be affected by the body's level of sodium, with serum levels rising due to low sodium intake and increased excretion with sodium supplementation (Krause & Mahan, 1984). Some tranquilizers may cause reduced acuity of the taste sensation (hypogeusia) or abnormal taste sensation (dysgeusia). However, this must be distinguished from zinc deficiency or viral infections, which may also alter the ability to taste.

Some of the psychotropic medications may cause tardive dyskinesia, which is characterized by involuntary movement of the face, mouth, and tongue and has been shown to cause dysphagia (Moss & Green, 1982). Anticholinergics, which are often used in conjunction with neuroleptics, may contribute to dysphagia by impairing the gag reflex (Craig & Richardson, 1982). This can lead to a high risk of aspiration (Weiden & Harrigan, 1986).

Anthropometric Measurements

Anthropometric measurements of body growth and composition are widely used to assess nutritional status and are particularly useful in the pediatric population because they are noninvasive and can be repeated over time. Growth in infants and young children is rapid and follows predictable patterns. Rates of growth have been referenced across age and sex (Hamill et al., 1979; National Center for Health Statistics, 1977), so it is possible to identify deviation from expected values. Anthropometry becomes a functional indicator of nutritional status when serial, longitudinal measures are made (Allen, 1990). Additionally, monitoring growth response following nutritional intervention provides information about the effectiveness of the intervention as well as whether previous intake was adequate (Allen, 1990).

Due to several limitations, however, assessment of growth and body composition using anthropometry should be used in combination with other predictors to assess nutritional status. Anthropometry is a relatively insensitive method and cannot detect short-term changes in nutritional status or identify specific nutrient deficiencies (Gibson, 1990). Furthermore, it cannot be used to determine whether abnormalities seen in growth are due to a specific nutrient deficiency, such as zinc, or from imbalances in protein or energy intake. Sources of error that can further limit the usefulness of anthropometry arise from examiner and instrument error and measurement difficulties (Gibson, 1990). These errors can be minimized with the use of trained personnel and repeated measures, using validated techniques, and ensuring that instruments are correctly calibrated.

Measuring growth in children with neurological or other developmental disorders associated with impaired feeding and swallowing can pose a challenge to the health care provider. Most reference data are derived from populations of children without disabilities, and their applicability to a population of children with neurological or other handicapping conditions is questionable. Measurement data must be collected in the same way as reference data that is being used for comparison (Hamill et al., 1979). However, in the population of children with feeding and swallowing disorders, this is not always possible. For example, a nonambulatory, 6-year-old child with cerebral palsy may require linear rather than standing measurement to monitor height. There are situations where a child may not achieve expected growth compared to a normal population but may be growing well given limitations resulting from their disability. These situations must be recognized and interpretation of growth data adjusted accordingly. Growth charts are available for some of these conditions, such as prematurity and low birth weight (Babson & Benda, 1976; Gairdner & Pearson, 1971), Down syndrome (Cronk, Crocker, Pueschel, Shea, Zackal, Pickens, et al., 1988; Ershow, 1986), Turner syndrome (Lyon, Preece, & Grant, 1985), skeletal dysplasias (Horton, Hall, Scott, Pyeritz, & Rimoin, 1982), and Prader Willi syndrome (Butler & Meaney, 1991).

Length and Height

Recumbent length is measured for children younger than 24 months and for children between 24 and 36 months who cannot stand unsupported or are too short to plot on 2- to 18-year-old growth charts. These children should be measured on a length board. Laying the child on an examination table and marking the paper at the head and foot, although commonly done in clinical settings, is not an acceptable method of measuring, particularly in a child

at risk for growth problems, because it greatly increases the measurement error. When positioning the child, avoid stimulating the plantar reflexes. These reflexes may be strong in young infants and children with neurological damage (Roche, 1979) and, if triggered, will make it difficult to maintain the foot flat against the footboard.

Children between 2 and 3 years of age can be measured either recumbent or in the standing position, depending on the child's postural control and ability to cooperate. It must be noted in the record, however, which method is used because recumbent length can be greater than stature by up to 2 centimeters in the youngest children and around 1 centimeter in children 4 to 5 years and older (Hamill et al., 1979). If there is concern about growth in a child at age 2, continued measurement of recumbent length plotted on the birth to 36-month growth chart would be appropriate for continuity up to age 3 years (Moore & Roche, 1987).

Children over 2 years of age who are able to stand independently are measured without shoes and in undergarments in a standing position using a stadiometer or portable anthropometer. With hypotonic or other neurologically impaired children, two people may be required to successfully complete a height measurement. It may be necessary to hold the child's ankles against the wall and stabilize the trunk by gently putting pressure on the chest. Note any circumstances that compromise reliability of the measurement in the record.

Special Anthropometric Techniques for Assessing Stature

Traditional anthropometric measurements are not always appropriate for children who are unable to stand and/or have joint contractures or scoliosis. Various methods for estimating height in a child with contractures who cannot straighten her body or stand appear in the literature. They include recumbent length, crown-rump length, sitting height, arm length, tibia length, arm span, knee height, and even photometric height estimation. These methods will be described and indications for their use will be discussed.

Recumbent Length

For a child over 3 years who is unable to stand, a recumbent length can be measured if a long enough length board is available. This measurement also requires two people, and its accuracy is decreased if the child has scoliosis or leg contractures. If the child is unable to lay flat due to contractures or scoliosis, a flexible tape measure can be used to obtain an estimated height. Beginning at the crown of the head, follow the spine down the back, around the hip to the back of the knee and down the leg to the heel. When scoliosis is present, measure the side opposite the scoliosis, and where there is a leg length discrepancy, use the longer side. If the measurement cannot be completed in one sequence, sections can be measured and totaled for an estimation of height. Although this method can be used in clinical practice to obtain serial measurements for monitoring growth when other methods are inappropriate, data validating this method as an accurate measurement for height are not available.

Crown-Rump Length

This method may be useful for children who are unable to stand or sit and for those with severe contractures of the legs. A length board is used with two people assisting to obtain the measurement. One person holds the child's head in place against the fixed headpiece. The legs are raised and held in position so that the thighs are at a 90° angle to the board. The reading is taken after the sliding footboard is brought up against the buttocks with firm pressure (Figure 9–1). Several readings are taken for accuracy (should be within ⅛ inch or 0.2 cm of each other) and then averaged together (Feucht, 1989; Roche, 1979. This measure-

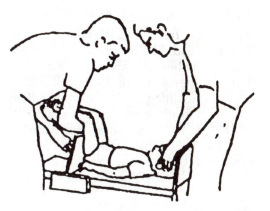

FIGURE 9–1. Crown-rump measurement (Adapted from Feucht [1989] with permission).

ment may be negatively affected by scoliosis or hip dislocation.

Sitting Height

Sitting height may be useful for a child who has severely deformed legs but is able to sit erect. For this measurement, a regular wall-mounted stadiometer can be fitted with a sitting base that slides into place in front of the stadiometer (see Figure 9–2). The buttocks, shoulders and head are in contact with the backboard while the child sits as straight as possible on the base. The

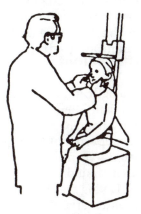

FIGURE 9–2. Sitting height measurement (Adapted from Feucht [1989] with permission).

hands should be resting on the thighs, the legs hanging freely, and the knees pointed straight ahead. The headboard is brought down to the head for measurement in the same manner as when doing a standing height. The sitting surface height is then subtracted from the reading to estimate sitting height. Reference charts are available for sitting height and crown-rump length; however, they are based on a British population (Tanner & Whitehouse, 1978).

Arm Span

Measurement of arm span may be used for individuals who are unable to sit or stand such as children with cerebral palsy or myelomeningocele (spina bifida). This measurement is taken from the tip of the middle finger of the right hand across the back to the tip of the middle finger of the left hand. The arms are in full extension and the measurement is done with a straight rod that has numbers etched on it. "There is an immobile tab at one end and a sliding tab at the other for the middle finger tips to touch (similar to an adjustable curtain rod)" (Brizee, 1988) (Figure 9–3). If this measurement tool is unavailable, the child can stand against a wall with arms outstretched and parallel to the floor. The middle finger of one hand rests against a right angle (in a corner) and a mark is made at the end of the middle finger of the other hand. The distance between these two points can then be measured with a steel tape (D. Sobel, personal communication). If necessary, this

measurement could also be performed with the child lying supine on the floor. Two people are required to properly position the child and perform the measurement. Measurement of arm span is not accurate in children with scoliosis or arm contractures.

In individuals with myelomeningocele, short stature is common especially for those with the highest spinal cord lesions (Rosenblum, Finegold, & Charney, 1983). In this patient population, arm span may be a more useful measure than length in evaluating linear growth. Arm span measurements were reported to be easier to obtain than measurements of length because children did not have to undress or remove orthopedic appliances.

In normal children, arm span has been found to correlate directly with stature on a 1:1 ratio (Feucht, 1989). According to Brizee (1988), after some adjustments, it can be used in place of height on the NCHS growth grids for children with decreased leg muscle mass due to spina bifida. The adjustments are as follows:

height (cm) =

0.9 × arm span for no leg muscle mass (high lumbar and thoracic level defects)

0.95 × arm span for partial loss of leg muscle mass (mid and low lumbar level defects)

1.0 × arm span for minimal or no loss of leg muscle mass (sacral level defects)

The estimated height obtained from the arm span may not be appropriate to use for determining energy needs or evaluating weight for height employing this calculation for body mass index (BMI). (For information on BMI, see Gibson, 1990; for reference data for children 6 years and older, see Must, Dallal, and Dietz, 1991.) If the disability causes short stature but does not affect growth of the arms, then arm span would be an indication of potential rather than current height. However, arm span measurement may be sequentially plotted over time to demonstrate growth.

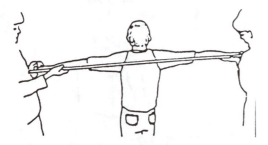

FIGURE 9–3. Arm-span measurement (Adapted from Brizee [1988] with permission).

Measures of Arm and Leg Segments

Various limb segment measures have been proposed for use in children with contractures or musculoskeletal deformities who are unable to stand or sit erect (Feucht, 1989). Segments such as the arms and legs have been used to indicate growth. These measuring techniques are relatively new, and for measurements to be accurate and meaningful, training to identify the specified landmarks is very important. In some cases special measuring equipment such as an anthropometer or sliding calipers is also necessary.

Spender et al. (1989) found that both upper-arm and lower-leg lengths were valid estimators of recumbent length or height of normal children. The smoothed 5th, 50th, and 95th percentile charts developed by these investigators may be used to assess linear growth in children with cerebral palsy, ages 3 to 18 years. An anthropometer must be used to measure upper-arm length, whereas lower-leg length can be measured using either a steel or plastic tape measure or an anthropometer (Figure 9–4).

Arm Length

Although arm span has been used in children with spina bifida (Brizee, 1988), Belt-Niedbala, Ekvall, Cook, Oppenheimer, and Wessell (1986) found that arm length was a more accurate indicator of growth in this population. A high spinal lesion may affect the width of the shoulders in an arm-span measurement, whereas arm growth does not appear to be affected in patients with myelomeningocele. In contrast to arm span measurement, accurate measurement of arm length may be obtained by one person rather than two. In addition, arm length can be measured while the child is recumbent or seated.

Upper-arm length has also been used to monitor growth. The upper arm is measured with a flexible tape while the child is standing, if possible with the arm hanging

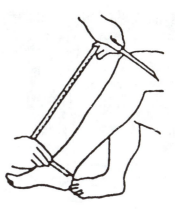

FIGURE 9-4. Lower leg length with anthropometer (Adapted from Feucht [1989] with permission).

at the side and with a 90° flexion at the elbow. Measure from the acromion process to the radialis. The length in centimeters can then multiplied by a factor to determine height (Belt-Niedbala et al., 1986) or the measurement directly plotted on growth charts recently developed by White and Ekvall (1993) based on normal children aged 2 to 18 years.

Knee Height

Measurement of knee height has been used primarily in the elderly, but recently this parameter has been applied to young adults with disabilities (Johnson & Ferrara, 1991). With the subject seated or in a supine position, sliding calipers are used to measure knee height on the left leg (Figure 9–5). The ankle and knee are each flexed in a 90° angle and the distance from the sole of the foot to the anterior surface of the thigh is the knee height. As described by Chumlea (1985):

> One blade of a sliding, broad-blade caliper is placed under the left heel, and the other blade is placed over the anterior surface of the left thigh above the condyles of the femur and just proximal to the patella. The shaft of the caliper is held parallel to the shaft of the tibia and pressure is applied to compress the tissues (p. 88).

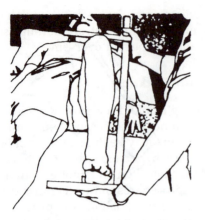

FIGURE 9–5. Knee height measurement
(Courtesy of Ross Laboratories).

Chumlea (1985) stated that knee height studied in an elderly population was more highly correlated with stature than length measurements of the ulna, thigh, tibia, or total arm length. However, knee height could not be accurately measured if the individual has leg or foot contractures that do not allow the 90° angle required.

The equations available for the estimation of stature from knee height reflect normal patterns of growth and development developed from the 1960–1970 National Health Examination Surveys of healthy individuals (Johnson & Ferrara, 1991). In determining whether these equations are applicable for persons with cerebral palsy, Johnson and Ferrara (1991) found reasonable accuracy for women over age 18 and only in men over age 18 without lower extremity cerebral palsy (LECP). Knee height did not predict stature accurately in women or men under age 18 or in men over 18 with LECP involvement. White and Ekvall (1993) have developed charts for assessing growth in normal children using knee height. However, there is still a need for validation of the knee height measurement in children with neurological impairment and physical disabilities.

Tibia Length

Tibia length was measured in 177 normal children aged 12–14 years and regression equations for determining height were ob-

tained by Zorab, Prime, and Harrison (1963). The equations are as follows:

> *Boys:*
> height (cm) = [2.92 × tibial length (cm)] + 49.84
>
> *Girls:*
> height (cm) = [2.53 × tibial length (cm)] + 67.22.

Gleason, Trahms, Okamota, and Worthington-Roberts (1983) found that, in a population of boys with Duchenne muscular dystrophy, stature estimated from arm span and tibial length correlated with actual height in the 6- to 9-year-olds. In ages 9–12 years and 12–17 years, estimated stature appeared to parallel normative curves for growth.

Photometric Height

Smith and Gines (1989) conducted a feasibility study for estimating height by using photographs of able-bodied persons seated in wheelchairs. Comparison of height estimation techniques included standing height, recumbent length, knee height, and photometric limb measurements. Standing height correlated significantly with recumbent length, knee height, and computed height based on the photograph measurements. The disadvantages of this method include the length of time necessary to obtain the measurement, the need for photographic equipment, and lack of validation in the pediatric population.

Weight

Infants and young children are weighed without clothes or diapers lying recumbent on a pan-type pediatric scale that is accurate to within 10 grams (Moore & Roche, 1987). Weight is plotted on the birth to 36 month chart.

Older children who can stand are weighed without shoes, in light undergarments using a beam-balance scale. Weight is plotted on the weight chart for children ages 2 to 18 years. Children with cerebral palsy and spina bifida may have braces which need to be removed prior to weighing.

Chair scales, table scales, wheelchair scales, and bed sling scales are available for measuring nonambulatory children and can be obtained through medical equipment supply companies or companies that specialize in scales.

Head Circumference

Head circumference is routinely measured and used as an indicator of brain growth in infants and young children (Morgan, 1990). Head circumference should be measured routinely in infants and children until they are 36 months of age (Moore & Roche, 1987). Reference data are available for children from birth to 18 years (Nellhaus, 1968). Malnutrition can adversely affect fetal and postnatal brain growth but so can a myriad of other insults and/or combined insults such as exposure to toxins.

Body Composition

Measuring body composition is a useful and important tool for assessing nutritional status. Acute episodes of malnutrition can be determined by indirect measurements of body fat, because fat is the main storage form of energy in the body. Consequently, changes in body fat content provide indirect evidence of changes in energy balance (Gibson, 1990). Lean body mass, which is composed largely of protein, can also be measured indirectly, providing information about body protein reserves which become depleted during chronic undernutrition (Gibson, 1990). Body composition can be assessed in a variety of ways. The reader is referred to Gibson (1990) for an overview of methods. Several of these methods have been described for use in a population of ill children (Pencharz, Vaisman, Azcue, & Stallings, 1990) and infants (Nichols, Sheng, & Ellis, 1990). The two methods most commonly encountered in clinical practice to assess body composition are measurements of arm circumference and skinfold thickness. These techniques are simple to perform, have been validated in

the pediatric population, require relatively inexpensive equipment, are non-invasive, and can be repeated over time.

Skinfold Thickness

Obtaining skinfold measurements in children with neurological and neuromuscular disorders may be difficult if the child is particularly hypersensitive to touch. These children have often undergone a variety of medical procedures and are fearful and anxious during examinations and procedures. Calipers are a strange looking device, and great care and sensitivity must be employed to obtain accurate measurements without causing the child undue stress. Depending on the child's cognitive level and temperament, it may be helpful to demonstrate the device by gently allowing the caliper jaws to close on the child's finger or a parent's arm. This also can heighten the child's anxiety, however; and a judgment must be made whether to attempt to do the measurements quickly and without demonstration.

Skinfold thickness is used to estimate the size of subcutaneous fat stores using calipers that measure the compressed double fold of fat plus skin. Various sites are used, and there is large variability depending on body weight, sex, race, and age (Robson, Bozin, & Soderstrom, 1971). In children with atrophied extremities, arm measurements generally can be done effectively using the least atrophied extremity. Triceps and subscapular skinfolds are most often used in children because reference data are available from the National Health and Nutrition Examination Survey I (1971–1975) (National Center for Health Statistics, 1981). Additionally, triceps and subscapular skinfold equations to estimate body fatness in children have been published (Slaughter et al., 1988). Using measurements of biceps and supra-iliac skinfolds, body fat may be calculated from equations validated by Weststrate and Deurenberg (1989).

Limited reference data are available for children with neurological or other handicapping conditions, and the importance of body fat in relation to particular disease states is unknown (Gibson, 1990). Recently, however, efforts have focused on assessing body composition in children with chronic illnesses and handicapping conditions (Thomas et al., 1990). Butler and Meaney (1991) have reported standards for triceps and subscapular skinfolds for Prader-Willi syndrome.

Although measurement of triceps skinfold appears to be a suitable assessment of body fat in children (Gibson, 1990), subscapular measurement will also provide an estimate of truncal fat stores. This information may be particularly important in the neurologically impaired population due to potential differences in body fat distribution and atrophied extremities. Body fat has been shown to be greater in children with myelomeningocele (Shepard, Roberts, Golding, Thomas, & Shapard, 1991) and in children with Prader-Willi syndrome (Butler & Meaney, 1991). In children with atrophied extremities, arm measurements can generally be done effectively using the least atrophied extremity.

Mid-Upper Arm Circumference and Mid-Arm Muscle Area

Mid-upper arm circumference and mid-arm muscle circumference can be used to estimate changes in body fat and muscle which are indirect indicators of energy and protein reserves (Frisancho, 1974). Mid-upper arm circumference is used in combination with the triceps skinfold to estimate arm muscle area and arm fat area. Reference data for infants and children are available from Frisancho (1981) for mid-upper arm circumference, arm muscle circumference, arm-muscle area, and arm fat area.

Interpretation of Anthropometric Measurements

Interpretation of growth data in children with feeding and swallowing disorders depends to a large extent on the underlying etiology of the disorder, the severity of oral-motor dysfunction, and the presence of other factors that impact on growth. Hamill et al. (1979) defined normal growth as generally represented by measurements of height and weight for age that plot between the 10th and 25th percentiles. Measurements between the 10th and 25th and the 75th and 90th percentiles may or may not be normal, depending on the pattern of serial measurements. Genetic abnormalities, handicapping conditions, chronic illness, or treatment may limit growth (Roche, 1979); therefore, when interpreting growth parameters in the population of children with feeding and swallowing disorders, it may be necessary to use specialized growth charts. Where available and applicable, it may also be necessary to adjust measurements for gestational age in premature infants, adjust for parental heights when one or both parents are tall or short, document previous growth data to recognize deviations (serial measurements), and utilize weight for height graphs.

When special measurement techniques are used, limitations in interpretation must be realized. Most of these techniques do not have standards or curves against which points can be plotted and compared. However, these techniques may be appropriate for serial measurements and for monitoring change over time as long as methods of measurement remain consistent. To this end, the method used should be clearly documented in the record.

Growth Curves

Growth curves available from the National Center for Health Statistics/Center for Disease Control (Hamill et al., 1979; National Center for Health Statistics, 1977) are considered adequate for monitoring growth in the normal pediatric population but may not as be useful for assessing growth in children with chronic disorders that affect growth attainment (Dibley, Goldsby, Staehling, & Trowbridge, 1987). The World Health Organization has recommended using the standard deviation score (Z-score) because it can be used for children in whom growth parameters fall outside of percentile ranges (Waterlow et al., 1977). The Z-score expresses the measured value in relation to the median reference value in standard deviation units, where Z = actual anthropometric value − median reference value/standard deviation (Dibley et al., 1987). This method has been used successfully in the population of developmentally delayed children to monitor changes in growth (Krick, 1986).

Crossing growth channels may be viewed as requiring intervention but according to Hamill et al. (1979), crossing percentiles with advancing age within the 25th and 75th percentiles is probably normal unless the relative deviation is progressively upward or downward before pubescence. A simultaneous decrease or increase in rate of height and weight gain indicates a normal growth pattern (Feucht, 1989). A change in rate of weight gain is usually the presenting sign of over- or undernutrition with effects on height seen in more chronic situations.

Weight for Height

Plotting weight for height can be an important tool in determining nutritional status because it gives an indication of whether weight is appropriate for a given length or height. Weight for height is a sensitive index of current nutritional status (Gibson, 1990) and can be used to differentiate between nutritional stunting, where weight may be appropriate for height, and wasting, where weight is low in relation to height (Gibson, 1990). Weight for height curves apply only to prepubescent children because during puberty marked changes in body proportions occur that are not measured and accounted for in the reference population (Hamill, et. al., 1979). During puberty, weight for stature is no longer independent of age (Gibson, 1990). Therefore, a child entering puberty should not be plotted on the weight for stature charts (Hamill, et al., 1979). Weight for height ratio tables are available for adolescents ages 12 to 17 years (National Center for Health Statistics, 1973).

In children with feeding and swallowing disorders, plotting weight for height is particularly important when the underlying etiology is known to be associated with abnormal body weight. In the older child with spina bifida, Down syndrome, or Prader-Willi syndrome, weight for age may fall within the 25th to 50th percentile but when plotted against height, may fall between the 90 to 95th percentile or above, suggesting that the child is obese.

In children with cerebral palsy, a weight for height ratio between the 10th and 25th percentile may be appropriate (Lucas, 1989) and is considered by some clinicians to reflect adequate nutriture in this population (Shapiro, Green, Krick, Allen, & Capute, 1986). In situations where under- or overnutrition is suspected based on weight for height measurements, skinfold measurements and upper arm circumference will provide an estimation of body fatness and muscle protein reserves. In children with cerebral palsy, Patrick, Boland, Stoski, and Murnay (1986) suggested that because there are no appropriate standards for weight to length ratio, measurement of skinfolds will identify children with deficient subcutaneous fat reserves.

Protein-Energy Malnutrition

Protein-energy malnutrition (PEM) can be classified based on anthropometric data. Although PEM is not commonly seen in ambulatory pediatric practices in the United States, it is a recognized condition in hospitalized children and in children with chronic disease (MacLean, 1987). Various criteria and classification methods for assessing the degree of malnutrition are available and include the Gomez Criteria (Gomez, 1956), Waterlow Classification (Waterlow, 1976), and the method of McLaren and Read (1972).

Physical Signs of Nutritional Status

Important clues about the macronutrient and micronutrient status of the child can be obtained from the physical examination. These clues must be interpreted carefully because they may not be specific for nutrient deficiency but rather caused by disease, medication use, or other environmental factors. Clinical signs of deficiency or malnutrition do not usually appear until there has been prolonged deprivation (Ross Laboratories, 1989). Clinical information should be used in conjunction with other information about body composition, biochemical status, and dietary intake. Clinical signs of possible nutritional significance can be found in Krause and Mahan (1984) and Ross Laboratories, (1989).

Dental Concerns

A dental examination is important for the child with feeding and swallowing difficulties. Problems with the gingiva and teeth may be caused by medications (especially phenytoin and carbamazepine), overreliance on soft foods, and poor oral hygiene resulting from hypersensitivity (Baer, 1976). Poor dentition and oral hygiene can affect the child's ability to consume adequate nutrients. Additionally, severely impaired chewing ability can result from misaligned jaws and teeth. Teeth that are abnormally developed may have increased susceptibility to decay. Bruxism, which is frequently seen in children with neurological impairment, involves clenching and grinding of the teeth. This may cause jaw pain and the teeth to become loose, misaligned, and eroded making it difficult to eat chewy foods (McKinney, Palmer, Dwyer, & Garcia, 1991a).

Gingival overgrowth occurs in approximately 50% of individuals receiving phenytoin on a long-term basis (Hughes, 1980). Excess gum tissue may trap food debris and delay eruption of permanent teeth (McKinney et al., 1991a). Surgical removal of the gingiva is sometimes needed, and good oral hygiene is essential in preventing infection and tooth decay. If food reinforcers are needed to help modify behavior, foods that stimulate the gums such as raw fruits and vegetables should be chosen over sweet, sticky snacks.

Carbamazepine may cause xerostomia (dry mouth) which is a reduction or absence of saliva (McKinney, Palmer, Dwyer, & Garcia, 1991b). Saliva helps to lubricate the oral tissues and inhibits both bacterial activity and adhesion to teeth and gums (McKinney et al., 1991a). Without saliva, chewing and swallowing become difficult, and there is an increased susceptibility to dental caries and other oral infections.

Baby Bottle Tooth Decay (BBTD), a disease seen primarily in children under 2 years of age, is characterized by rampant caries (Johnsen & Nowjack-Raymer, 1989). One of the contributing factors is putting the child to bed with a bottle containing sweetened liquids (juice, soft drink, or sugar water) or milk. BBTD may be an issue for children with feeding and swallowing problems due to the increased time needed to finish a feeding, feeding in a reclined position, frequent feedings, and prolonged use of a bottle.

Feeding Evaluation

An observational feeding evaluation can be conducted by the nutritionist in conjunction with a speech pathologist, physical therapist, or occupational therapist to assess diet and texture adequacy, oral motor skills, positioning during feeding/eating, and need for adaptive equipment for eating or self-feeding. This information will be the basis for the formulation of a comprehensive treatment plan and may suggest areas where goals can be implemented.

Observation of the feeding process as well as the foods eaten is equally important. The child's behavior and the interaction and communication with his parents around mealtimes provide a complete picture along with subtle information that would not be available from an interview (Baer, 1976; Satter, 1990).

Nutritional Therapy

Estimating Calorie and Nutrient Needs

Total energy expenditure is the sum of energy expended at rest, in physical activity, and through thermogenesis (National Research Council, 1989). Several factors affect energy expenditure and must be taken into account when estimating energy needs. They are age, sex, body size and composition, genetics, physiologic state, coexisting pathological conditions, and ambient temperature (National Research Council, 1989).

Estimating calorie, nutrient, and fluid needs of children with feeding and swallowing disorders depends on the child's nutritional status and degree of under- or overnutrition, level of activity, and any underlying medical condition that may dictate specific increases or restrictions in calories and nutrients.

Calorie needs can be estimated in several ways. Using the Recommended Dietary Allowance (RDA) for weight and age alone will overestimate calories in a child who is overweight and may not provide sufficient calories for catch-up growth in a child who is stunted or underweight for height. Kilocalories per centimeter of height is a useful criteria to base estimated needs in a child whose physical growth deviates from the norm (Pipes & Glass, 1989). Table 9–1 lists these values. Using several methods and providing a range within which calorie needs are expected to fall is more useful than providing a single level based on weight alone.

Children with feeding and swallowing disorders requiring nutritional rehabilitation may have energy and protein needs in excess of normal to achieve catch-up growth. One method of calculating catch-up growth requirements utilizes ideal body weight and provides a margin for catch-up growth (Peterson, Washington, & Rathbun,

TABLE 9–1. Estimating calorie needs for children based on weight and height.

Child's Age in Years	Weight (Kcal/kg)	Height (Kcal/cm)
0.0–0.5	108	10.8
0.5–1.0	98	12.0
1–3	102	14.4
4–6	90	16.1
7–10	70	15.2
Male		
11–14	55	16.0
15–18	45	17.0
Female		
11–14	47	14.0
15–18	40	14.0

Source: Adapted from National Research Council (1989). *Recommended dietary allowances* (10th ed.). Washington, DC: National Academy Press.

1984) in a child whose weight for height is less than the 10th percentile (Table 9–2). For children with cerebral palsy, Shaddix (1991) has provided guidelines for Kcal/cm height depending on degree of involvement (Table 9–3). A child with mild cerebral palsy is an independent walker; moderate involvement defines a child who can walk with support or crawls; while severe involvement is a non-ambulatory child (Russman & Gage, 1989). Athetoid refers to involuntary, purposeless movements of the limbs (Shaddix, 1991) which increases calories irrespective of ambulatory status.

Estimating basal energy needs and adding a factor for activity level and existing stress factors can be accomplished using several methods depending on the age of the child. Correction factors for modifying standard methods have been published which take into account level of physical activity and disease state. (See National Research Council, 1989, and Boston Children's Hospital, 1987, for correction factors.)

Increasing Calories

In children identified as being underweight, high calorie, nutrient dense foods should

TABLE 9–2. Methods for calculating calorie needs for catch-up growth.

Method	Protocol
Boston Children's Hospital Method (Peterson, Washington, & Rathburn, 1984)	1. Plot height and weight on NCHS growth charts.
	2. Determine at what age present weight would be 50th percentile. This is the weight age.
	3. Determine ideal weight (50th percentile for present age).
	4. Multiply recommended calories for weight age (see Table 9–1) × ideal weight. Divide by actual weight to determine predicted kcal/kg for catch-up growth.
	$$\frac{(\text{kcal/kg for weight age}) \times (\text{ideal weight in kilograms})}{\text{actual weight in kilograms}}$$
Method of MacLean, de Romana, & Masse (1980)	1. Using the weight for height growth chart, determine the 50th percentile weight for actual height. This is the ideal body weight.
	2. Multiply 120 kcal × the ideal body weight. Divide by actual weight to obtain kcal/kg for catch-up growth.
	$$\frac{(120 \text{ kcal/kg}) \times (\text{ideal body weight for actual height})}{\text{actual weight (kg)}}$$

Source: From Peterson, Washington, & Rathburn. (1984). Team management of failure to thrive. *Journal of the American Dietetic Association, 84*(7), p. 814, used with permission.

TABLE 9–3. Estimating calorie needs based on height and degree of involvement.

Involvement	Calorie Needs (kcal/cm height)
Mild-Moderate	13.9
Severe	11.1
Athetoid	13.9*

*Plus kcal for energy expenditure

Source: From Shaddix, T. E. (1991). Nutritional implications in children with cerebral palsy. *Nutrition Focus, 6*(2), p. 2, used with permission.

be provided. The volume of food will need to be slowly increased as tolerance to larger quantities is achieved. Texture level must be appropriate for the child's level of oral motor function and self-feeding skills.

In the infant, formulas can be concentrated to provide up to 30 calories per ounce. Formula modification may increase protein intake and renal solute load. This alteration can lead to dehydration if sufficient fluid (free-water) is not provided. The hydration status of the infant should be closely monitored when using highly concentrated formulas. Concentrating the formula by adding less water generally can be achieved safely up to 26 calories per ounce without providing excessive protein. Further calories should be added as carbohydrate (e.g., glucose polymers, Polycose) and/or fat (MCT oil or a liquid vegetable oil). In children where aspiration is a concern, oil should not be added to formula because it may be aspirated and result in a lipoid pneumonia. Oil can be safely added to solid foods.

In children over 1 year of age, a high calorie beverage can be provided for nutritional supplementation. Commercial products offer a distinct advantage for the gastrostomy-tube fed child because they are convenient, provide complete nutrition, and have a low risk of contamination. Children with PEM receiving an enteral formula for 8 to 35 days demonstrated weight gain and an increase in serum proteins (Morales et al. 1991). Most children receiving nutrition via the oral route will accept an enteral formula such as PediaSure®, or any other formula or beverage change, when it is gradually introduced by mixing with the current formula and slowly increasing the concentration until full strength is achieved. This method will also improve tolerance to the new product. Many enteral formulas are expensive and may be beyond the financial means of some families. Most are available for eligible children through the Women Infants and Children (WIC) program. Alternatives to enteral formulas include "shakes" with such products as Carnation Instant Breakfast, fruit, dry baby cereal, and oil. These thicker beverages may be easier for the child with impaired swallowing to handle. Wheat germ, nonfat dry milk powder, cooked eggs, cream cheese, cream, and full fat yogurt will add additional calories and nutrients to food.

In the overweight child, provision of a variety of low calorie, nutritious foods in regularly timed meals and snacks should be stressed. Exercise and activity should be encouraged. For nonambulatory or physically handicapped children, consultation with the occupational therapist or speech-language pathologist will be required to design a specific program for individual children to ensure that exercise and activity are undertaken safely.

Meal Patterning

Meal patterning includes the feeding/eating environment as well as the foods offered to the child. Eating difficulties may make mealtime unpleasant and, therefore, discourage adequate intake. The environment can be structured, however, to minimize discomfort and focus on the positive aspects of eating.

A comfortable, quiet setting with minimal distractions should be provided to focus attention on eating and decrease the risk of choking. This may mean turning off the television or radio and minimizing interruptions during the meal so full attention can be given to eating. Special positioning may be required to facilitate safe oral intake.

A specific area should be designated for eating so the child learns that she is to eat when in this area. When possible the child should sit at the dinner table with the rest of the family to learn acceptable mealtime behavior and social skills. Eating should not take place while the child is running around the house or sitting in front of the television. For a child who is difficult to feed, a trained consistent person should do the feeding so the child does not have to continually adjust and adapt to different feeding styles.

Meals and snacks should be offered at regular and consistent intervals to take advantage of the child's hunger. Lowenberg (1989) pointed out that a good appetite is promoted by serving meals at the same time each day. A schedule that is compatible with the family routine will probably work best, keeping in mind that if young children are fatigued, they usually do not eat well. An example of a feeding schedule is breakfast at 7 a.m., lunch at 12 noon, and dinner at 5 p.m., with between meal snacks at approximately 9:30 a.m., 2:30 p.m., and before bed. Young children may need to eat small amounts of food more frequently, but meal and snack times should be scheduled at least 2 hours apart so the child will develop an appetite.

Allow a reasonable amount of time for the child to complete the meal without rushing and then end the meal. Give positive reinforcement for desirable behavior and praise the child's successes. In learning self-feeding skills, encourage as much independence as the child is capable of. Use of small, manageable, and unbreakable utensils or adaptive equipment may foster progress. The dishes should be unbreakable and not tip over easily; glasses or cups should be easy to hold (Pipes, 1992).

Young children learn about their environment by touching, smelling, and tasting. Where food is involved this exploration may become messy so be prepared by covering the floor, using a bib, or whatever it takes so the child has the opportunity to make mistakes as he or she learns. For a child with motor problems, achieving independent self-feeding skills and the associated feeling of accomplishment and pride are more important than neatness. Independence may also result in weight gain and improved nutritional status despite some spillage (Hull & Kidwell, 1988).

Parents should not make eating or not eating an issue with the child, and the child should not be forced to eat. Children quickly learn that they can control their parents by accepting or rejecting food (Pipes & Glass, 1989). If attention is given to the child's refusal to eat, he or she learns that this is a way of attaining parental attention. Mealtime and eating should be positive experiences not a battle. In a study of normal preschool children 26 to 62 months of age who were presented with wholesome food, daily energy intake was relatively constant although consumption was highly variable from meal to meal (Birch, Johnson, Andresen, Peters, & Schulte, 1991). It is not unusual for 2- to 6-year-old children to have a variable appetite or go on "food jags." A food jag is defined as wanting to eat the same food at every meal or refusal to eat previously accepted foods (Lucas, 1992). If the refusal escalates so that a whole category of foods or a texture level is rejected, consultation with a dietary and oral motor specialist would be indicated.

Young children generally prefer simple, uncomplicated foods (Lowenberg, 1989). Because they tend to eat small amounts frequently, both snacks and meals must be nutritious as they will be contributing nutrients as well as calories for energy. It is better to offer small rather than large portions. This makes it easier for the child to accomplish the goal of eating everything and then asking for second helpings if still hungry.

Attention should be given to the way new foods are offered to young children. When an unfamiliar food is presented for the first time, the child may refuse to eat it. If this occurs, it is best not to pressure the child to eat it, but to offer the food again at another time. As the child becomes familiar with the new food, she will probably decide to try it. Another strategy is to offer a very small portion of a new food along with a favored food or to offer the new food when the child is hungriest. Involve the child in choosing food for the meal and/or in the preparation of the food when possible.

When a child is unable to eat enough food to supply the calories and nutrients required for maintenance and growth, a nasogastric or gastrostomy tube may be recommended. If the child is able to safely eat a small amount by mouth, this should be encouraged to provide oral stimulation for the continued development of oral motor skills (Pipes & Glass, 1989). In gastrostomy fed children, a correlation with successful transition to oral feeding was found when some oral intake was maintained (Isaacs, 1991). To ensure adequate intake, continuous feeds could be given at night with oral feeding during the day.

Bolus Modification

Texture

Once the decision has been made to proceed with oral feeding, the optimal texture of the food must be determined. Texture involves both viscosity and consistency of the food item. Viscosity refers to the "thickness" or "thinness" of the material (Coster & Schwarz, 1987). Thick items include cooked cereal, milkshakes, pudding, and mashed potatoes. Thin items include water, juices, and pureed canned fruit. Consistency refers to how smooth or coarse the texture is. Examples of food with smooth consistency are yogurt, pudding, infant cereals, and strips of cooked vegetables; tapioca pudding, crackers, meats, and rice are foods with coarse texture.

Textures should be gradually increased in a progressive manner as the child moves from sucking liquids to consumption of pureed foods and on to table foods (Feucht, 1988). See Table 9–4 for texture levels of foods commonly consumed. Keeping the child on strained or pureed foods for too

TABLE 9–4. Increasing texture levels within groups of foods.

	Milk		**Cereals**
Fine	Fresh milk	Fine	Infant cereals
↓	Yogurt	↓	Instant hot cereals
	Soft ice cream		Cold cereal soaked in milk
	Milk pudding		Add raisins to cereal
	Custard, tapioca		Finger foods (i.e., graham crackers,
Coarse	Cheddar cheese chunks	Coarse	cheerios, dry toast)

	Vegetables		**Finger Foods**
Fine	Mashed table vegetables: potatoes, cooked carrots, peas (These can be mashed with a fork.)	Fine	Strips of cooked vegetables (i.e., green beans, carrots, broccoli)
↓		↓	French fries
	Coarsely chopped (diced) table vegetables (baked or boiled potatoes, carrots, beets, baked beans, etc.)		Banana slices
			Cheese slices
			Cookies, crackers
Coarse	Raw tomatoes, carrots, celery, lettuce		Cheetos
			Soft breadsticks or toast
			Meat sticks (chopped)
		Coarse	Pretzels (thin sticks)

	Fruits
Fine	Pureed or strained
↓	Small pieces of soft, fresh fruit — peaches, pears, oranges (You may choose to mash at first.)
	Small pieces of peeled raw, ripe fruit — apples, oranges, grapefruit
	Dried prunes, apricots, raisins may be cut up and cooked
	Finger fruits — peeled apple sections, halves of oranges or pears. As the child becomes
Coarse	more proficient, the skins may be left on.

	Eggs and Meat
Fine	Eggs, soft, poached, scrambled, hard poached
↓	Hard poached — mash with fork
	Hard boiled — mashed and gradually leave more lumps
	Finely ground meat — hamburger, tuna, turkey, chicken
	Tender meat or chicken bits
	Ground meat patties may be given to suck and chew
Coarse	Tender bits of steak

	Snack Foods		**Starches**
Fine	Peanut butter	Fine	Pasta
↓	Marshmallows	↓	Macaroni
	Cheetos (soft ones)	Coarse	Rice
	Crackers		
	Pop Tarts		
Coarse	Cookies		

Source: From Linden, J., Burch, J., & Cross, K. A. (1991, May). School and hospital collaboration on nutritional services to malnourished children with multiple handicaps. Workshop presented at AAMR Annual Meeting, Washington, DC.

long will increase the chance of resistance to textured foods when they are introduced. The child may refuse to eat or eat only small amounts which may not meet his nutritional requirement.

As members of the interdisciplinary team, the child's occupational and/or speech therapist should be involved in determining readiness skills for increased texture. Shaddix and Barnacastle (1986) have developed some guidelines for the progression of food textures. The selection of foods appropriate for each stage of oral motor development are listed in Table 9–5.

TABLE 9–5. Guidelines for the progression of food textures.

Level 1: Pureed Foods

- Avoid the use of commercially prepared strained (baby) foods. The taste difference will make the transition to table foods more difficult.
- Puree regular table foods to the consistency of strained foods by using a household blender. Allow several weeks for the child to adapt to the change in taste.
- Progress to Level 2 when the child displays a predominant sucking action during feeding, but cannot move food to the sides of the mouth using the tongue.

Level 2: Thickened Pureed Foods

- Thicken pureed foods in order to facilitate certain tongue and jaw movements which are unnecessary to ingest thinner foods. Nutritious thickeners include mashed potatoe flakes, wheat germ, bread crumbs, or dry baby cereals. Thicker pureed foods may also be produced by using less blender action.
- Include other nutritious foods such as oatmeal or cream of wheat, mashed potatoes, mashed banana, applesauce, or yogurt.
- Progress to Level 3 when the child begins to display vertical (up and down) chewing.

Level 3: Ground Foods

- Grind regular table foods by using a small baby food grinder, or a food chopper, both of which may be purchased at most deprtment stores. A household food processor may be used for grinding larger quantities of food.
- Include ground meats with broth or gravy, ground or mashed cooked vegetables and fruits, scrambled egg, mashed soft-boiled egg, egg salad, cottage cheese, pimento cheese, or prepared meat salads.
- Offer foods designed to stimulate biting and chewing such as toasted bread strips or crusts, dried fruits, cheese strips, cooked vegetable pieces, and strips of meat. Note that the child may have difficulty with raisins, grapes, or meats which require shearing and tearing.
- Progress to Level 4 when the child begins to move foods from side to side by using the tongue.

Level 4: Chopped Foods

- Obtain textures for this stage by chopping meats, fruits, and vegetables into small bite-size pieces by using a knife rather than the blender, food processor, or baby food grinder. Meats, fruits, and vegetables would be cut into bite-size pieces.
- Include chopped meats and casseroles, chopped cooked vegetables, chopped fruits, grilled cheese or chopped meat sandwiches, and finely chopped slaw or salad.
- Progress to Level 5 when the child has a mature rotary chew and freely moves food from side to side in the mouth. However, some children with dysphagia may never progress to this advanced level.

Level 5: Coarsely Chopped Foods

- Include small pieces of chopped meats, crispy fruits and vegetables, coarsely chopped salad and slaw, and cornbread.

Source: From Shaddix, T., & Barnacastle, N. (1986). *Nutritional care for the child with developmental disabilities — Oral motor development and feeding techniques.* Birmingham, AL: United Cerebral Palsy of Greater Birmingham.

The consistency of liquids offered is also important in oral motor development. A large amount of liquid may be lost during feeding, placing the child at risk for dehydration or inadequate nutrient intake. Thicker liquids may be easier for a child to handle than thinner ones. The thicker, heavier liquids may provide greater tactile stimulation and also pass more slowly from the mouth to the throat allowing more time to swallow (Feucht, 1988). Progression of liquids begins with those easiest to handle and progresses to the most difficult as oral motor skills improve. Guidelines have been presented by Shaddix and Barnacastle (1986) (see Table 9–6).

Thickeners

Foods and/or liquids may need to be thickened during the progression of oral motor skills to ensure adequate intake and decrease the risk of aspiration. Thickened liquids may be needed temporarily, for example, in the case of a child with Down syndrome who has delayed feeding skills. Thickeners will help in the transition to a more mature feeding level. However, significantly abnormal oral motor patterns, as seen in a child with cerebral palsy, may require thickened foods and beverages for an indefinite time. Patients diagnosed with neurogenic oropharyngeal dysphagia, which is usually the case in children with cerebral palsy, typically have more difficulties with liquids and a tendency to aspirate (Horner & Massey, 1991).

Various commercial products are available to use as thickeners. Starch-based thickeners are metabolized as a carbohydrate, and 98% of the water is released. Gum-based products bind water, and because gums are not digestible by the body, this water is unavailable (representative from Milani Foods, personal communication). Some of the products also supply various amounts of calories and added nutrients. The water and calorie needs of the child should be considered when choosing which product to use. Dried infant foods can also be used as a thickener, but less water is available because the dried product requires fluid to be reconstituted. Thickening with protein foods such as yogurt requires more fluid for digestion than carbohydrate foods such as cereal (Feucht, 1988). Another consideration when using infant cereals as a thickener is the total daily iron intake of the child. Because most cereals are fortified with iron, there is a possibility of iron excess depending on how much cereal is used for thickening in addition to the child's iron intake from the rest of the diet and supplements.

Stanek, Hensley, and Van Riper (1992) studied 13 frequently used thickening agents to determine amounts needed for thickening, cost, effect on volume, and effect on energy and nutrient intake. Several commercial products and a variety of common foods were used. Commercial agents were found to be the best thickeners to achieve low and medium viscosity for three test liquids (water, apple juice, and milk) whereas baby rice

TABLE 9–6. Comparative difficulties of liquids from easiest to most difficult.

Level 1: Heavy, Milky Liquids

- Milk thickened with baby cereal, blenderized fruit or yogurt
- Milkshakes
- Cooked cereals thinned with milk, such as oatmeal, cream of wheat, etc.

Level 2: Heavy, Clear Liquids

- Fruit blended in own juice
- Blended fruit drinks, such as fruit slush and sherbets

Level 3: Thin, Milky Liquids

- Milk
- Cream soup (thinned)

Level 4: Thin, Clear Liquids

- Water
- Bouillon/broth
- Fruit juices
- Soft drinks
- Tea

Source: From Shaddix, T., & Barnacastle, N. (1986). *Nutritional care for the child with developmental disabilities — Oral motor development and feeding techniques.* Birmingham, AL: United Cerebral Palsy of Greater Birmingham.

cereal was best at the high viscosity level. Baby cereal was also the least expensive and baby apple flakes the most expensive.

Adequate fluid intake is a concern when thickeners are used because they may bind part of the fluid making it unavailable to hydrate the body. For a child who has difficulty swallowing liquids or routinely consumes thickened beverages, assessment of fluid needs versus intake is important to prevent dehydration. Additionally, water needs are increased when losses are greater than usual such as during episodes of fever, vomiting or diarrhea, and for excessive drooling.

Adaptive Equipment

Improvement in self-feeding skills has been associated with the improvement in nutritional status (Hull & Kidwell, 1988). To enhance safe swallowing and promote the acquisition of independent feeding skills, specially adapted eating utensils and special positioning techniques may be necessary. Occupational therapy is the discipline that usually assesses which pieces of equipment would enhance the feeding process for a specific individual, and occupational therapists may also provide various techniques needed for the child to learn self-feeding skills. Evaluation of the child for proper positioning or for specialized seating equipment during meals is carried out by the physical therapist.

Spoons are available with a variety of modifications to facilitate independent feeding. They may have built-up or angled handles of various sizes and textures to facilitate grasp. Various bowl sizes are available which may be coated with nylon or plastic to prevent damage where bite reflex is a problem. A rocker or roller knife with a curved blade allows for one-handed cutting. If grasp on a utensil cannot be maintained, a universal cuff, which is a strap that fits over the hand and has a pocket to hold the eating utensil, may be used.

Plates come in various sizes with high sides or a combination of high and low sides or lipped edges to aid in maneuvering the food onto the eating utensil. Plate guards are available that can be clamped onto regular dinner plates. Suction cups or nonslip mats called dycem, anchor the plate and keep it from sliding around.

Glasses are available in different diameters, with or without handles, with rounded bottoms to prevent tipping or wide bases for stability and to encourage returning the glass upright rather than on its side. Spouted tops or covers minimize spillage and allow more control for independent drinking or in directing liquids to one side of the mouth if the child is fed.

In addition to eating utensils, adaptive equipment related to proper positioning is also important for success in the feeding environment. Proper positioning will minimize the effect of abnormal muscle reflexes and facilitate swallowing, prevent aspiration of food, and allow for socialization (Poleman & Peckenpaugh, 1991). Positioning equipment may include a lap tray, footrest, harness for trunk support, and so forth. If the child must eat in bed, wedges and pillows may be used to support her in an upright position.

Proper positioning for eating includes head and trunk as upright as possible, feet adequately supported, hips and knees flexed to approximate a 90° angle, head tipped slightly forward, and arms centered close to the body and resting comfortably on the lap (Poleman & Peckenpaugh, 1991). When the child's positioning is secure, she can focus all her energy on safely ingesting food or on learning how to feed herself.

References

Adams, C. F. (1988). *Nutritive value of American foods* (Handbook No. 456). Washington, DC: Agricultural Research Service, United States Department of Agriculture.

Allen, A. M. (1991). *Powers and Moore's Food Medication Interactions* (7th ed.). Tempe, AZ: Ann Moore Allen.

Allen, L. H. (1990). Functional indicators and outcomes of undernutrition. *Journal of Nutrition, 120,* 924–932.

American Dietetic Association. (1988). *Manual of clinical dietetics.* Chicago, IL: American Dietetic Association.

American Dietetic Association. (1992). Position of the American Dietetic Association: Nutrition in comprehensive program planning for persons with developmental disabilities. *Journal of the American Dietetic Association, 92*(5), 613–615.

Babson, S. G., & Benda, G. I. (1976). Growth graphs for the clinical assessment of infants of varying gestational age. *Journal of Pediatrics, 89*(5), 814–820.

Baer, M. T. (1976). Nutrition. In R. B. Johnston & P. R. Magrab (Eds.), *Developmental disorders: Assessment, treatment and education* (pp. 315–340). Baltimore: University Park Press.

Baranowski, T., Sprague, D., Baranowski, J. H., & Harrison, J. A. (1991). Accuracy of maternal dietary recall for preschool children. *Journal of the American Dietetic Association, 91,* 669–674.

Belt-Niedbala, B. J., Ekvall, S., Cook, C. M., Oppenheimer, S., & Wessel, J. (1986). Linear growth measurement: A comparison of single arm lengths and armspans. *Developmental Medicine and Child Neurology, 28*(3), 319–324.

Birch, L. L., & Deysher, M. (1986). Caloric compensation and sensory specific satiety: Evidence for self-regulation of food intake by young children. *Appetite, 7,* 323–331.

Birch, L. L., Johnson, S. L., Andresen, G., Peters, J. C., & Schulte, M. C. (1991). The variability of young children's energy intake. *New England Journal of Medicine, 324*(4), 232–235.

Blyler, E., & Lucas, B. (1987). Nutrition in comprehensive program planning for persons with developmental disabilities: Technical support paper. *Journal of the American Dietetic Association, 87*(8), 1069–1074.

Boston Children's Hospital. (1987). *Pediatric nutrition handbook.* Available from Department of Nutrition and Food Service, The Children's Hospital, 300 Longwood Avenue, Boston, MA.

Breningstall, G. N. (1990). Carnitine deficiency syndromes. *Pediatric Neurology, 6*(2), 75–81.

Brizee, L. (1988). Nutrition concerns associated with spina bifida. *Nutrition News, 3*(4), 1–4.

Broquist, H. P. (1988). "Vitamin-like" molecules, carnitine. In M. E. Shils & V. R. Young (Eds.), *Modern nutrition in health and disease* (pp. 453–458). Philadelphia: Lea & Febiger.

Butler, M. G. & Meaney, F. J. (1991). Standards for selected anthropometric measurements in Prader-Willi syndrome. *Pediatrics, 88*(4), 853–860.

Byrd-Bredbenner, C. (1988). Computer nutrient analysis software packages: Considerations for selection. *Nutrition Today, 23,* 13–21.

Catto-Smith, A. G., Machida, H., Butzner, J. D., Gall, D. G., & Scott, R. B. (1991). The role of gastroesophageal reflux in pediatric dysphagia. *Journal of Pediatric Gastroenterology and Nutrition, 12,* 159–165.

Chumlea, W. C., (1985). Methods of assessing body composition in nonambulatory persons. In *Body composition assessments in youth and adults, 6th Ross Conference* (pp. 86–90). Columbus, OH: Ross Laboratories.

Cole, H. S., Lopez, R., Epel, R., Singh, B. K., & Cooperman, J. M. (1985). Nutritional deficiencies in institutionalized mentally retarded and physically disabled individuals. *American Journal of Mental Deficiency, 89*(5), 552–555.

Coster, S. T., & Schwarz, W. H. (1987). Rheology and the swallow-safe bolus. *Dysphagia, 1*(3), 113–118.

Craig, T. J., & Richardson, M. A. (1982). Swallowing, tardive dyskinesia, and anticholinergics. *American Journal of Psychiatry, 139*(7), 1083.

Cronk, C., Crocker, A. C., Pueschel, S. M., Shea, A. M., Zackal, E., Pickens, G., & Reen, R. B. (1988). Growth charts for children with Down syndrome: 1 month to 18 years of age. *Pediatrics, 81*(1), 102–110.

Czajka-Narins, D. M. (1992a). The assessment of nutritional status. In L. K. Mahan and M. T. Arlin (Eds.), *Krause's food, nutrition, and diet therapy* (8th ed., pp. 293–313). Philadelphia: W. B. Saunders.

Czajka-Narins, D. M. (1992b). Minerals. In L. K. Mahan & M. T. Arlin (Eds), *Krause's food, nutrition, and diet therapy* (8th ed., pp 110–114). Philadelphia: W. B. Saunders.

Danford, D. E., Smith, J. C., Jr., & Huber, A. M. (1982). Pica and mineral status in the mentally retarded. *American Journal of Clinical Nutrition, 35*(5), 958–967.

D'Arcy, P. F., & McElnay, J. C. (1985). Drug interactions in the gut involving metal ions. *Reviews on Drug Metabolism and Drug Interactions, 5*(2/3), 83–108.

Dibley, M. J., Goldsby, J. B., Staehling, N. W., & Trowbridge, F. L. (1987). Development of normalized curves for the international growth reference: Historical and technical considerations. *American Journal of Clinical Nutrition, 46,* 736–748.

Eck, L. H., Klesges, R. C., & Hanson, C. L. (1989). Recall of a child's intake from one meal: Are parents accurate? *Journal of the American Dietetic Association, 89,* 784–789.

Education of All Handicapped Children Act of 1975. P.L. No. 94-142, 89 STAT. 773 (codified as amended at 20 USC secs. 1410, 1405, 1406, 1411–1420 [1982]).

Ershow, A. G. (1986). Growth in black and white children with Down syndrome. *American Journal of Mental Deficiency, 90*(5), 507–512.

Farnan, S. (1988). Nutrition and feeding of children with cleft lip/palate. *Nutrition News, 3*(2), 1–4.

Feucht, S. (1988). Guidelines for the use of thickening agents in foods and liquids. *Nutrition News, 3*(6), 1–5.

Feucht, S. (1989). Assessment of growth. *Nutrition Focus, 4*(6), 1–8, 10.

Frisancho, A. R. (1974). Triceps skin fold and upper arm muscle size norms for assessment of nutritional status. *American Journal of Clinical Nutrition, 27,* 1052–1058.

Frisancho, A. R. (1990). *Anthropometric Standards for the Assessment of Growth and Nutritional Status* (pp. 47–52). Ann Arbor: The University of Michigan Press.

Gairdner, D., & Pearson, J. (1971). A growth chart for premature and other infants. *Archives of Disease in Childhood, 46,* 783–787.

Gebhardt, S. E., & Matthews, R. H. (1981). *Nutritive value of foods* (Home and Garden Bulletin No. 72) Washington, DC: Human Nutrition Information Service, United States Department of Agriculture.

Gibson, R. S. (1990). *Principles of nutritional Assessment,* New York: Oxford University Press.

Gleason, C. S., Trahms, C. M., Okamota, G., & Worthington-Roberts, B. S. (1983). Nutritional assessment in boys with physical deformities: Stature estimation. *Federation Proceedings, 42*(4), 1044.

Goggin, T., Geough, H., Biosessar, A., Crowley, M., Baker, M., & Callaghan, N. (1987). A comparative study of the relative effects of anticonvulsant drugs and dietary folate on the red cell folate status of patients with epilepsy. *Quarterly Journal of Medicine, 65* (247), 911–919.

Gough, H., Bissesar, H., Goggin, T., Higgins, D., Baker, M., Crowley, M., & Callaghan, N.

(1986). Factors associated with the biochemical changes in vitamin D and calcium metabolism in institutionalized patients with epilepsy. *Irish Journal of Medical Science, 155* (6), 181–189.

Gomez, F., Galvan, R. R., & Frenk, S. (1956). Mortality in second and third degree malnutrition. *Journal of Tropical Pediatrics, 2,* 77.

Grant, A., & DeHoog, S. (1991) *Nutritional assessment and support* (4th ed., pp. 99–152). Seattle, WA: Grant & DeHoog.

Guthrie, H. A., & Crocetti, A. F. (1985) Variability of nutrient intake over a three-day period. *Journal of the American Dietetic Association, 85*(3), 325–327.

Hahn, T. J. (1976). Bone complications in anticonvulsants. *Drugs, 12,* 201–211.

Hahn, T. J., & Avioli, L. V. (1984). Anticonvulsant-drug-induced mineral disorders. In D. A. Roe & T. C. Campbell (Eds.), *Drugs and nutrients — The interactive effects* (pp. 409–427). New York: Marcel Dekker.

Hamill, P. V. V., Drizd, T. A., Johnson, C. L., Reed, R. B., Roche, A. F., & Moore, W. M. (1979) Physical growth: National Center for Health Statistics percentiles. *American Journal of Clinical Nutrition, 32,* 607–629.

Holmes, G. L. (1987). *Diagnosis and management of seizures in children* (p. 87). Philadelphia: W. B. Saunders.

Horner, J., & Massey, E. W. (1991). Managing dysphagia: Special problems in patients with neurologic disease. *Postgraduate Medicine, 89*(5), 202–213.

Horton, W. A., Hall, J. G., Scott, C. I., Pyeritz, R. E., & Rimoin, D. L. (1982). Growth curves for height for diastrophic dysplasia, spondyloepiphyseal dysplasia congenital, and pseudoachrondroplasia. *American Journal of Diseases of Children, 136*(4), 316–319.

Hughes, J. R. (1980). Epilepsy: A medical overview. In B. P. Herman (Ed.), *A multidisciplinary handbook of epilepsy.* Springfield, IL: Charles C. Thomas.

Hull, A. (1993). Children with chronic congenital heart disease and renal disease. In S. Ekval (Ed.), *Pediatric nutrition in chronic disease and developmental disorders* (pp. 279–287). New York: Oxford Press.

Hull, M. A., & Kidwell, J., (1988). Feeding skills and weight gain in institutionalized adults with severe handicaps. *Developmental Disabilities and Psychiatric Disorders Newsletter, 7*(2), 6–8.

Hurwitz, A., Robinson, R. G., Vats, T. S., Whittier, F. C., & Herrin, W. F. (1976). Effects of antacids on gastric emptying. *Gastroenterology, 71*(2), 268–273.

Individuals with Disabilities Education Act. P.L. No. 101-476, 104 STAT. 1103 (1990) (codified as amended at 20 U.S.C. secs. 1400–1485).

Individuals with Disabilities Education Act Amendments of 1991. P.L. No. 102-119, 105 STAT. 587 (1991) (codified as amended at 20 U.S.C. secs. 1400–1485).

Isaacs, J. S. (1991). Assessment of neurologically impaired children fed by gastrostomy. *Journal of the American Dietetic Association Supplement, 91*(9), A-45.

Johnsen, D., & Nowjack-Raymer, R. (1989). Baby bottle tooth decay (BBTD): Issues, assessment, and an opportunity for the nutritionist. *Journal of the American Dietetic Association, 89*(8), 1112–1116.

Johnson, R. K., & Ferrara, M. S. (1991). Estimating stature from knee height for persons with cerebral palsy: an evaluation of estimation equations. *Journal of the American Dietetic Association, 91*(10), 1283–1284.

Kalisz, K., Ekvall, S., & Palmer, S. (1978). Pica and lead intoxication. In S. Palmer & S. Ekvall (Eds.), *Pediatric nutrition in developmental disorders* (pp. 150–155). Springfield, IL: Charles C. Thomas.

Kastner, T., Friedman, D. L., & Pond, W. S. (1992). Carbomazepine-induced hyponatremia in patients with mental retardation. *American Journal on Mental Retardation, 96*(5), 536–540.

Klein, G. L., Florey, J. B., Goller, V. L., Larese, R. J., & Van Meter, Q. L. (1977). Multiple vitamin deficiencies in association with chronic anticonvulsant therapy. *Pediatrics, 60* (5), 767.

Klesges, R. C., Klesges, L. M., Brown, G., & Frank, G. C. (1987). Validation of the 24-hour dietary recall in preschool children. *Journal of the American Dietetic Association, 87*(10), 1383–1385.

Krause, M. V., & Mahan, L. K. (1984). *Food, nutrition, and diet therapy* (7th ed., pp. 200–203). Philadelphia: W. B. Saunders.

Krick, J., & VanDuyn, M. A. F. (1984). The relationship between oral-motor involvement and growth: A pilot study in a pediatric population with cerebral palsy. *Journal of the American Dietetic Association, 84*(5), 555–559.

Krick, J. (1986). Using the Z score as a descriptor of discrete changes in growth. *Nutritional Support Services, 8*(8), 14–21.

Lahr, M. B. (1985). Hyponatremia during carbamazepine therapy. *Clinical Pharmacology and Therapeutics, 37*(6), 693–696.

Larkin, F. A., Metzner, H. L., & Guire, K. E. (1991). Comparison of three consecutive-day and three random-day records of dietary intake. *Journal of the American Dietetic Association, 91*, 1538–1542.

Lee, J. J. K., Lyne, E. D., Kleerekoper M., Logan, M. S., & Belfi, R. A. (1989). Disorders of bone metabolism in severely handicapped children and young adults. *Clinical Orthopaedics and Related Research, 245*, 297–302.

Levitsky, D. A. (1984). Drugs, appetites and body weight. In D. A. Roe and T. C. Campbell (Eds.), *Drugs and nutrients — The interactive effects* (pp. 375–408). New York: Marcel Dekker.

Lifshitz, F., & Maclaren, N. K. (1973). Vitamin D-dependent rickets in institutionalized mentally retarded children receiving long-term-anticonvulsant therapy: 1. A survey of 288 patients. *Journal of Pediatrics, 83*(4), 612–620.

Linden, J., Burch, J., & Cross, K. A. (1991, May). School and hospital collaboration on nutritional services to malnourished children with multiple handicaps. Workshop presented at AAMR Annual Meeting, Washington, DC.

Lowenberg, M. E. (1989). Development of food patterns in young children. In P. L. Pipes (Ed.), *Nutrition in infancy and childhood* (4th ed., pp. 143–159). St. Louis, MO: Times Mirror/Mosby.

Lucas, B. (1989). Failure-to-thrive: The child with developmental disabilities. *Nutrition News, 4*(2), 1–5.

Lucas, B. (1992). Nutrition in childhood. In L. K. Mahan & M. T. Arlin (Eds.), *Krause's food, nutrition, and diet therapy* (8th ed., pp. 217–231). Philadelphia: W. B. Saunders.

Lyon, A. J., Preece, M. A., & Grant, D. B. (1985). Growth curve for girls with Turner syndrome. *Archives of Disease in Childhood, 60*, 932–935.

MacLean, W. C., de Romana, G. L., & Masse, E. (1980). Nutritional management of chronic diarrhea and malnutrition. *Journal of Pediatrics, 97*(2), 316–323.

MacLean, W. C. (.987). Protein-energy malnutrition. In R. I. Grand, J. L. Stuphen, W. H. Dietz (Eds.), *Pediatric nutrition, theory and practice* (pp. 421–431). Stoneham, MA: Butterworth Publishers.

Mahan, L. K., & Arlin, M. (1992). Interactions between drugs and nutrients. In L. K. Mahan & M. T. Arlin (Eds.), *Krause's food, nutrition and diet therapy* (8th ed., pp. 431–440). Philadelphia: W. B. Saunders.

Mattes, J. A., & Gittelman, R. (1983). Growth of hyperactive children on maintenance regimen of methylphenidate. *Archives of General Psychiatry, 40*(3), 317–321.

McElnay, J. C., Uprichard, G., & Collier, P. S. (1982). The effect of activated dimethicone and a proprietary antacid preparation containing the agent on this absorption of phenytocin. *British Journal of Clinical Pharmacology, 13*(4), 501–505.

McKinney, L. A., Palmer, C. A., Dwyer, J. T., & Garcia, R. (1991a). Common dentally related nutrition concerns of children with special needs: Part 1. *Topics in Clinical Nutrition, 6*(2), 70–75.

McKinney, L. A., Palmer, C. A., Dwyer, J. T., & Garcia, R. (1991b). Managing dentally related nutrition concerns of children with special needs: Part 2. *Topics in Clinical Nutrition, 6*(2), 76–85.

Medical Economics Data. (1993). *Physicians' desk reference* (47th ed.). Montvale, NJ: Medical Economics Data Production Company.

Moffat, V. (1984). In G. T. McCarthy et. al. (Eds.), *The physically handicapped child* (pp. 133–137). London: Faber & Faber.

Moore, W. M., & Roche, A. F. (1987). *Pediatric anthropometry* (3rd ed.). Columbus, OH: Ross Laboratories.

Morales, E., Craig, L. D., & MacLean, W. C. (1991). Dietary management of malnourished children with a new enteral feeding. *Journal of the American Dietetic Association, 91*(10), 1233–1238.

Morgan, B. L. G. (1990). Nutrition and Brain Development. In S. M. Pueschel & J. A. Mulick (Eds.), *Prevention of developmental disabilities* (pp. 261–286). Baltimore: Paul H. Brookes.

Moss, H. B., & Green, A. (1982). Neuroleptic-associated dysphagia confirmed by esophageal manometry. *American Journal of Psychiatry, 139*(4), 515–516.

Murray, J. J., & Healy, M. D. (1991). Drug-mineral interactions: A new responsibility for the hospital dietitian. *Journal of the American Dietetic Association, 91*(1), 66–70, 73.

Must, A., Dallal, G., & Dietz, W. H. (1991). Reference data for obesity: 85th and 95th percentiles of body mass index (wt/ht^2) and triceps skinfold thickness. *American Journal of Clinical Nutrition, 53*, 839–846.

National Center for Health Statistics. (1973). Height and weight of youths 12 to 17 years United States (Series 11, No. 124, DHEW Publication No. 73-1606). Washington, DC: Government Printing Office.

National Center for Health Statistics. (1977). Growth curves for children birth–18 years (Series 11, No. 16, DHEW Publication No. 78-1650). Washington, DC: Government Printing Office.

National Center for Health Statistics. (1981) Anthropometric measurements 1–74 years (DHHS Publication No. PHS81-16690. Washington, DC: Government Printing Office.

National Research Council. (1989). *Recommended dietary allowances* (10th ed.). Washington, DC: National Academy Press.

Nellhaus, G. (1968). Head circumference from birth to 18 years. *Pediatrics, 41*(1, Part 1), 106–114.

Nichols, B. L., Sheng, H., & Ellis, K. J. (1990). Infant body composition measurements as an assessment of nutritional status. In S. Yasumura, J. E. Harrison, K. G. McNeill, A. D. Woodhead, & F. A. Dilmanian (Eds.), *Advances in in vivo body composition studies* (pp. 1–14). New York: Plenum Press.

Nieman, D. C., Butterworth, D. E., Nieman, C. N., Lee, K. E., & Lee, R. D. (1992). Comparison of six microcomputer dietary analysis systems with the USDA nutrient data base for standard reference. *Journal of the American Dietetic Association, 92*(1), 48–56.

Opala, G., Winter, S., Vance, C., Vance, H., Hutchison, H. T., & Linn, L. S. (1991). The effect of valproic acid on plasma carnitine levels. *American Journal of Diseases of Children, 145*, 999–1001.

Patrick, J., Boland, M., Stoski, D., & Murray, G. E. (1986). Rapid correction of wasting in children with ceberal palsy. *Developmental Medicine and Child Neurology, 28*(6), 734–739.

Pencharz, P. B., Vaisman, N., Azcue, M., & Stallings, V.A. (1990). Body compartment changes in sick children. In S. Yasumura, J. E. Harrison, K. G. McNeill, A. D. Woodhead, & F. A. Dilmanian (Eds.), *Advances in in vivo body composition studies* (pp. 31–38). New York: Plenum Press.

Pennington, J. A. (1989). *Bowes and Church's food values of portions commonly used* (15th ed.). Philadelphia: J. B. Lippincott.

Peterson, K., Washington, J. S., & Rathburn, J. (1984). Team management of failure-to-thrive. *Journal of the American Dietetic Association, 84*(7), 810–815.

Pipes, P. L. (1992). Nutrition in infancy. In L. K. Mahan & M. T. Arlin (Eds.), *Krause's food, nutrition, and diet therapy* (8th ed. pp. 177–192). Philadelphia: W. B. Saunders.

Pipes, P. L., & Glass, R. P. (1989). Nutrition and feeding of children with developmental delays and related problems. In P. L. Pipes, *Nutrition in infancy and childhood* (4th ed., pp. 361–386). St. Louis, MO: Times Mirror/Mosby.

Poleman, C. M., & Peckenpaugh, N. J., (1991). *Nutrition essentials and diet therapy* (6th ed., pp. 375–397). Philadelphia: W.B. Saunders.

Potosky, A. L., Block, G., & Hartman, A. M. (1990). The apparent validity of diet questionnaires is influenced by number of diet-record days used for comparison. *Journal of the American Dietetic Association, 90,* 810–813.

Putnam, P. E., Orenstein, S. R., Pang, D., Pollack, I. F., Proujansky, R., & Kocoshis, S. A. (1992). Cricopharyngeal dysfunction associated with Chiari malformations. *Pediatrics, 89*(5/1), 871–876.

Rebouche, C. J. (1992). Carnitine function and requirements during the life cycle. *The FASEB Journal, 6*(15), 3379–3386.

Robson, J. R. K., Bazin, M., & Soderstrom, R. (1971). Ethnic differences in skin-fold thickness. *American Journal of Clinical Nutrition, 24,* 864–868.

Roche, A. F. (1979). Growth assessment of handicapped children. *Dietetic Currents, 6*(5), 25–30.

Roche, A. F., Guo, S., & Moore, W. M. (1989). Weight and recumbent length from 1 to 12 mo of age: Reference data for 1-mo increments. *American Journal of Clinical Nutrition, 49,* 599–607.

Rogers, B., Stratton, P., Victor, J., Kennedy, B., & Andres, M. (1992). Chronic regurgitation among persons with mental retardation: A need for combined medical and interdisciplinary strategies. *American Journal of Mental Retardation, 96*(5), 522–527.

Roe, D. A. (1985). Drug-induced nutritional deficiencies (2nd ed., pp. 153–172, 249–259). Westport, CT: AVI Publishing.

Roe, D. A. (1989). *Diet and drug interactions.* New York: Van Nostrand Reinhold.

Rosenblum, M. F., Finegold, D. N., & Charney, E. B. (1983). Assessment of stature of children with myelomeningocele and usefulness of armspan measurement. *Developmental Medicine and Child Neurology, 25*(3), 338–342.

Ross Laboratories. (1989). *Nutritional assessment: What is it? How is it used?*, G593. Columbus, OH: Ross Laboratories.

Russman, B. S., & Gage, J. R. (1989). Cerebral palsy. *Current Problems in Pediatrics, 29*(2), 70–111.

Safer, D. J., Allan, R. P., & Barr, E. (1972). Depression of growth in hyperactive children on stimulant drugs. *New England Journal of Medicine, 287*(5), 217–220.

Said, H. M., Redha, R., & Nylander, W. (1989). Biotin transport in the human intestine: Inhibition by anticonvulsant drugs. *American Journal of Clinical Nutrition, 49*(1), 127–131.

Satter, E. (1990). The feeding relationship: Problems and interventions. *The Journal of Pediatrics, 117*(2, Part II), S181–S191.

Shaddix, T. E. (1991). Nutritional implications in children with cerebral palsy. *Nutrition Focus for Children with Special Health Care Needs, 6*(2), 1–6.

Shaddix, T., & Barnacastle, N. (1986). *Nutritional care for the child with developmental disabilities — Oral motor development and feeding techniques.* Birmingham, AL: United Cerebral Palsy of Greater Birmingham.

Shapiro, B. K., Green, P., Krick, J., Allen, D., & Capute, A. J. (1986). Growth of severely impaired children: Neurological versus nutritional factors. *Developmental Medicine and Child Neurology, 28*(6), 729–733.

Shepard, K., Roberts, D., Golding, S., Thomas, B. J., & Shepard, R. W. (1991). Body composition in myelomeningocele. *American Journal of Clinical Nutrition, 53,* 1–6.

Slaughter, M. H., Lohman, T. G., Boileau, R. A., Horswill, C. A., Stillman, R. J., VanLoan, M. D., & Bemben, D. A. (1988). Skinfold equations for estimation of body fatness in children and youth. *Human Biology, 60*(5), 709–723.

Smith, C. H., & Bidlack, W. R. (1984). Dietary concerns associated with the use of medication. *Journal of the American Dietetic Association, 84*(8), 901–914.

Smith, D., & Gines, D. (1989). Photometric height estimation compared with traditional measures. *Journal of the American Dietetic Association, 89*(2), 254.

Spender, Q. W., Cronk, C. E., Charney E. B., & Stallings, V. A. (1989). Assessment of linear growth of children with cerebral palsy: Use of alternate measures to height or length. *Developmental Medicine and Child Neurology, 31*(2), 206–214.

Springhouse Corporation. (1989). *Nursing 89 drug handbook.* Springhouse, PA: Springhouse Corporation.

Stanek, K., Hensley, C., & Van Riper, C. (1992). Factors affecting use of food and commercial agents to thicken liquids for individuals with swallowing disorders. *Journal of the American Dietetic Association, 92*(4), 488–490.

Stein, A. D., Shea, S., Basch, C. E., Contento, I. R., & Zybert, P. (1991). Variability and tracking of nutrient intakes of preschool children based on multiple administrations of the 24-hour dietary recall. *American Journal of Epidemiology, 134,* 1427–1437.

St. Jeor, S. T., Gutherie, H. A., & Jones, M. B. (1983). Variability in nutrient intake in a 28-day period. *Journal of the American Dietetic Association, 83*(2), 155–162.

Tanner, J. M., & Whitehouse, R. H. (1984). *Standards for sitting height (crown-rump) and subischial leg length from birth to maturity: British children 1978.* Ref. 61 & 62. (Available from author, Castlemead Publications, Swains Mill, 4A Crane Mead, Ware, Herts. SG129PY, England.)

Taylor, M. L., Kozlowski, B. W., Baer, M. T., Blyler, E. M., & Trahms, C. M. (1982). Anticonvulsant therapy and differences in iron parameters in developmentally delayed children. *Federation Proceedings 41*(4), 953.

Thomas, B. J., Shepherd, R. W., Holt, T. L., Shepherd, K., Greer, R., & Cleghorn, G. J. (1990). Body composition studies in cystic fibrosis and myelomeningocele. In S. Yasumura, J. E. Harrison, K. G. McNeill, A. D. Woodhead, & F. A. Dilmanian (Eds.), *Advances in in vivo body composition studies* (pp. 23–29). New York: Plenum Press.

Thommessen, M., Heiberg, A., Kase, B. F., Larsen, S., & Riis, G. (1991). Feeding problems, height, and weight in different groups of disabled children. *Acta Pediatrica Scandinavica, 80*(5), 527–533.

Thommessen, M., Riis, G., Kase, B. F., Larsen, S., & Heiberg, A. (1991). Energy and nutrient intakes of disabled children: Do feeding problems make a difference? *Journal of the American Dietetic Association, 91*(12), 1522–1525.

Tluczek, A., & Sondel, S. (1991). *Project SPOON: Special program of oral nutrition for children with special needs.* (Available from Office of University Publications, University of Wisconsin Children's Hospital, 600 Highland Avenue, Madison, WI 53792.)

Tolman, K. G., Jubiz, W., Sanella, J. J., Madsen, J. A., Belsy, R. E., Goldsmith, R. S., & Freston, J. W. (1975). Osteomalacia associated with anticonvulsants drug therapy in mentally retarded children. *Pediatrics, 56*(1), 45–51.

Treiber, F. A., Leonard, S. B., Frank, G., Musante, L., Davis, H., Strong, W. B., & Levy, M. (1990). Dietary assessment instruments for preschool children: Reliability of parental responses to the 24-hour recall and a food frequency questionnaire. *Journal of the American Dietetic Association 90*(6), 814–820.

Valli, C., Schalthess, H. K., Asper, R., Escher, F., & Hacki, W. H. (1986). Interaction of nutrients with antacids: A complication during enteral tube feeding. *Lancet, 1*(8483), 747–748.

Van Acker, R. (1991). Rett syndrome: A review of current knowledge. *Journal of Autism and Developmental Disorders, 21*(4), 381–406.

Veldee, M. S., & Peth, L. D. (1992). Can protein-calorie malnutrition cause dysphagia? *Dysphagia, 7*(2), 86–101.

Wallach, J. (1986). *Interpretation of diagnostic tests* (4th ed., pp. 124–125). Boston, MA: Little, Brown.

Waterlow, J. C. (1976). Classification and definition of protein-energy malnutrition. In G. H. Beaton & J. M. Bengoa (Eds.), *Nutrition in preventative medicine: The major deficiency syndromes, epidemiology, and approaches to control* (pp. 530–550). Geneva, Switzerland: World Health Organization.

Waterlow, J. C., Buzina, R., Keller, W., Lane, J. M., Nichamon, M. Z., & Tanner, J. M. (1977). The presentation and use of the height and weight data for comparing the nutritional status of groups of children under the age of 10 years. *Bulletin of the World Health Organization, 55*(4), 489–498.

Weiden, P., & Harrigan, M. (1986). A clinical guide for diagnosing and managing patients with drug-induced dysphagia. *Hospital and Community Psychiatry, 37*(4), 396–398.

Weststrate, J. A., & Deurenberg, P. (1989). Body composition in children: Proposal for a method for calculating body fat percentage from total body density or skinfold-thickness measurements. *American Journal of Clinical Nutrition, 50,* 1104–1115.

White, T. K., & Ekvall, S. W. (1993). Acromial radiale (upper arm) length and knee height growth chart, 2–18 years. In S. W. Ekvall (Ed.), *Pediatric nutrition in chronic diseases and developmental disorders* (p. 489). New York: Oxford Press.

Wodarski, L. A. (1990a). An interdisciplinary nutrition assessment and intervention protocol for children with disabilities. *Journal of the American Dietetic Association, 90*(11), 1563–1568.

Wodarski, L. A. (1990b). Hypercholesterolemia in children with developmental disabilities.

Journal of the American Dietetic Association, Supplement, 90(9), A-77.

Yassa, R., Natase, C., Camille, Y., Henderson, M., Belzile, L., & Beland, F. (1987). Carbamazepine, diuretics, and hyponatremia: A positive interaction. *Journal of Clinical Psychiatry, 48*(7), 281–283.

Zorab, P. A., Prime, F. J., & Harrison, A. (1963). Estimation of height from tibial length. *Lancet, 1*(7274), 195–196.

Videofluoroscopy of Swallowing in Pediatric Patients: A Component of the Total Feeding Evaluation

10

CHAPTER

Jane E. Benson, M.D.

Maureen A. Lefton-Greif, Ph.D., CCC-SP

Swallowing enhances nutrition while simultaneously imperiling the airway, a paradox easily solved by the neurologically normal individual. In a dysphagic person, concern for preservation of the airway and prevention of pneumonia often becomes paramount. Prior to the 1970s, patients who could not swallow properly were managed as though they had an incurable disease, palliated by gastrostomy or nasogastric tube feedings (Groher, 1984). Since then, however, technological advances have paralleled attitudinal changes among clinicians and radiologists alike:

> Dysphagia is not a disease. Rather it is a symptom of a disease that may be affecting any part of the swallowing tract from the mouth to the stomach (Donner, 1986, p. 1).

> Active intervention with dysphagic patients, including carefully planned diagnostic evaluations and subsequent management and rehabilitative techniques, often assists a patient's return to normal feeding and swallowing (Groher, 1984, p. xi).

With the promise of therapy came the need for more complete, precise evaluation. Swallowing involves the complex interaction of many muscles and tissues that are not observable clinically without severe distortion of the process. Fluoroscopy enables the clinician and radiologist to evaluate oral, pharyngeal, laryngeal, and cervical esophageal function in true physiologic action (Logemann, 1983). Originally recorded as individual frames on a long strip of radiographic film (cine-fluoroscopy), the advent of video recorders has greatly enhanced the performance and review of these studies. Videofluoroscopy offers insights into both diagnosis and therapy: It defines the swallowing problem, the patient's spontaneous response to the deficit, and factors contributing to aspiration so that appropriate management can be implemented to reduce the potential for airway compromise. As an added benefit, the radiographic dose per minute of examination time is lower with videofluoroscopy (Beck & Gayler, 1990).

Pediatric videofluoroscopy (VF) differs in scope from the standard upper gastrointestinal (UGI) examination and in content from the modified barium study (MBS) used in adults. The UGI examination encompasses the pharynx, but generally is more concerned with the anatomy and physiology of the esophagus, stomach, and duodenum. For example, questions concerning esophageal stricture, ulcer disease, reflux, and esophagitis are addressed in UGI examination. Only liquid contrast is used. Infants and young children are usually examined supine with no attempt to duplicate feeding postures, and a clinical therapist is not present. The adult MBS (Ekberg, 1992; Groher, 1984; Jones, Kramer, & Donner, 1985; Logemann, 1983; Logemann 1986a) utilizes limited bolus sizes presented in systematic increments that are swallowed on command, which is not a program that can be generalized to a population of suckling infants or children who will not swallow unfamiliar foods.

The pediatric VF examination combines components of diagnostic and rehabilitation studies used in adults with techniques unique to the feeding styles of individual children (Beecher, 1988; Kramer, 1989). Elements of diagnosis and therapy are used in the same examination (Linden, 1989; Logemann, 1986a) to attain several goals:

1. Define the nature and pathophysiology of the swallowing impairment.

2. Provoke the system to try to recreate the dysphagia complaint.

3. Identify adaptations that facilitate the child's "best" performance so that a management protocol can be developed.

General Considerations

Patient Referral and Selection

Because VF is invasive in the sense that it employs radiation, one must ensure that the choice of examination matches the child's clinical problem as well as his physical abilities. Suspicion of aspiration or other airway compromise during feeding may prompt the child's pediatrician or another clinician to request an evaluation with VF. The child may cough, choke, or become apneic when feeding, have repeated bouts of pneumonia or asthma, or

make "gurgly" sounds when vocalizing. All of these signs suggest the possibility that oral contents (food or saliva) enter the airway. In a child with feeding difficulty or food refusal, VF may also help assess the interaction and competency of the structures of the oropharynx in shaping and accomplishing a swallow.

Consideration must be given to whether VF is appropriate for a child's limitations. VF is a participatory exercise. The child must be able to cooperate sufficiently to stay in a chair and to swallow what is given to him or her. A child with uncontrolled, ballistic movements might injure her- or himself when placed within the confines of the fluoroscopic unit: a completely somnolent child might be exposed to lengthy periods of radiation with little benefit. If the child has a history of aspiration, choking, or seizures, nursing assistance with suctioning apparatus, pulse oxymeter, and oxygen should be arranged in advance. If the child has an indwelling nasogastric or tracheostomy tube, thought must be given to how these might change swallow performance or even render the examination inconclusive. Temporary feeding tubes are usually removed prior to evaluation.

In general, VF is an appropriate tool for evaluation of children who require an objective account of either pharyngeal phase functioning or the interface between oral and pharyngeal phase functioning, which are not readily observable from a clinical examination alone. According to Sonin (Sonin, Somers, Austin, & Bester, 1988):

> Several critical observations can only be made after videofluoroscopy: observations of velopharyngeal function, laryngeal elevation and closure, pharyngeal motility, pharyngeal transit time, pooling in the valleculae and pyriform sinuses, the number of swallows necessary to clear material, presence of aspiration, and the timing of aspiration in relation to the swallow. (p. 135)

Coordination of VF with clinical assessment will determine an evaluation and management program. Finally, VF can examine the value of rehabilitation strategies (Linden, 1989; Linden-Castelli, 1991; Logemann, 1986a, Sorin et al., 1988).

Patient Preparation and Timing of Examination

Before coming for VF, the child should have a complete clinical evaluation to assess medical and social history, developmental stage, neurologic impairment, and feeding and nutritional status. From this, the clinician can derive an examination agenda tailored to the child's needs, including where the impairment may be, what substances the child might swallow easily, and what foods with which to challenge him.

Every effort must be made to avoid circumstances that might degrade the child's performance. The child should be in good health, with any seizure activity under control. He or she should have had no recent distressing procedures that might be associated with the VF suite. A person familiar to the child should be available to feed him or her during the examination; if the child's regular caretaker is pregnant or cannot attend, a backup person with whom the child can interact must be provided. The parents or caretakers must be taught about the VF process and what to expect, because their comfort level with the procedure will directly influence that of the child. The choice of contrast materials should try to mimic his or her personal preferences in food tastes.

Equipment and Room Set-Up

A standard, tiltable fluoroscopic table with image intensifier and video monitor are needed to perform the examination. To record the study, a videotape recorder should be wired into the monitor so that viewing through the fluoroscope and tape recording are simultaneous. Many units have a built-in clock or timer, a useful feature for referencing individual frames or sequences. The playback device should include a "search" mode that allows slow motion play as well as freeze frame and frame-by-frame tape movement, both forward and backward. The examiners should be able to review the tape at intervals during the examination, to decide how best to continue. The optional addition of a microphone and an audio track lends another dimension to the record of the examination: Commands and comments of the examiners can be recorded by an ambient microphone, while a device taped to the patient's cricoid cartilage in the midline will pick up the sounds of swallowing as well as quality of vocalizations.

VF is performed with the fluoroscopic table in the erect position, with the child placed between the tabletop and the image intensifier. The table footplate may be used to support a baby carrier or a small seat modified so that it bolts firmly to the table surface and footplate. If a free-standing chair is used, the footplate is detached from the table.

The choice of chair or holder should be appropriate to the age and size of the child and should approximate the kind of seating positioning the child is accustomed to at feeding time. The chair should provide supportive restraints for the child as needed: lap and shoulder belts, footrest, and head cushion. The back and seat should be adjustable in height and angle, and there should be side supports for the head to minimize head turning. The goal is to duplicate the child's home feeding situation, so that he or she feels comfortable and more willing to cooperate, while ensuring proper positioning for videotaping. The chair should be radiolucent (i.e., made of wood or plastic), at least in the region of the head and shoulders. Many seating alternatives are commercially available (car seats, infant carrier, MAMA Chair®[1], wheelchair inserts) or can be constructed (Figure 10–1).

---

[1] Multiple Application Multiple Articulation Seating System, MAMA System, Inc., Oconomowoc, WI.

Feeding Equipment and Bolus Selection

One of the goals of the evaluation is to define the characteristics of foods and liquids and specific adaptations to the feeding circumstance that enable the child to experience safe and efficient feeding. It

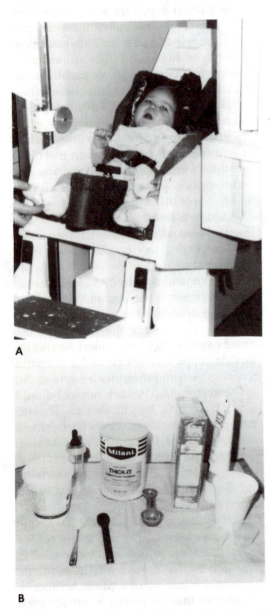

FIGURE 10–1. A. Child in MAMA Chair®, in lateral position, ready for feeding study. **B.** Examples of contrast and thickening agents assembled for feeding study.

is equally important to have a provocative imaging evaluation that mimics the child's decompensation patterns. In the pediatric patient, bolus selection addresses both issues. The pre-examination evaluation should have identified bolus characteristics in both categories. These can then be modified using variables such as viscosity, homogeneity of texture, temperature and resistance to separation into particles, all of which affect oral manipulation (Siebens & Linden, 1985).

VF and clinical assessment of oral stage function provide similar findings. Whereas bedside evaluation qualitatively estimates oral transit time, VF quantifies it (Sorin et al., 1988). Therefore, bolus types that require excessively long oral manipulation should be avoided, so as not to prolong the radiation exposure.

The caregiver might be asked to bring types of food the child enjoys as well as those that might encourage system decompensation. The foods are then made radiopaque. Barium sulfate powder is the imaging agent of choice for VF. It combines well with water, juice, or other foods and can be mixed to any desired consistency, yet is dense enough to be seen fluoroscopically even in very small amounts. This ensures that a tiny fleck of barium in the airway will be detected even though it may not provoke symptoms.

Standardization of textures is desirable so that sequential studies on one patient or multiple patients' performances can be compared. In practice, however, it is difficult to make standard foods that are palatable to all patients, and the examination period often becomes a time for culinary improvisation. Textures can be created by mixing barium with the patient's familiar foods, or it can be offered alone. Barium sulfate is commercially available in several standard forms (powder, low-density liquid, high-density liquid, paste) which can then be modified in measurable ways: thinned with water, thickened with rice cereal or Thick-it®, used to coat solids such as crackers. More devious methods of hiding the radiopaque additive (replacing the white cream in Oreo® cookies or Twinkies®, masquerading as mayonnaise in a tuna fish sandwich) result in foods that are less standard, but are more likely to be eaten. Recording the "recipes" used for the patient in the exam record can be helpful when planning a follow-up examination.

Feeding utensils should be the same as those used at home (e.g., bottle, nipple, cup, spoon, or straw). Occasionally a child with oral stage difficulties may require special modification of a feeding utensil to help isolate and evaluate the pharyngeal stage. For example, a pacifier may be adapted by inserting a nasogastric tube connected to a syringe. With an older child, a larger syringe may be used alone or with a feeding tube. These adaptations are tailored to the needs of the child and to address the youngster's overall diagnostic and management requirements.

Radiation Dose Considerations

The dose (i.e., the amount of radiant energy deposited in the tissues) received by the patient, and other personnel is determined by several variables, most of which are controllable, although some are not (Beck & Gayler, 1990). The brand of radiographic equipment and the weight or size of the child are examples of uncontrollable factors. The duration of examination and the amount of surface area exposed are controllable. Maximum permissible radiation exposure limits have been suggested by the National Institute of Health (NIH) Guidelines of Radiation Safety as 5 rem/year for all diagnostic procedures in the adult (over 18 years) and "for those under 18 years, a 10% reduction from this level is recommended" (Sonies, 1991, p. 189). Common sense dictates that examination time be kept to a minimum. In practice, this can be difficult when a child is not cooperative. Careful preparation is very important and should include coaching of the patient, selection of palatable foods, and adherence to a plan of clearly devel-

oped hypotheses formulated during pre-VF evaluation. Additional strategies include sampling of random swallows over a prearranged volume or time period, choosing textures that minimize oral manipulation, scheduling the patient after a nap to avoid the interference of fatigue, and conducting the examination at mealtime to increase the incentive.

Surface exposure can be minimized through shielding, distance, and collimation. The child's lower body can be protected by a lead apron or by a lead glove taped to the side of the chair or holder. All other persons in the examination room must wear lead aprons and, when handling or feeding the patient during fluoroscopy, lead gloves. When not interacting directly with the patient, they should stand as far as possible from the source of the x-ray beam within the fluoroscopy table. Radiant energy diminishes proportional to the square of the distance from the source.

The benefits of collimation (diminishing the beam diameter using internal sliding lead plates) are twofold: Dose is diminished, and image is sharpened. The ocular lens and the thyroid gland are the most radiosensitive tissues in the field. Unfortunately, shielding this region is impossible, because the child frequently moves during the examination, forcing the imaging field to "follow," and the thyroid lies very close to the larynx, an area of clinical interest. The image should be collimated to include only the mouth, pharynx, and cervical esophagus and trachea, with centering over the mandibular rami in younger children or over the pyriform sinuses in older children. In infants, the image field may need some posterior expansion with centering over the auditory canals to smooth the contrast range and avoid overexposure of the trachea. Magnifying the image may make the swallow easier to interpret, but it also increases the dose by 50 to 100%. Limiting fluoroscopic time to that necessary to record pertinent swallows is the best way to keep the dose within acceptable boundaries. Use the video playback to study a few swallows in greater depth, rather than recording more swallows.

Women who are or may be pregnant should be encouraged to leave the room or watch from a remote monitor. If there is a question as to whether a female patient is sexually active, the examination should be performed during the first 10 days of her menstrual cycle.

Conducting the Examination

As much preparation as possible should be done before the patient is brought into the fluoroscopy suite to minimize exposure to noise and bustle. The fluoroscopy table should be elevated, the chair readied, the videotape recorder set up and tested, and the feeding textures and utensils assembled and set out on a table or stand. Only then should the child be brought in, seated, and made comfortable. Changes in room lighting should be made gradually, dimming only to the level required to see the image intensifier, not to so dark a level that the child is frightened or feeding is difficult. Children may experience some uneasiness when the image intensifier is positioned next to them and they find themselves in a more confined space. Positioning the parent or caretaker in front of the child to speak, hold hands, or otherwise provide distraction is helpful. Some children respond well to music or to a special toy brought from home.

If more than one substance is to be offered, a selection of lead letters or numbers should be available to tape to the face of the image intensifier and include in the image. This will eliminate confusion when the tape is reviewed. If the video recorder has an audio track, commentary from the examiners describing the substance, mode of presentation, and patient reaction will be very useful during review.

Substances should be offered sequentially, and approximately three swallows of each should be recorded. If the child is a suckle feeder, a rhythmic "run" of swallows should be recorded, if achieved. A recent study (Lazarus et al., in press) demonstrated that at least an 80% accuracy level of pharyngeal stage parameters can be obtained by imaging three swallows in normal adults and stroke patients. To date, data are not available concerning the number of swallows needed to accurately predict aspiration potential. It is possible that the sampling size of the suckle feeder should be greater than that observed with controlled bolus sizes.

The image should remain centered, rather than moving with the bolus. The mode of presentation (cup, syringe, nipple, spoon) and approximate amount swallowed should be noted. If the history indicates that swallowing difficulty increases as feeding progresses, additional swallows "off-camera" can be given, then several more swallows recorded. Generally, it is a good idea to progress from substances that the patient is known to tolerate to those with which he or she may have trouble (Beecher, 1988; Logemann, 1983, 1986a). The decision regarding the order in which to present different textures should be made on the basis of the comprehensive clinical assessment completed prior to the imaging study. Additionally, during the study, "on-line" decisions are made about the progression of consistencies based on review of previously recorded swallow patterns.

Maintaining the patient in the lateral position is extremely important because this is the only projection where penetration and aspiration can be reliably observed (Logemann, 1986a). The changing interrelationships among the structures comprising the upper aerodigestive tract during each swallow are also best assessed with this view.

The frontal projection occasionally is useful to demonstrate abnormalities in posterior pharyngeal function that lateralize, and that may be amenable to head-turning maneuvers. The clinical examination and past medical history should enable the examiner to make some predictions about the possibility of unilateral impairments prior to the imaging study. In this position, the patient is turned to face the image intensifier, his head is turned to the side to be given a mouthful of contrast, then turned forward again to swallow. For best visualization of the pharynx, the head must be extended during the swallow to move the mandible out of the way. Difficulty in the infant patient stems from shortness of the neck, which prevents hyperextension, and the mechanical issue of how to administer liquid to a suckle-feeder without obscuring the field with the bottle. One solution is to fill the child's mouth through a feeding tube attached to a syringe, with liquid delivery via gentle hand pressure, either continuously or in measured increments. Another practical problem may be encountered if the patient's knees stop the image intensifier's descent before the head can be brought into view. This can sometimes be solved if the patient can stand or sit directly on the fluoroscopy table footplate and be supported from the side with legs abducted. This position may be impossible for some patients because of spasticity or the need for extensive head support, although tilting the table back can be helpful for the latter.

During the examination, the child's condition should be continually assessed. Penetration or aspiration of barium into the trachea does not mean that the study should be terminated; rather, the study should move on to the next phase with a change in bolus size, consistency, manner of presentation, body positioning, or oral stimulation. Modification of swallowing maneuvers may be attempted in the older child who is either cognitively intact or able to imitate gestures (e.g., cough). Medical or behavioral decompensation of the patient should signal the premature end of the examination; that is, if the patient chokes or coughs unduly and becomes upset, or if oxygen saturation by pulse oxymetry diminishes and extensive suctioning of the patient is required, or if the patient becomes resistant to further feeding and begins to cry or struggle. The child's caretakers often have the best idea of normal feeding behavior and whether observed changes during the exam become extraordinary. Otherwise, the evaluation should be terminated if the persistence of current behavioral or swallowing patterns would not significantly change the management plan.

Reviewing the Videotape

Immediately following the evaluation, the videotape should be reviewed by the radiologist and the clinician, in both real time and slow motion/stop frame. Involving the caretakers in this process increases their understanding of the procedure and promotes compliance with therapy regimens. Parameters of the evaluation must be recorded for future reference; sample checklists are illustrated in Tables 10–1, 10–2, 10–3, and 10–4 and are used for each of the variables manipulated in the study (e.g., textures, volume). Information gained from the examination should be shared with the referral source and integrated into the child's overall assessment.

Interpretation

One of the more difficult developmental tasks of childhood is the progression from suckle feeding to the bite-and-chew pattern of mature feeding (Bosma, 1992). This must go on as the child's face and neck grow and lengthen: The larynx drops away from the nasopharynx; and the relationship formed by the mouth, pharynx, and esophagus changes from an oblique angle to a right angle (Hast, 1970; Kramer, 1985; Lieberman, 1975; Newman, 1992). There is loss of the "natural" airway protection of the infant where the laryngeal aditus is covered by the base of the tongue during the swallow contraction. At each stage of development, however, the mouth, pharynx, and esophagus must maintain an integrated continuity that ensures both the smooth transfer of food and complete airway protection. This has been de-

TABLE 10–1. Documentation necessary for analyzing videofluoroscopic assessment of feeding and swallowing function in the pediatric patient.

Examination Environment
Imaging plane
Imaging field
Magnification

Patient Setup
Positioning equipment
Position of patient
Person feeding patient
Bolus characteristics
Special feeding utensils
Special feeding directions
Monitoring or suctioning equipment

Respiratory Status
Specify status (e.g., WNL/stable)
Tracheostomy (+/− valve)
Ventilatory dependency
Suctioning required
Read-outs from monitoring equipment (e.g., pulse oxygen, respiratory, or heart rate)

Patient's State
Alert
Active, not crying
Crying
Drowsy to varying degrees of sleep

Risk of Airway Compromise
Specific bolus characteristics (e.g., size, texture, temperature)
When airway entrance occurred in relation to the swallow contraction
Response to the airway contamination (e.g., cough, respiratory changes, cyanosis)
Estimate of amount entering airway
Frequency of airway threat

TABLE 10–2. Checklist for oral phase of videofluoroscopy.

Leakage from mouth	_____	Nasopharyngeal reflux	_____
Residue: _____	_____	Poor posterior tongue thrust	_____
Reduced A/P movement	_____	Suckle/Suck: Swallow ratio	_____
Incomplete contact of tongue to palate	_____	Swallows to clear (No.)	_____
Poor bolus formation	_____		
Poor bolus transfer	_____		
Piecemeal deglutition	_____		
Lingual movements to clear (No.)	_____	Delayed oral transit time	_____
Insufficient/delayed velar elevation/retraction	_____	Oral transit time (msec.)	_____
		Swallow initial time (msec.)	_____

TABLE 10–3. Checklist for pharyngeal stage of videofluoroscopy.

Spillage over tongue base	_____	Clearance of airway (Yes/No)	
Valleculae (pre-swallow)		With subsequent swallows	_____
Pooling/**S**tasis	_____	With cough	_____
Pyriform sinuses (pre-swallow)		Aspiration (**Pre/Po**st swallow)	_____
Pooling/**S**tasis	_____	Pharyngeal peristalsis	
Delayed swallow onset (msec.)	_____	**W**eak/**A**bsent	_____
Failure to initiate swallow	_____	Post swallow residue	
Hyoid movement (Ant./Up)		Valleculae	_____
Delayed/**R**educed/**A**bsent	_____	Pyriform sinuses	_____
Epiglottis (Note: _____)	_____	Cough response	
Laryngeal elevation		Not assessed	_____
Delayed/**R**educed/**A**bsent	_____	Delayed	_____
Laryngeal penetration		Absent	_____
Pre/**D**uring/**Po**st swallow	_____		
Airway penetration			
To ventricle (____/____ swallow)	_____	Pharyngeal transit time (msec.)	_____
To vocal cords (____/____ swallow)	_____	Pharyngeal clearance time (msec.)	_____
To trachea (____/____ swallow)	_____	Total swallow time	_____

TABLE 10–4. Checklist for esophageal phase of videofluoroscopy.

Cricopharyngeal sphincter		Gastroesophageal reflux	
Delayed opening	_____	During modified barium evaluation:	
Short opening phase	_____	_____ No _____ Yes	
Premature close	_____	to level of _____	
		During UGI series:	
Anatomic changes	_____	_____ No _____ Yes	
Functional changes	_____	to level of _____	

scribed as a series of five steps, outlined in Table 10–5 (Buchholz, 1985).

A prototypical "normal" swallow does not truly exist. Besides the developmental forces at work, a competent swallow is one that continually adapts to the demands of the substance being swallowed. This flexibility also allows compensatory function of one element in the sequence to counterbalance deficiency in another area, as when a deficiency of the pharyngeal palate is compensated for by greater convergence of the pharyngeal constrictor muscles (Buchholz, 1985). Each swallow, then, must be evaluated along a continuum of normality. The video record is indispensable for this task, because a different element in the complex interplay of tissues and surfaces that comprises each swallow can be observed on each replay, making swallowing abnormality easier to recognize. In the video swallow, this is usually evident when contrast material appears where it should not be or outlines abnormal structures. Figures 10–2 to 10–4 show a normal suckle-swallow as well as exam-

TABLE 10–5. Normal pharyngeal function during swallow.

1. Control of the junctions of the mouth and pharynx as accomplished by the actions of the tongue and pharyngeal palate.

2. Closure of the palatal pharyngeal isthmus.

3. Active propulsion of the bolus through the pharynx by pharyngeal constrictor muscles with assistance from the coordinated activity of the palate, tongue, hyoid muscles, and larynx.

4. Airway protection as a result of the epiglottis tilting downward and the closure of the laryngeal complex.

5. Cricopharyngeal relaxation and opening to allow for bolus passage.

Source: From Buchholz, D. W., Bosma, J. F., & Donner, M. W. (1985). Adaptation, compensation, and decompensation of the pharyngeal swallow. *Gastrointestinal Radiology, 10,* 235–239, with permission.

ples of some of the abnormalities described in the next two sections.

Oral Phase Abnormalities

Oral stage function affects the efficiency of bolus formation and transport to the posterior portion of the oral cavity. The following patterns can interfere with function: leakage from the mouth, piecemeal deglutition, multiple sucks to initiate a swallow, insufficient or delayed velar movement (elevation and/or retraction), nasopharyngeal reflux, and a poor posterior tongue thrust.

In a suckling infant, deficient tongue apposition to the palate can result in poor expression of contrast from the nipple and spreading of contrast over the lingual surface and under the tongue. When the palate and posterior pharyngeal wall fail to oppose completely or in a timely manner relative to the transport of the bolus between the oral and pharyngeal cavities, there is nasopharyngeal reflux. In small amounts, this can occur normally in premature or even full-term babies (Kramer, 1985), but it should not occur repetitively, or in amounts that compromise nasal breathing, particularly in the infant who is an obligate nose-breather. Nasopharyngeal masses also can interfere with palatal elevation. Suckling causes contrast to accumulate in either the posterior oral cavity or in the vallecula prior to swallow, but should not be seen beyond this point (Newman, Blickman, Hillman, & Jamarillo, 1991). A swallow response is said to be delayed when the contrast "hesitates" or accumulates in the pyriform sinuses prior to the swallow contraction.

A child in transitional feeding may have tongue protrusion that extrudes a portion of the bolus during oral manipulation; with the development of better lip closure and tongue tip elevation, spill ceases (Sivit, 1990). The tongue should lateralize the bolus toward the teeth, but contrast should not appear under the tongue. Lingual movements should be

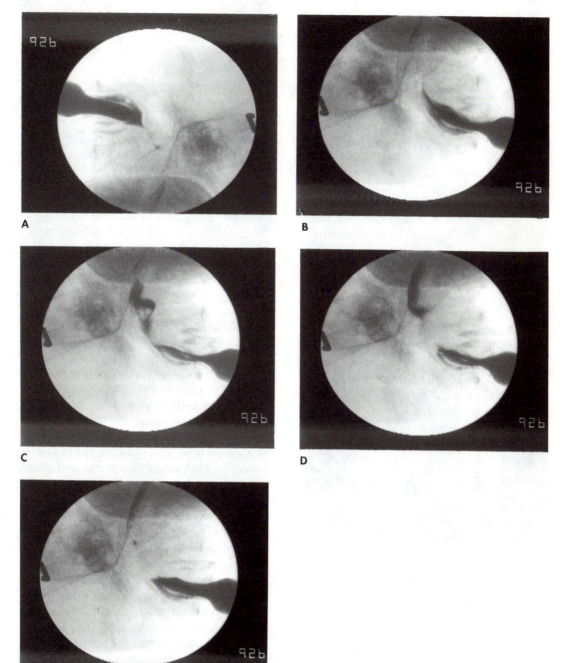

FIGURE 10–2. Patient 1, semi-reclining, lateral projection. Video frames of a normal infant suck-swallow. Frames are 1/6 second apart. **A.** Suckle begins as the posterior tongue drops, followed by the soft palate which keeps the faucial isthmus closed. Contrast is drawn into the mouth. **B.** Tongue tip elevates, expressing more contrast from the nipple, beginning the peristaltic wave that carries the bolus through the faucial isthmus toward the valleculae. **C.** Tongue is flattened against the hard palate; soft palate has risen to block the nasopharynx; bolus has been delivered to the valleculae and pyriform sinuses; superior aspect of posterior pharyngeal wall begins anterior movement. **D.** Pharyngeal peristalsis continues, forcing bolus down through the open upper esophageal sphincter. **E.** Tongue flattens; nipple re-expands; faucial isthmus remains closed; bolus tail seen in esophagus; fleck of barium remains in valleculae.

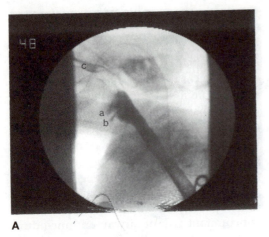

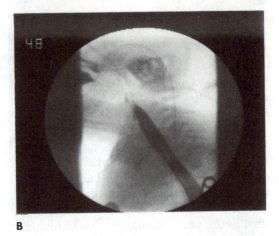

A   **B**

FIGURE 10–3. Patient 2, semi-reclining, lateral projection. Pharyngeal phase of swallow. Frames are 1/6 second apart. **A.** Contrast in valleculae (*a*). Epiglottal undercoating (*b*). Nasopharyngeal airway (outlined by NG tube) is still open due to incomplete palatal closure and there has been nasopharyngeal reflux (*c*). **B.** Contrast is gone from laryngeal aditus as bolus continues down the esophagus. New bolus is forming. Contrast remains in nasopharynx.

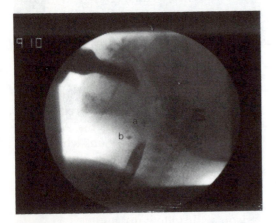

FIGURE 10–4. Patient 3, semi-reclining, lateral projection. Single frame from early esophageal phase of swallow. Flecks of contrast in the valleculae (*a*) and in the subglottic trachea (*b*). Patient has not coughed, and is continuing to suckle.

Pharyngeal Phase Abnormalities

Specific attention is directed toward recording of episodes of frank airway compromise as well as predictive patterns of dysfunction. The structures comprising the pharynx are assessed for structural integrity as well as the relative timing relationships with other structures and bolus movement. Parameters that may predispose the patient to airway compromise include delivery of the bolus into the pharynx prior to airway closure, a delay in pharyngeal swallow onset, and contrast penetration (i.e., contrast entering the ventricle or upper airway during swallow) even with extrusion during swallow contraction, if the episodes are seen on half or more of the imaged swallows.

Contrast can enter the airway prior to, during, or after the swallow contraction, through muscular or respiratory action, and gain access to any level of the respiratory tract (Logemann, 1983, 1986a). Normally, the epiglottis tilts down to cover the larynx during swallow. However, if contrast arrives prematurely in the pharynx through poor oral control, or if the pharynx fails to empty with swallow, the epiglottis may be seen outlined by contrast.

quick and efficient, and the oral cavity should be cleared of all residue following the delivery of the bolus to the pharynx. Adequate bolus formation does not demonstrate spreading of contrast over the lingual surfaces. Transport of the bolus to the posterior portion of the oral cavity should not require multiple lingual "pumping" gestures reminiscent of suckle feeding.

This may take the form of simple "undercoating" which clears as the swallow passes over it; or with successive levels of dysfunction, there may be true penetration of contrast to the level of the laryngeal ventricle, the vocal cords, or the trachea (Kramer, 1985). Undercoating may be seen in suckling babies, especially with the first swallow, although it should not be a repetitive event. Contrast may also appear at any of these levels because of aspiration, the inhaling of residual contrast from the pharynx. The persistence of contrast in the pharynx may be due to insufficiency in the pharyngeal stripping wave, premature arrival of contrast from the oral cavity, or reflux from the esophagus due to cricopharyngeal spasm or incoordination (Fisher, Painter, & Milmoe, 1981).

It is important to note the presence and timing of cough or any other sign associated with aspiration. Sometimes the child demonstrates changes in color, respiratory function, upper aerodigestive tract noises, and/or vocal quality that are more subtle than those characteristic of adults. Failure to manifest any of these signs in the face of documented airway contamination is know as "silent aspiration."

Esophageal Phase Structure and Function

The upper portion of the esophagus is imaged during the examination, and occasional findings will be of interest. The cricopharyngeal sphincter may be dysfunctional, displaying delayed opening, a short opening phase, or premature closure. Prominence of the sphincter may be seen in patients with gastroesophageal reflux or with Arnold-Chiari malformation, although the functional significance of this finding is unclear (Putnam et al., 1992). Retrograde movements of contrast in the esophagus may signal dismotility, distal obstruction, or gastroesophageal reflux and should prompt the request of an UGI.

Conclusion

Videofluoroscopy is a valuable tool to examine a dysphagic child. Oral, pharyngeal, and cervical esophageal stage function can be assessed. Oral stage function defines characteristics that either enhance or prevent efficient bolus formation and transport to the posterior portion of the oral cavity. Evaluation of pharyngeal stage structure and function addresses the propulsion of the bolus through the pharynx and its passage into the esophagus and the concomitant risk of airway entrance during any portion of the swallow sequence. Anatomic and functional deviations of the cervical esophagus are identified, along with the relationship of bolus passage to the opening and closing of the cricopharyngeal sphincter. Although radiation dose must be a consideration, the ability to see the complex muscular mechanisms at work and to capture them in a real-time format for later study and review is a benefit that outweighs the risk.

The clinical examiner must judge the reliability of these findings in relation to the child's presenting problems. Any procedural or situational variations which may have influenced the outcome must be reported. Terminology must be standardized and reports must be comprehensive to allow for meaningful interpretation and comparison with follow-up studies.

Finally, the videofluoroscopic evaluation is only a single component of the comprehensive evaluation of a child with a feeding and swallowing impairment. Its results must be integrated with the child's overall medical, developmental, and cognitive status to address the clinical complaints and produce an appropriate management plan.

References

Beck, T. J., & Gayler, B. W. (1990). Image quality and radiation in swallowing. *Dysphagia, 5*(3), 118–128.

Beecher, R. B. (1988, February). *Videofluoroscopic swallow studies with the pediatric patient: What, who, when, why, how, what to do.* Paper presented at the meeting of the Illinois Speech-Language-Hearing Association, Chicago, IL.

Bosma, J. F. (1992). Development and impairments of feeding in infancy and childhood. In M. E. Groher (Ed.), *Dysphagia: Diagnosis and management,* (2nd ed., pp. 107–141). Boston: Butterworth-Heinemann.

Buchholz, D. W., Bosma, J. F., & Donner, M. W. (1985). Adaptation, compensation, and decompensation of the pharyngeal swallow. *Gastrointestinal Radiology, 10,* 235–239.

Donner, M. W. (1986). Editorial. *Dysphagia, 1*(1), 1–2.

Ekberg, O. (1992). Radiologic evaluation of swallowing. In M. E. Groher (Ed.), *Dysphagia: Diagnosis and management,* (2nd ed., pp. 163–195). Boston: Butterworth-Heinemann.

Feinberg, M. J., & Ekberg, O. (1991). Videofluoroscopy in elderly patients with aspiration: Importance of evaluating both oral and pharyngeal stages of deglutition. *American Journal of Roentgenology, 165,* 293–296.

Fisher, S. E., Painter, M., & Milmore, G. (1993). Swallowing disorders in infancy. *Pediatric Clinics of North America, 28*(4), 845–853.

Groher, M. E. (Ed.). (1984). *Dysphagia: Diagnosis and management.* Stoneham, MA: Butterworth.

Groher, M. E. (Ed.). (1992). *Dysphagia: Diagnosis and management* (2nd ed.). Boston: Butterworth-Heinemann.

Hast, M. H. (1970). The developmental anatomy of the larynx. *Otolaryngologic Clinics of North America, 3,* 413–438.

Jones, B., Kramer, S. S., & Donner, M. W. (1985). Dynamic imaging of the pharynx. *Gastrointestinal Radiology, 10,* 213–224.

Kramer, S. S. (1985). Special swallowing problems in children. *Gastrointestinal Radiology, 10,* 241–250.

Kramer, S. S. (1989). Radiologic examination of the swallowing impaired child. *Dysphagia, 3,* 117–125.

Lazarus, C., Logemann, J. A., Rademaker, A. W., Kahrilas, P. J., Pajak, T., Lazar, R., & Halper, A. (in press). Effects of bolus volume, viscos-ity and repeated swallow in normals and stroke patients. *Archive of Physical Medicine and Rehabilitation.*

Lieberman, P. (1975). *On the origins of language.* New York: Macmillian.

Linden, P. (1989). Videofluoroscopy in rehabilitation for swallowing dysfunction. *Dysphagia, 3,* 189–191.

Linden-Castelli, P. (1991). Treatment strategies for adult neurogenic dysphagia. *Seminars in Speech and Language, 12*(3), 255–260.

Linden, P., & Siebens, A. A. (1983). Dysphagia: Predicting laryngeal penetration. *Archives of Physical Medicine and Rehabilitation, 64,* 281–284.

Logemann, J. A. (1983). *Evaluation and treatment of swallowing disorders.* San Diego: College-Hill Press.

Logemann, J. A. (1986a). *Manual for the videofluorographic study of swallowing.* San Diego: College-Hill Press.

Logemann, J. A. (1986b). Treatment of aspiration related to dysphagia: An overview. *Dysphagia, 1,* 34–36.

Newman, L. A., Cleveland, R. H., Blickman, J. G., Hillman, R. E., & Jaramillo, D. (1991). Videofluoroscopic analysis of the infant swallow. *Investigative Radiology, 26,* 870–873.

Newman, L. A. (1992). *Oral and pharyngeal swallowing in infancy.* Unpublished doctoral dissertation. Boston University, Sargent College, Boston, MA.

Putnam, P. E., Orenstein, S. R., Pang, D., Pollack, I. F., Proujansky, R., & Kocoshis, S. A. (1992). Cricopharyngeus dysfunction associated with Chiari malformation. *Pediatrics, 89*(5 Part 1), 871–876.

Sivit, C. (1990). Role of the pediatric radiologist in the evaluation of oral and pharyngeal dysphagia. *Journal of Neurology and Rehabilitation, 4,* 103–110.

Sonies, B. C. (1991). Instrumental procedures of dysphagia diagnosis. *Seminars in Speech and Language, 12*(3), 185–197.

Sorin, R., Somers, S., Auston, M., & Bester, S. (1988). The influence of videofluoroscopy on the management of the dysphagic patient. *Dysphagia, 2,* 127–135.

Other Diagnostic Tests Used for Evaluation of Swallowing Disorders

Jane E. Benson, M.D.
David N. Tuchman, M.D.

The only diagnostic test routinely used in clinical evaluation of the swallowing mechanism in infants and children is the videofluoroscopic study. Other modalities are available; however, these tests are investigational in nature, not widely available, poorly standardized, or not well tolerated by patients in this age group. A brief discussion to acquaint the reader with additional techniques follows.

Ultrasonography

Ultrasound has become an important imaging modality in the pediatric population. It uses no injected or unpalatable contrast material or injurious radiation and has the added advantage of being portable and relatively inexpensive. Advances in technology have decreased the size of transducers so that even the smallest infant can be imaged.

Principles

Sonography relies on the propagation of sound energy through fluid or semi-fluid matter (such as blood and tissues) and de-

tection of reflections from specular interfaces, points at which the transmitting quality of the tissue changes. The send/receive time interval is coded as distance, and the strength of the returning signal is seen as brightness. All signal information is compiled into an image on a monitor which, with today's real-time scanners, is updated many times per second. The image represents a slice of tissue with depth and width (the vertical and horizontal dimensions of the screen) but with only a millimeter or two of thickness. Depth of penetration is determined by the transducer frequency, while the orientation represented horizontally on the screen changes as the examiner rotates the transducer through sagittal, coronal, and oblique planes. Sound travels best through fluids and homogeneous soft tissues. Fat is a poor sound transmitter because it is a complex tissue with many septations. Sound will not pass through bone or air and will be completely reflected.

Technique

Most infants and children can be imaged using a 5 megahertz transducer, although tiny premature infants may need the resolution afforded by a 7.5 megahertz instrument. The send/receive modules are arranged in the transducer in a straight line ("linear array") or in a fan-shape ("sector array"). The transducer can be placed beneath the chin (submental approach) (Figure 11–1a) or on the cheek (transbuccal approach). The latter position works only in infants with unerupted teeth. Sector array rather than linear array fits best into these positions, affording the widest view through the smallest sonographic window. Some resolution is lost at the margins of the fan-shaped image field, but the important structures are optimally seen. Water-soluble jelly establishes fluid continuity between the transducer and the skin.

With the submental approach, the tongue can be visualized in coronal and sagittal planes. Static and interactive anatomy of the oropharynx has been described in adults using this format (Shawker, Sonies, & Stone, 1984a, 1984b; Shawker, Sonies, Stone, & Baum, 1983; Sonies, Parent, Morrish, & Baum, 1988); infants also have been imaged in this way (Bosma, Hepburn, Josell, & Baker, 1990; Smith, Erenberg, Nowak, & Franken, 1985; Weber, Woolridge, & Baum, 1986). The transbuccal approach looks at the tongue and buccal surfaces in the transverse or coronal planes (Smith et al., 1985). As a point of reference for measurement, the hyoid bone (ossified to varying degrees, depending on patient age) can be included in the imaging plane as a shadow on the submental view. To see the tongue interact with the palate and buccal surfaces, the oral cavity must be filled with fluid, with the exclusion of air bubbles. A suckling infant accomplishes this well (Figure 11–1b); an older child can be given liquids from a straw or syringe.

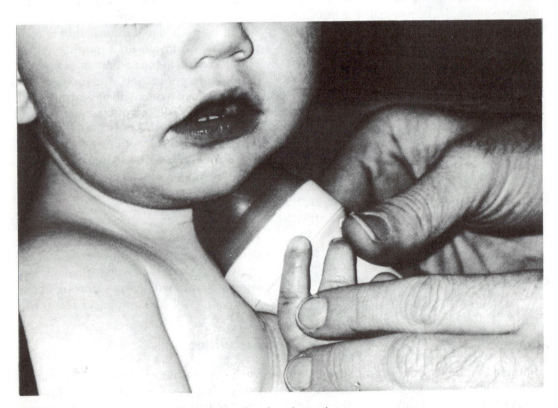

FIGURE 11–1a. Ultrasound transducer positioned in the submental region.

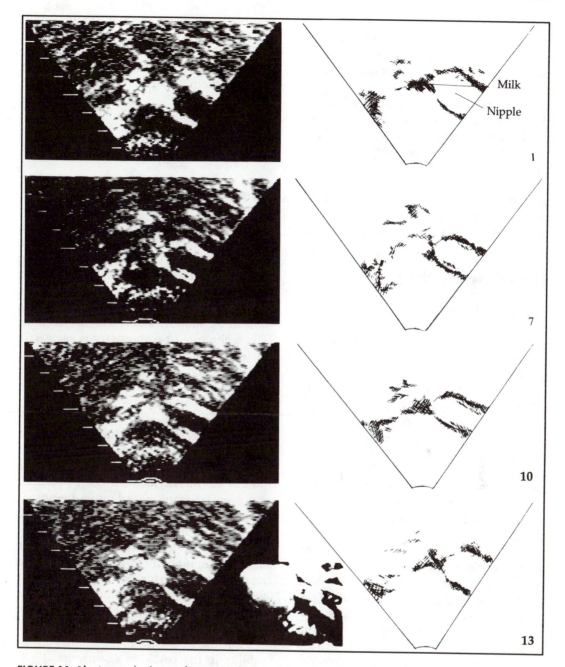

FIGURE 11–1b. Longitudinal view of tongue and nipple during one suckle cycle. Frames each represent 1/30 second, taken at indicated intervals.

Advantages and Limitations

Unlike fluoroscopy, which gives three-dimensional information in one image, ultrasound is limited to a single two-dimen-sional plane at a time. Thus, when looking at the tongue and palate in the sagittal mid-line, one cannot see what the lateral bor-ders of the tongue are doing at the same moment. On the other hand, imaging in multiple planes for prolonged periods is not injurious to the patient and is usually well-tolerated. Finding consistent landmarks for orientation and measurement can be difficult, but qualitative observations concerning tongue motion, palatal elevation, and buccal compression can be made.

Although the oral cavity is visualized best, the pharynx can sometimes be seen by angling the transducer. The oropharynx can be included in the same image in babies and small children. Because the trachea is an air-filled space, fluid penetration or aspiration cannot be visualized with ultrasound.

Clinical Applications

The complex, three-dimensional interactions of the tissues of the oral cavity are only beginning to be appreciated. Normative data remain to be standardized (Sonies et al., 1988; Weber et al., 1986), but qualitative studies have uncovered interesting differences in the appearance of the oral phase of swallowing between normal subjects and those with cerebral palsy (Kenny, Casas, & McPherson, 1989), post-polio syndrome (Sonies et al., 1990), cystinosis (Sonies et al., 1990), and prematurity (Bu'Lock, Woolridge, & Baum, 1990). On screen, real-time measurements of tongue thickness and excursion are possible, and timing of events can be easily derived with an in-line clock.

Because of its completely noninvasive character, sonography has potential for development as a diagnostic discipline in children, particularly as a complement to the barium swallow. Subtle difficulties with the oral phase of swallow, especially if they develop gradually during the course of a feed, might best be addressed with this modality when prolonged fluoroscopy would be injurious. Assessment of swallow skills in the premature nursery might precede the institution of full feeding. Assessment of tongue action in children with speech impediments might include an instructional "biofeedback" element where the child attempts to duplicate normal tongue action by watching his own on the monitor screen. New clinical challenges confront us daily; ultrasound is yet another tool with which to meet them.

Manometry

General Principles

Manometry is a technique that quantifies force of contraction of the muscular wall of the gut. Manometry is not an imaging study, but rather a test of function, enabling the clinician to measure motor activity of muscle by measuring the strength, speed, direction and duration of muscle contraction. The technique of manometry is reviewed in detail in standard gastroenterology texts including Malagelada, Camilleri, and Stanghellini, (1986); Hogan and Dodds (1989); Richter and Castell (1989); and Scott (1991).

Older manometric methods used air-filled balloons and nonperfused water-filled catheters. However, these systems do not accurately reflect pressure changes in a hollow viscous organ such as the proximal gut. Newer techniques of measuring pressures use low compliance, water-perfused systems and intraluminal pressure transducers. The water-perfused system, when used in the intestine, measures the force needed by the perfusate to "push" the gut wall away from the recording side hole of a flexible recording catheter (the "yield pressure"). This type of equipment is generally available in most centers and has applicability in the pediatric age group.

The most accurate method for measuring gastrointestinal pressures involves using intraluminal pressure transducers. These devices directly measure pressures in the lumen and eliminate the need for water perfusion. This system has rapid response characteristics exceeding those necessary for accurate recording in the proximal gastrointestinal tract. Disadvantages include limited versatility due to fixed placement of the transducers inside the catheter and expense of the system. Intraluminal pressure transducers are used mainly in research settings.

Manometric Recording of the Upper Esophageal Sphincter

It is well established that during deglutition there is significant axial movement of the upper esophageal sphincter. Because the manometry catheter may remain relatively fixed during swallowing, decrease in sphincter pressure may be an artifact and represent movement of the pressure sensor out of the high pressure zone. Accordingly, many investigators use a sleeve device (commonly termed a "Dent" sleeve) to measure pressure in the upper sphincter. In addition, the pressure profile of the upper esophageal sphincter is asymmetric; that is, pressures tend to be higher in the posterior-lateral directions. Therefore, orientation of the recording device must be taken into account during upper esophageal manometry. Finally, each component of the recording system (catheter, transducer, perfusion system) must be able to respond to rapidly occurring motor events and pressure changes in the striated muscle portion of the proximal esophagus. This is in contrast to the smooth muscle of the distal esophagus where events occur more slowly.

Application of Manometry

Usual indications for use of manometry include diagnosis of esophageal motility disorders such as achalasia (failure of the lower esophageal sphincter to relax following deglutition, absence of peristalsis in the esophageal body) and systemic disorders affecting gastrointestinal motor function such as scleroderma and chronic idiopathic intestinal pseudo-obstruction.

Manometry may also be used to investigate the function of the upper esophageal sphincter (UES). UES pressure, response of the UES to swallowing, and timing between pharyngeal contraction and UES relaxation may be measured. Manometry may be particularly helpful in instances where videofluoroscopic imaging demonstrates impaired or absent transit of contrast from the hypopharynx to the esophagus. When this occurs, it may be difficult to distinguish between a sphincter that fails to relax versus a sphincter that relaxes but fails to open. Failure of upper esophageal sphincter relaxation, termed cricopharyngeal achalasia, may be documented using manometry. A relaxing, but nonopening, sphincter may result from poor pumping action of weakened pharyngeal musculature that is unable to deliver the hypopharyngeal bolus through the valve. In this instance, manometry may confirm relaxation of the UES; whereas contrast studies demonstrate inadequate pharyngeal pumping action.

Electromyography

Modalities such as videofluoroscopy, ultrasonography, and manometry do not directly assess the activity of individual muscles. Electromyography (EMG) is a technique that enables the investigator to assess the myoelectric activity of muscle. To obtain accurate recordings, good contact is required between probe and muscle. A variety of probe devices are available including suction cups, clips, and electrode needles. Electromyographic recording of muscles of the swallowing apparatus has been reviewed by Palmer (1989). At present, this technique is not indicated for routine clinical evaluation of swallowing function in children and remains a research tool.

Nuclear Scintigraphy

The technique of nuclear scintigraphy involves swallowing a liquid or solid that is labeled with a radiopharmaceutical. Technetium-99m, the radionuclide used in swallowing and esophageal scintigraphic studies, is not absorbed after oral administration, and does not become attached to gastrointestinal mucosa. Using a gamma counter, images of esophagus and portions of the oropharynx and stomach are obtained. Using computer processing, regions of interest and selection of time intervals are generated which allow measurement of transit time and estimation of intraluminal volumes. During these studies, exposure to radiation is less than during analogous fluoroscopic procedures. Problems include poor resolution of the image and poor localization. The technique of nuclear scintigraphy has been reviewed by Cowan (1989) and others.

In the gastrointestinal tract, scintigraphy has been used mainly for evaluating esophageal function. Recently, scintigraphy has also been used in adults to assess transit of a liquid bolus through the oropharynx (Hamlet, Muz, Patterson, & Jones, 1989; Holt et al., 1990; Humphreys et al., 1987). Silver et al. (1991) attempted to use nuclear scintigraphy for detecting and quantifying aspiration. Unfortunately, this technique proved to have poor sensitivity for detecting aspiration during swallowing in known aspirators. At present, clinical experience with this technique as a test of swallowing function in children is limited, and it should be used as an investigational tool.

References

Bosma, J. F., Hepburn, L. G., Josell, S. D., & Baker, K. (1990). Ultrasound demonstration of tongue motions during suckle feeding. *Developmental Medicine and Child Neurology, 32,* 223–229.

Bu'Lock, F., Woolridge, M. W., & Baum, J. D. (1990). Development of coordination of sucking, swallowing and breathing: Ultrasound study of term and preterm infants. *Developmental Medicine and Child Neurology, 32,* 669–678.

Cowan, R. J. (1989). Radionuclide evaluation of the esophagus in patients with dysphagia. In D. W. Gelfand, & J. E. Richter (Eds.), *Dysphagia: Diagnosis and treatment* (pp. 127–158). New York: Igaku-Shoin.

Hamlet, S. L., Muz, J., Patterson, R., & Jones, L. (1989). Pharyngeal transit time: Assessment with videofluoroscopy and scintigraphic techniques. *Dysphagia, 4,* 4–7.

Hogan, W. J., & Dodds, J. (1989). Gastroesophageal reflux disease (reflux esophagitis). In M. H. Sleisenger, & J. S. Fordtran (Eds.), *Gastrointestinal disease* (pp. 594–619). Philadelphia: W. B. Saunders.

Holt, S., Miron, S. D., Diaz, M. C., Shields, R., Ingram, D., & Bellon, E. M. (1990). Scintigraphic measurement of oropharyngeal transit in man. *Digestive Diseases and Sciences, 35,* 1198–1204.

Humphreys, B., Mathog, R., Rosen, R., Miller, P., Muz, J., & Nelson, R. (1987). Videofluoroscopic and scintigraphic analysis of dysphagia in the head and neck cancer patient. *Laryngoscope, 97,* 25–32.

Kenny, D. J., Casas, M. J., & McPherson, K. A. (1989). Correlation of ultrasound imaging of oral swallow and ventilatory alterations in cerebral palsied and normal children: Preliminary observations. *Dysphagia, 4,* 112–117.

Malagelada, J. R., Camilleri, M., & Stanghellini, V. (Eds.). (1986). *Manometric diagnosis of gastrointestinal motility disorders.* New York: Thieme.

Palmer, J. B. (1989). Electromyography of the muscles of oropharyngeal swallowing: Basic concepts. *Dysphagia, 3,* 192–198.

Richter, J. E., & Castell, J. A. (1989). Esophageal manometry. In D. W. Gelfand, & J. E. Richter (Eds.), *Dysphagia: Diagnosis and treatment* (pp. 83–114). New York: Igaku-Shoin.

Scott, B. (1991). Motility studies. In W. A. Walker, P. R. Durie, J. R. Hamilton, J. A. Walker-Smith, & J. B. Watkins (Eds.), *Pediatric gastrointestinal disease* (pp. 1324–1330). Philadelphia: B. C. Decker.

Shawker, T. H., Sonies, B., Hall, T. E., & Baum, B. F. (1984). Ultrasound analysis of tongue, hyoid, and larynx activity during swallowing. *Investigative Radiology, 19*(2), 82–86.

Shawker, T. H., Sonies, B. C., & Stone, M. (1984a). Soft tissue anatomy of the tongue and floor of the mouth: An ultrasound demonstration. *Brain and Language, 21,* 335–350.

Shawker, T. H., Sonies, B. C., & Stone, M. (1984b). Sonography of speech and swallowing. In R. C. Sanders & M. Hill (Eds.), *Ultrasound annual.* New York: Raven Press.

Shawker, T. H., Sonies, B., Stone, M., & Baum, B. J. (1983). Real-time ultrasound visualization of tongue movement during swallowing. *Journal of Clinical Ultrasound, 11,* 485–490.

Silver, K. H., Van Nostrand, D. V., Kuhlemeier, K. V., & Siebens, A. A. (1991). Scintigraphy for the detection and quantification of subglottic aspiration: Preliminary observations. *Archives of Physical Medicine and Rehabilitation, 72,* 902–910.

Smith, W. L., Erenberg, A., Nowak, A., & Franken, E. A. (1985). Physiology of sucking in the normal term infant using real-time ultrasound. *Radiology, 156,* 379–381.

Sonies, B. C., Eckman, E. F., Andersson, H. C., Adamson, M. D., Kaler, S. G., Markello, T. C., & Gahl, W. A. (1990). Swallowing dysfunction in nephropathic cystinosis. *New England Journal of Medicine, 323* (9), 565–570.

Sonies, B. C., Parent, L. J., Morrish, K., & Baum, B. J. (1988). Durational aspects of the oral-pharyngeal phase of swallow in normal adults. *Dysphagia, 3,* 1–10.

Weber, F., Woolridge, M. W., & Baum, J. D. (1986). An ultrasonographic study of the organization of sucking and swallowing by newborn infants. *Developmental Medicine and Child Neurology, 28,* 19–24.

Pulmonary Complications of Impaired Swallowing

12

CHAPTER

Susanna A. McColley, M.D.
John L. Carroll, M.D.

Mechanisms of Airway Protection

That passages are shared by the respiratory and digestive systems makes pulmonary aspiration of oral and gastric contents seem inevitable. In fact, aspiration of oropharyngeal contents appears to be a common event in healthy humans. Huxley, Viroslav, Gray, and Pierce (1978), using a technique that introduced small (1 ml) aliquots of radiolabeled liquid into the oropharynx during sleep, found tracer in the lungs in 45% of healthy adult subjects. A variety of airway protective mechanisms exist that limit aspiration and prevent it from causing disease. These mechanisms are summarized in Table 12–1. A review of normal airway protective mechanisms, emphasizing changes in airway protective mechanisms during growth and development, is presented to enhance understanding of pulmonary aspiration syndromes in infants and children.

Upper Airway Defense Mechanisms

The air and food passages arise from the hypopharynx together. The glottis and cricopharyngeus muscle are intimately related, with the cricoid cartilage serving as a fulcrum for the activity of both structures and as the main supporting structure for the tracheoesophageal septum. During swallowing, coordination of vocal cord closure with cricopharyngeal opening is the chief mechanism protecting the lower airways from contamination by food (Tucker, 1985). Palatal elevation and epiglottic tilt aid in propagation of food away from the airway and into the esophagus (Carpenter, 1989; Ogura, Kawaski, & Takenouchi, 1964).

The larynx is the most important structure protecting the lower airways from contamination. It is richly supplied with sensory receptors that respond to both mechanical and chemical stimuli via afferent pathways in the superior laryngeal

TABLE 12–1. Airway protective mechanisms.

I. Mechanisms preventing airway contamination
   A. Upper airway defense mechanisms
      1. laryngeal closure or cough in response to laryngeal
         or pharyngeal stimulation
      2. coordination of laryngeal closure and swallowing
      3. coordination of breathing and swallowing
   B. Lower airway defense mechanisms
      1. cough
      2. mucociliary clearance

II. Responses to lower airway contamination
   A. Clearance of particulate matter
      1. mucociliary clearance
      2. phagocytosis
   B. Clerance of bacteria
      1. mucociliary clearance
      2. antibody binding
      3. phagocytosis
      4. intracellular killings

nerve. Laryngeal closure occurs when the laryngeal epithelium is touched. Changes in airway pressure or flow also influence laryngeal aperture size, the aperture widening during inspiration and narrowing during expiration. Chemical irritants, such as acidic fluids, cause laryngeal closure in immature animals (Boggs & Bartlett, 1982; Kovar, Selstam, Cattenton, Stahlman, & Sundell, 1979). Newborns develop sustained apnea when water is placed on the larynx (Downing & Lee 1975; Johnson, Salisburg, & Storey, 1975). This response diminishes with age; it is replaced by cough, which serves as a major defense against aspiration throughout life (Bartlett, 1985).

Coordination of Breathing and Swallowing

Swallowing develops as early as 11 weeks gestation; sucking movements follow between 18 and 20 weeks, and the coordination of the two is acquired by term (Bosma, 1985; Diamant, 1985). Preterm infants have been noted to make inspiratory ef-

forts during swallowing (Wilson, Thach, Brouillette, & Abu-Osba, 1981). In these infants, swallows are initiated throughout the respiratory cycle; when swallows interrupt any phase of respiration, inspiratory efforts occur after airflow is interrupted (Figure 12–1). These inspiratory efforts, called "swallow-breaths," are postulated to serve a role in removing air from the pharynx, but may also make infants more vulnerable to aspiration. Bamford, Taciak, and Gewold (1992) found that term neonates also exhibited swallowing during all phases of respiration during suckle feeding. Inspiration and expiration were equally likely to precede swallowing, whereas expiration more frequently follows swallowing. In these infants, runs of repetitive swallows occurred more frequently than isolated swallows (Figure 12–2). The number of swallows contained in such runs increased with age. Respiratory rate and tidal volume were reduced during suckle feeding, and transient oxyhemoglobin desaturation occurred frequently. Thus, little coordination between breathing and swallowing was discernible, with swallowing

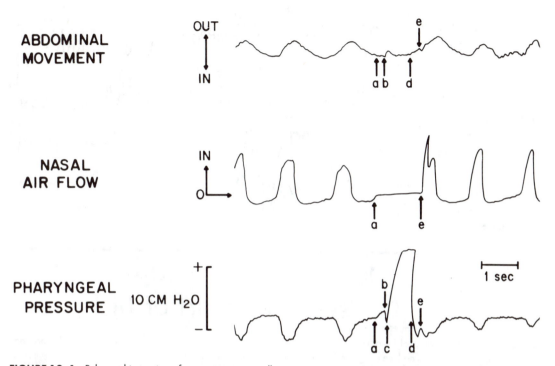

FIGURE 12-1. Polygraphic tracing of a spontaneous swallow interrupting expiration to show interaction of swallow and respiratory events. At **A**, airway closes in midexpiration at swallow onset; **B** marks onset of "swallow-breath," indicated by a brief outward abdominal movement; **C** marks beginning of pharyngeal pressure peak; at **D**, pharyngeal pressure falls; and at **E**, airway opens and inspiratory flow commences. (Reproduced with permission from Wilson, S. L., Thach, B. T., Brouillette, R. T., & Abu-Osba, 1980. Coordination of breathing and swallowing in human infants. *Journal of Applied Physiology, 50,* 851–858.)

often being maintained at the expense of respiration.

Few studies have examined the development of coordinated sucking, swallowing, and respiration in infants and children beyond the neonatal period. Available studies indicate that these processes mature over time (Bosma, 1985). In adults, swallowing during feeding occurs almost exclusively during expiration (Smith, Wolkove, Colacone, & Kreisman, 1989). This probably represents the end-point of maturation of coordinated swallowing and breathing, serving an important role in preventing pulmonary aspiration.

Swallowing occurs both during and apart from feeding. Adequate swallowing during feeding protects the airway from contamination by food; however, nonfeeding swallows may also be important in

clearance of pharyngeal secretions and regurgitated stomach contents (Thach & Menon, 1985). These nonfeeding swallows may be especially important in limiting aspiration of pharyngeal contents during sleep.

Lower Airway Defense Mechanisms

Although the upper airway serves a primary role in preventing pulmonary aspiration, the lower airways are equipped with several mechanisms that serve to clear aspirated material. These include cough, mucociliary clearance, and cell-mediated clearance of bacteria and other foreign substances.

Cough occurs when pharyngeal or laryngeal receptors are stimulated; it prevents foreign materials from entering the lower airways. In the lower airways, cough serves

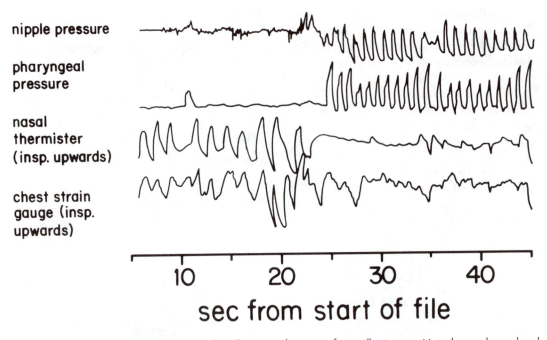

nipple pressure

pharyngeal pressure

nasal thermister (insp. upwards)

chest strain gauge (insp. upwards)

10   20   30   40

sec from start of file

FIGURE 12–2. Recordings of breathing and swallowing at the onset of a swallowing run. Note the regular oral and pharyngeal pressure waves and the irregular slow breathing as the swallow run starts. (Modified and reproduced with permission from Bamford, O., Taciak, U., & Gewald, I. H., 1992. The relationship between rhythmic swallowing and breathing during suckle feeding in term neonates. *Pediatric Research, 31*, 619–624.)

to expel foreign matter or abnormal secretions. This is mediated by receptors that are concentrated at the carina and bronchial bifurcations. Cough is a complex event that requires intact sensory pathways, central nervous system processing, and coordinated neuromuscular activity. It consists of a variable inspiratory phase, thought important in producing a high expiratory flow rate by increasing lung volume, a compressive phase, with glottic closure and onset of expiratory muscle activity; and an expiratory phase, which produces high flow rates leading to expulsion of material within the airways (Leith, 1985). Patients with impaired cough due to muscle weakness are at risk for lower airway contamination because of failure of clearance of aspirated contents from the airways. Furthermore, in patients with chronic aspiration syndromes, cough is often absent or inadequate, leading to repeated penetration of oral contents into the trachea and lower airways.

Whether this defect in cough is a cause or result of chronic aspiration is unclear.

Mucociliary function is important in the physical matter and in the provision of humoral and cellular constituents that defend the lower airways from infection. The respiratory epithelium is made up of ciliated columnar cells and goblet cells in a ratio of approximately 5:1. The cilia contain contractile elements and beat in a coordinated manner on both individual and adjacent cells. The cilia lie within periciliary fluid, a product of transepitheleal ion and water transport. This fluid supports a layer of mucus, secreted by submucosal glands and goblet cells, that moves towards the larynx as the cilia beat. Small foreign particles are trapped within the mucus layer and thus transported out of the lower airways. Mucus contains macromolecules, including immunoglobins and enzymes, that are important in defending the lower airway from infection (Wanner, 1985).

The pulmonary macrophage is the most abundant and important phagocytc cell found in the airways. Its membrane contains specific receptors for opsonic proteins, including immunoglobulin G, immunoglobulin E, and serum complement. These opsonins bind bacteria and facilitate phagocytosis. Immunoglobulin G is the predominant immunoglobulin in the distal airways; immunoglobulin A, the predominant immunoglobulin in the proximal airways, has not been found to have a receptor on the pulmonary macrophage. After phagocytosis, bacterial killing occurs through the activity of lysozyme and other hydrolytic enzymes.

Pulmonary macrophages arise from bone-marrow-derived circulating monocytes. Coincident with the extracellular release of surfactant into the alveoli prior to birth, an influx of pulmonary macrophages occurs. Scavenging of excess surfactant appears to be an important function of the pulmonary macrophage in the neonate; however, the presence of surfactant within macrophages appears to inhibit bacterial killing. This may contribute to the increased susceptibility of neonates to pulmonary infection.

Macrophages release chemotactically active substances that attract polymorphonuclear leukocytes. These and other inflammatory cells, which are recruited from the vascular space, aid in phagocytosis and bacterial killing. Pulmonary macrophage chemotactic factors also elicit release of lysosomal enzymes from recruited polymorphonuclear leukocytes; these enzymes cause local destruction of pulmonary tissue, inactivation of complement, and decreased activity of alpha-1 antiprotease. This inflammatory response may result in irreversible injury to pulmonary tissue.

Pulmonary lymphocytes, a small but important constituent of airway cells, are required for normal pulmonary macrophage activity. B-lymphocytes interact with bacterial antigens and, with assistance from helper T-cells, transform into plasmacytes that secrete antibody. Antibody, in turn, binds to bacteria to promote phagocytosis. Lymphocytes arise from the bone marrow; T-cells differentiate within the thymus. Helper T-cell activity and immunoglobulin G secretion are incompletely developed at birth, while immunoglobulin M secretion is fully mature (Fick, 1985).

Airway Responses to Aspiration

There are three mechanisms by which impaired swallowing may lead to respiratory disease. The first is the entry of oropharyngeal contents, consisting of food and/or saliva, into the airway during or between swallows. This is direct aspiration (DA). The second is the entry of gastric contents into the airway, or aspiration of gastric contents (AGC). This may occur as a result of gastroesophageal reflux (GER/AGC) or vomiting. GER without aspiration of gastric contents has also been implicated as a cause of or contributor to respiratory disease. In the following discussion, GER refers to GER without AGC. Although these processes may represent a continuum of impaired swallowing and may exist at different times in the same subject, their consequences will be discussed separately for clarity.

Apnea

The term *apnea* refers to a cessation of air movement into and out of the lungs. This may occur due to lack of respiratory muscle activity, called *central apnea*, or due to upper airway obstruction with continued respiratory efforts, called *obstructive apnea*. Episodes of apnea may have components of both central and obstructive apnea; these episodes are called *mixed apnea*. Brief episodes of apnea occur in normal infants and children; pathologic apnea is characterized by long duration, prolonged hypoxemia, or bradycardia.

Apnea appears to occur more commonly in response to DA in infants than in older children and adults. This is probably a consequence of laryngeal reflex activity previously discussed. Nasal receptors may also play a role. Apnea has been shown to result from nasopharyngeal reflux during feeding and to resolve with feeding techniques that avoid such reflux (Plaxico & Loughlin, 1981). Brief, self-resolving episodes of apnea have been noted to occur in healthy term neonates during feeding (Matthew, Clark, & Pronske, 1985); an exaggeration of this response, or its occurrence beyond the neonatal period, has been hypothesized as a factor in pathologic apnea or sudden infant death syndrome (SIDS).

GER has been described in infants with pathologic apnea and apparent life-threatening events (ALTE), formerly called "near-miss SIDS." Apnea and cyanosis have been found to be temporally related to acid reflux or regurgitation in infants with near-miss SIDS (Herbst, Book, & Bray, 1978) and apnea of prematurity and idiopathic prolonged apnea (Menon, Schefft, & Thach, 1985). Apnea has been shown to occur during acid perfusion of the esophagus in infants with a history of apnea and lung disease (Herbst, Minton, & Book, 1979), and to cease or decrease in frequency with medical or surgical therapy for GER (Herbst et al., 1978, 1979). Significant hypoxemia has been found in relation to GER during sleep in infants with a history of ALTE (See et al., 1989), even in the absence of apnea. Laryngospasm due to laryngeal chemoreceptor reflexes has been proposed as the etiology for apneic episodes, which are most often obstructive in nature. However, reflexes arising from the esophagus, pharynx, or trachea cannot be excluded based on methods used in these studies.

Lower Respiratory Tract Sequelae of Aspiration of Gastric Contents

Mendelson (1946) first brought attention to the effects of AGC in his report of this syndrome complicating obstetrical anesthesia. Two distinct processes were identified. The first, aspiration of solid material, occurred only rarely and resulted in laryngeal or bronchial obstruction, leading to suffocation or massive atelectasis. The second, aspiration of liquid stomach contents, led to an immediate "asthmatic-like syndrome," with cyanosis, tachycardia, dyspnea, wheezes, and rales. Massive pulmonary edema often ensued. To explore the pathology of this process, hydrochloric acid, vomitus, neutralized vomitus, or saline were administered intratracheally to rabbits. Rabbits given hydrochloric acid or vomitus developed the asthmatic-like syndrome. Pulmonary edema, subpleural hemorrhage, emphysematous blebs, bronchiolar necrosis, and exudate were present on pathologic examination. In contrast, administration of saline or neutralized vomitus caused a period of labored respiration and cyanosis, with spontaneous recovery within hours and without significant pathologic changes.

Although aspiration of liquids at pH less than 2.5 is associated with the most acute and profound pulmonary damage, aspiration of liquids at any pH has been found to cause significant damage. Aspiration of gastric liquid at a pH of 4.0 or higher causes acute pulmonary inflammation (Bond, Stoetling, & Gupta, 1979; Schwartz et al., 1980), and even experimental inhalation of antacid agents (Editorial, 1980; Gibbs, Schwartz, Wynne, Hood, & Kuck, 1979) and liquid at a neutral pH leads to pulmonary damage (Alexander, 1968). Aspiration of food particles alters the inflammatory response, leading to an influx of polymorphonuclear leukocytes and granuloma formation (Moran, 1951).

Single episodes of aspiration of small volumes of acidic liquid produce fewer acute changes, but still lead to interstitial pneumonitis, interstitial thickening, and pulmonary fibrosis (Moran, 1955). Additional evidence suggests that the aspirate need not reach the lower airways for lower airway responses to occur. Stimulation of tracheal irritant receptors may lead to bronchoconstriction through vagal pathways (Fillenz & Widdicombe, 1977; Widdicombe, 1954; Zimmerman, Ulmer, & Weller, 1979). In cats, tracheal instillation of only 0.05 ml of 0.2 N hydrochloric acid evokes a significant increase in total lung resistance; this change does not occur with instillation of saline (Tuchman et al., 1984). In humans with asthma or bronchitis, inhaled citric acid produces a similar increase in lung resistance; radiolabeling of the citric acid solution shows that it remains within the trachea (Simonsson, Jacobs, & Nadel, 1967). These and other findings have lead to the hypothesis that *microaspiration*, defined as aspiration of very small volumes of gastric contents, can lead to recurrent or chronic respiratory symptoms in the absence of acute or dramatic symptoms.

Respiratory Responses to Esophageal Acidification

Although microaspiration has been advanced as an explanation for pulmonary symptoms related to GER, other reports have suggested that GER may cause or exacerbate lung disease in the absence of AGC.

Reflux of acid into the distal esophagus may stimulate mucosal receptors that alter pulmonary mechanics via vagal reflexes. Acid perfusion of the esophagus has been shown to increase total lung resistance in dogs and in humans with esophagitis (Mansfield, Hameister, Spaulding, Smith, & Glab, 1981; Mansfield & Stein, 1978; Spaulding, Mansfield, Stein, Sellner, & Gremillion, 1982). Infusion of acid into the esophagus causes an increase in total lung resistance in cats and in humans with asthma; however, the magnitude of this increase is much less than that observed with tracheal acidification (Mansfield & Stein, 1978; Tuchman et al., 1984). Although it is possible that some microaspiration occurred during these studies, the potential of esophageal acidification alone

to cause or worsen respiratory symptoms clearly exists and merits further study.

Clinical Manifestations

Respiratory disorders and their associated disorders of swallowing are summarized in Table 12–2.

Apnea and Apparent Life-threatening Events

An apparent life-threatening event (ALTE) is described by the National Institutes of Health (1987) as:

> An episode that is frightening to the observer and that is characterized by some combination of apnea, color change, marked change in muscle tone, choking, or gagging. In some cases, the observer fears that the infant has died. (p. 4)

A number of studies have demonstrated a temporal relationship between apnea and GER in infants with a history of ALTE or observed apnea (Herbst et al., 1978, 1979; MacFayden, Hendry, & Simpson, 1983; Menon et al., 1984, 1985); in fact, GER is the most common abnormality diagnosed in infants presenting with ALTE (Jeffrey, Rahilly, & Read, 1983; Kahn, Montauk, & Blum, 1987; Trowitzsch, Meyer, Schluter, Buschatz, & Andler, 1992). Spitzer, Boyle, Tuchman, and Fox (1984) described a specific syndrome of sudden apnea: staring, rigid or opisthotonic posture, and color change following feeding during wakefulness. Concurrent obstructive apnea and GER were demonstrated by polygraphic monitoring. It is notable that most of the infants described in these studies did not have a history of frequent emesis that might otherwise lead to the diagnosis of GER. Further evidence for an association between GER and apnea is provided by studies demonstrating resolution of recurrent apneic episodes after medical or

TABLE 12–2. Respiratory presentations of swallowing impairment.

Respiratory Symptom	Associated Swallowing Abnormalities
Apnea and apparent life-threatening events	Direct aspiration Gastroesophageal reflux
Acute aspiration pneumonitis	Aspiration of gastric contents
Chronic lower respiratory tract disease	
Cough, wheeze, hoarseness	Direct aspiration Gastroesophageal reflux with aspiration of gastric contents Gastroesophageal reflux alone (controversial)
Recurrent pneumonia	Direct aspiration Gastroesophageal reflux with aspiration of gastric contents
With underlying lung disease	Direct aspiration Gastroesophageal reflux with aspiration of gastric contents Gastroesophageal reflux alone (controversial)

surgical treatment for GER (Herbst et al., 1979; Leape, Holder, Franklin, Amoury, & Ashcraft, 1977; Ramenofsky & Leape, 1981).

It should be noted that GER has never been proven to be temporally associated with an ALTE. The above studies inferred that GER-associated apnea and ALTE are related. Several studies have disputed this relationship; for example, Ariagno, Guilleminault, Coroblan, Owen-Boeddiker, and Baldwin (1983) reported no relationship between GER and apneic events in infants undergoing simultaneous recording of esophageal pH and respiratory parameters for near-miss SIDS. Methodologic limitations to this and other studies have been discussed (Putman, Ricker, & Orenstein, 1992). Available evidence suggests that a relationship between GER, apnea, and ALTE exists, and that treating GER may prevent recurrence of ALTE. GER is not the only cause of ALTE, and demonstrating the relationship of GER to apnea or ALTE in a given subject is often difficult. Therefore, infants presenting with this

syndrome should have a careful history, physical examination, and laboratory tests as needed to exclude systemic infection, central nervous system abnormalities, or metabolic disorders.

Acute Aspiration Pneumonitis

Despite widespread recognition of the risk of aspiration of gastric contents and the use of measures to decrease its incidence, acute aspiration pneumonitis remains a significant cause of morbidity and mortality. Aspirated gastric acid travels through the tracheobronchial tree in seconds, causing a rapid onset of diffuse damage. It occurs most frequently in patients who are unconscious due to illness, injury, or anesthesia; patients with endotracheal or tracheostomy tube placement; and patients with debilitating diseases, especially neuromuscular diseases that cause swallowing impairment. Patients in intensive care units and those undergoing emergency surgery are at particularly high risk. A high volume and low pH of gastric contents increase the risk of aspiration. Because gastric volume and acidity decrease with age, children theoretically are at high risk.

Respiratory distress, dry cough, and hypoxemia are the initial manifestations of acid aspiration. Rales may be heard in the early stages, but decrease as widespread pulmonary consolidation occurs. Severe hypoxemia occurs as edema progresses. The clinical picture is often that of the adult respiratory distress syndrome. Hypotension may occur; hypercapnia is unusual, except when particulate matter is aspirated. Purulent sputum may later develop, indicating the presence of bacterial superinfection.

The chest roentgenogram shows bilateral airspace diseases that range from irregular opacities to bilateral complete consolidation ("white-out"). Perihilar and basal regions are most involved. Findings may be asymmetric, probably dependent on the patient's position at the time of the aspiration event. Roentgenographic changes improve rapidly over a variable time period lasting one to several days.

The mortality rate is very high (Wynne et al., 1979). Complete resolution of pulmonary abnormalities occurs in most survivors; however, recovery may be prolonged, and some patients develop chronic respiratory insufficiency.

Chronic Lower Respiratory Tract Disease

Direct aspiration, GER, and GER/ACG are common causes of chronic or recurrent respiratory disease in infants and children. It is well-recognized that children who have undergone surgical repair of esophageal atresia and those with stable or progressive neurological diseases are at particularly high risk (Byrne, Campbell, & Ashcraft, 1983; Chrispin, Friedland, & Waterson, 1966; Shermeta, Whitington, Seto, & Haller, 1977; Whittington, Shermeta,

Seto, Jones, & Hendrix, 1977). However, even otherwise normal children may develop significant respiratory disease due to impaired swallowing. This may occur due to isolated developmental abnormalities of the cricopharyngeus muscle (Diamant, 1985). In otherwise normal children, the diagnosis is often delayed because no recognized risk factor is evident and because aspiration episodes are subtle or "silent." Early diagnosis and treatment have the potential of preventing chronic lung disease in this otherwise healthy population.

Symptoms include cough, wheezing, and congestion. Parents frequently describe "rattling in the chest." Apnea, stridor, or hoarseness may coexist. Some patients develop recurrent episodes of fever and dyspnea. Rhonchi and rales are noted on physical examination, and atelectasis or infiltrates are seen on chest roentgenogram (Figure 12–3) (Berquist, Rachelefsky, Kadden, Siegel, et al., 1991; Christie, O'Grady, & Mack 1978; Danus, Casar, Larrain, & Pope, 1976; Euler et al., 1979; Hoyaux, Forget, Lambrechts, & Geubelle, 1985). In some of these patients, aspiration leads to bacterial pneumonia, which may be recurrent. Severe complications, such as lung abscess or empyema (Figure 12–4) may result. Other patients have less dramatic but chronic symptoms, such as cough and wheeze. In fact, infants and young children with chronic aspiration syndromes often present with wheezing that is unresponsive to bronchodilator therapy.

A history of coughing or choking during feeding, recurrent regurgitation or emesis, or irritability is suggestive of respiratory disease due to impaired swallowing. However, quite often, infants and children with respiratory disease due to chronic DA or GER do not have symptoms of feeding difficulty or frequent emesis that suggest these processes. Nocturnal cough is often present (Euler et al., 1979). Chest auscultation during and after feeding may reveal adventitial sounds that were decreased or absent prior to feeding. Absence of these findings does not rule

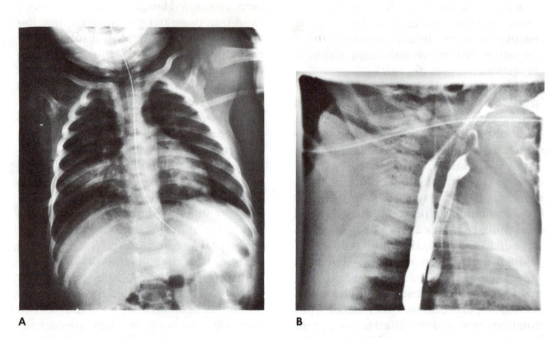

FIGURE 12–3. A. Right upper lobe pneumonia in a 5-month-old boy. **B.** Esophagram reveals direct aspiration during each swallow. (Courtesy of Dr. George Taylor.)

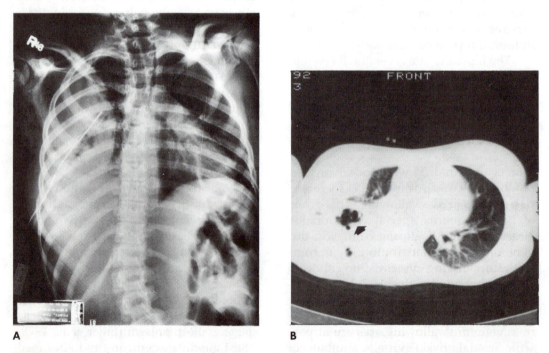

FIGURE 12–4. A. Chest roentgenogram and **B.** CT scan revealing empyema and lung abcess (*arrow*) in a 13-year-old girl with a history of mental retardation and gastroesophageal reflux. (Courtesy of Dr. George Taylor.)

out DA or GER as a cause of lung disease. These processes should be strongly suspected in any infant or child with unexplained chronic or recurrent respiratory disease.

Less common but important clinical presentations of chronic aspiration syndromes are severe, progressive chronic lung diseases. Diffuse pulmonary fibrosis has been described in adults (Mays, Dubois, & Hamilton, 1976; Pearson & Wilson, 1971); bronchiolitis obliterans (Hardy, Schidlow, & Zaeri, 1988) and chronic lipoid pneumonia (Fisher, Roggli, Merten, Mulvihill, & Spock, 1992) have been described in children. The latter has been described in children with underlying immunodeficiency, cardiac disease, or other medical conditions. In these children, nodular opacities were demonstrated on chest roentgenogram, and lung biopsy pathology showed features of endogenous lipoid pneumonia, cholesterol granulomas, and pulmonary alveolar proteinosis. The 63% mortality rate noted in this report underscores the need for aggressive diagnosis and therapy in children presenting with this clinical picture.

Underlying Respiratory Disease Complicated by Impaired Swallowing

Infants and children with underlying respiratory disease appear to be at increased risk for impaired swallowing. This group of patients merits special consideration because of the diagnostic confusion that may result from attributing symptoms to the underlying disease. Subjects with bronchopulmonary dysplasia (BPD), asthma, and cystic fibrosis (CF) appear to be at high risk for respiratory complications of impaired swallowing, particularly of GER. Several physiologic alterations occur in these disorders that may predispose patients to GER. First, pulmonary hyperinflation causes an alteration in diaphragm

configuration that may reduce lower esophageal sphincter (LES) pressure. Second, increased abdominal pressure during coughing promotes GER. Finally, medications used to decrease bronchomotor tone may also decrease LES pressure. Children with lung disease may be more vulnerable to the effects of GER, ACG, or DA. The resultant inflammatory and bronchoconstrictive responses are more likely to cause significant impairment of pulmonary function in patients who have underlying inflammation, increased mucous production, and hyperreactivity of the tracheobronchial tree.

Premature infants with BPD have a high prevalence of GER (Hrabovsky & Mullet, 1986). Although GER is common in infants (Vandeplas & Sacre-Smits, 1987) the finding of clinical improvement after antireflux therapy (St. Cyr, Ferrara, Thompson, Johnson, & Foker, 1989) indicates that GER contributes to lung disease in these patients. Infants born prematurely are also at high risk for impaired swallowing due to neurologic injury; this may lead to additional pulmonary damage through DA or GER/AGC. Although epidemiologic studies to address the incidence of impaired swallowing in BPD are not available, clinical experience suggests that swallowing impairment is a significant problem in this population. Infants and young children with severe BPD, or BPD that appears to be worsening rather than improving over time, should undergo assessment for impaired swallowing.

Gastroesophageal reflux occurs more commonly in children with asthma than in otherwise healthy children (Gustafsson, Kjellman, & Tibbling). This appears to be particularly significant in children with nocturnal or early morning wheezing (Davis, Larsen, & Grunstein, 1983). Many patients have symptoms or a positive Bernstein test (reproduction of a symptom, usually chest pain, during acid perfusion of the esophagus) suggestive of esophagitis. Although theophylline has been shown to decrease LES pressure in normal subjects (Berquist, Rachelefsky, Kadden, Siegel, Katz, et al., 1981), the use of theophylline or metaproterenol has not been shown to increase GER in children with asthma (Berquist et al., 1984). Thus, a decrease in bronchodilator therapy is probably not indicated on the basis of nocturnal or morning symptoms alone. However, in children with severe refractory asthma, a history compatible with esophagitis should be sought. Even in the absence of a positive history, diagnostic evaluation for GER should be considered, particularly when nocturnal and morning symptoms are prominent.

GER has been noted in CF both as an incidental finding (Guide to Diagnosis, 1979; Matseche, Go, & Di Magno, 1977) and as a cause of gastrointestinal bleeding (Bendig, Seilheimer, Wagner, Ferry, & Harrison, 1982). Children with CF have symptoms of GER more frequently than their unaffected siblings (Scott, O'Loughlin, & Gall, 1985). GER may contribute to poor appetite and malaise as well as to respiratory symptoms. It is important to note that, even in children with GER, nighttime nasogastric tube feedings do not impair pulmonary function (Scott et al., 1985). This important modality of nutritional rehabilitation should not be withheld due to suspicion of GER. The contribution of GER to the progression of CF lung disease has not been investigated.

Evaluation

Initial evaluation consists of the history and physical examination and a chest roentgenogram to evaluate the presence of lower respiratory tract disease. A number of other diagnostic tools are available to aid in the diagnosis of respiratory abnormalities due to aspiration and GER. Three general strategies are employed. The first is to document the presence of impaired swallowing and/or GER and infer that these processes cause or contribute to the respiratory process. The second is to docu-

ment the presence of pulmonary pathology due to aspiration. The third is to document a temporal relationship between GER or DA events and respiratory symptoms or changes in pulmonary function. The last strategy is most satisfactory but also most difficult to achieve. In difficult cases, a trial of therapy designed to bypass the upper airway during feeding and/or to prevent GER may be indicated as a diagnostic test.

Radiographic Studies

Demonstrating that oral or gastric contents enter the lower airways is a frequent method of linking aspiration to respiratory symptoms. This can be accomplished by demonstrating contamination of the lower airways by a radioopaque substance or radioactive tracer given by mouth or tube feeding.

The barium esophagram is a useful initial procedure in the diagnosis of respiratory disease due to impaired swallowing. The finding of isolated laryngeal penetration of contrast material, or episodes of GER not associated with aspiration, may not allow confirmation of a relationship between aspiration and pulmonary symptoms. As a single study, a barium esophagram is inadequate to exclude the diagnosis of GER. However, demonstration of contrast material within the trachea and bronchi strongly suggests that enough material can be aspirated to cause significant respiratory disease. Furthermore, the barium esophagram is useful in evaluating anatomic abnormalities that lead to impaired swallowing and aspiration, such as a vascular ring or H-type tracheoesophageal fistula. In patients with suspected GER, the barium esophagram should be combined with an upper GI series to rule out anatomic obstruction to gastric emptying. In patients who are fed via nasogastric or gastrostomy tube, a barium study through the tube may reveal high-grade GER, sometimes with airway contamination (Figure 12–5).

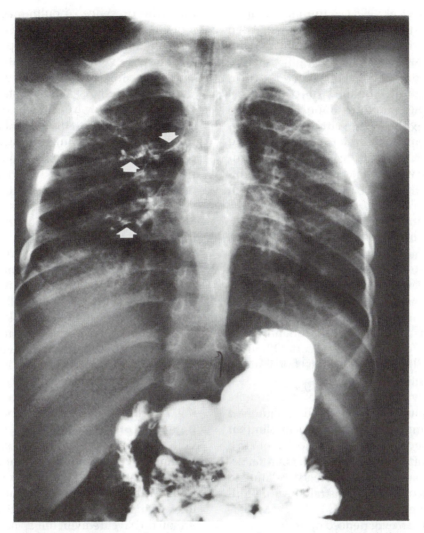

FIGURE 12–5. Barium introduced via gastrostomy tube is present in the bronchial tree (*arrows*) in a 3-year-old boy with respiratory disease following neurologic injury and percutaneous endoscopic gastrostomy tube placement.

Videofluoroscopy, discussed in Chapter 10, gives more information regarding the presence of impaired swallowing than a standard barium esophagram. This study is appropriate as an initial evaluation in children with suspected DA during feeding, because it is more sensitive in detecting both aspiration of small quantities of pharyngeal contents and abnormalities of swallowing that may lead to intermittent aspiration. Anatomic abnormalities also may be assessed using this method. The decision to perform a standard esophagram versus a videofluoroscopic study must be based on the degree to which DA is suspected, the availability of highly trained personnel, and the time and cost involved. In children with history and physical examination findings suggesting DA during feeding, use of videofluoroscopy as an initial procedure appears justified. In contrast, when findings are suggestive of GER or if aspiration disorders are being considered in evaluating lung disease of obscure etiology, a standard esophagram is a satisfactory initial procedure.

Radionuclide milk scanning is performed by adding a radioactive tracer to milk or infant formula. After the milk is taken, a gamma camera is used to image the thorax both immediately and over several (up to 24) hours. Appearance of tracer in the lungs is diagnostic of pulmonary aspiration. "Milk scans" may be more sensitive than the barium esophagram in detecting pulmonary aspiration in infants and children (McVeagh, Howman-Giles, & Kemp, 1987). The chief disadvantages are that meticulous care must be taken to ensure that skin and clothing are not contaminated with tracer, thus giving a false positive result, and the time and patient cooperation required.

Fiberoptic Bronchoscopy with Bronchoalveolar Lavage

Bronchoalveolar lavage (BAL) is a method of obtaining lower airway cell samples that has been evaluated as a diagnostic tool in a number of pulmonary disorders. In recurrent aspiration, lipid material related to dietary fat can be demonstrated within pulmonary macrophages. BAL should be performed by an experienced operator. A flexible instrument should be used to allow entry into distal airways. In children, 5–10 ml aliquots of 0.9% sodium chloride are introduced through the instrument, then suctioned after 5–10 seconds. Specimens are pooled, centrifuged, and stained with oil Red O. Quantitative methods are preferable to simple qualititative demonstration in assessing results (Davis, Larsen, & Grunstein, 1983).

The finding of numerous lipid laden macrophages (LLM) strongly suggests aspiration-related pulmonary disease. However, some LLM may be present in health and in other pulmonary disorders. Nussbaum, Maggi, Mathis, and Galant (1987) evaluated children with respiratory dis-

ease with and without GER as documented by esophageal pH monitoring, barium esophogram, and esophagoscopy. It should be noted that none of the children in either study group had DA. LLM were demonstrated by BAL in 85% of children with GER but also in 19% of children without GER. Furthermore, in the presence of acute or chronic bronchopulmonary infection, cells obtained by BAL may be predominantly neutrophils, making demonstration of LLM difficult. Thus, although demonstration of numerous LLM is indicative of aspiration-related pulmonary disease, lack of LLM may be misleading. The paucity of studies of LLM in BAL specimens from children further underscores the uncertainty in use of this procedure as a sole diagnostic test for aspiration-related respiratory disease. It may be useful in combination with esophagoscopy in patients with suspected esophagitis and respiratory symptoms related to GER.

Polygraphic Monitoring and Esophageal pH Studies

Attempting to document a temporal relationship between GER with or without aspiration and respiratory symptoms is most likely to be successful in infants and children who have frequent but episodic symptoms. Establishing causation requires simultaneous demonstration of episodes of GER and the associated respiratory abnormality. Currently available techniques for noninvasive monitoring allow simultaneous recording of esophageal pH, heart and respiratory rates, airflow, and oxyhemoglobin saturation at bedside over several hours. Further data, such as EEG sleep staging and end tidal carbon dioxide concentrations, can also be obtained when patients are studied in the polysomnography laboratory. Finding simultaneous GER and apnea, bradycardia, or oxygen desaturation is strong evidence that these processes are related. However, frequently no abnormal respiratory events are discerned. Because of the time and cost involved, and the difficulty in interpreting negative results, this type of study is best used in patients with symptoms that are very severe, very frequent, or both. Infants with ALTE requiring resuscitation meet these criteria, because a high percentage may have another episode of ALTE and treating GER may prevent recurrence. Infants and children with frequently observed episodes of apnea or nocturnal wheezing are also good candidates. In contrast, subjects who have sporadic respiratory symptoms are less likely to demonstrate diagnostic abnormalities during recording.

There is limited experience using the pH probe study without simultaneous respiratory monitoring to predict respiratory symptoms. Different patterns of GER may exist in infants with GER who do and do not have respiratory symptoms. Sleep-related GER occurs in infants with GER and ALTE but not in those with GER manifested by persistent emesis (Newman et al., 1989). Children with GER-related respiratory disease have more GER during sleep than children with respiratory disease unrelated to GER (Holly, Jolley, Tunell, Johnson, & Sterling, 1991). Thus, pH probe studies may be useful in instances where simultaneous monitoring of esophageal pH and respiratory parameters is not available, as well as in the many infants and children with respiratory disease who have symptoms of GER, such as frequent emesis and irritability.

Therapeutic Trial

There are often clinical situations in which chronic respiratory disease and some degree of DA/GER coexist, yet the relationship between these processes is not clear. Demonstrating the relationship between respiratory symptoms and swallowing dysfunction is often necessary for therapeutic decision making. In these cases, a trial of nasogastric tube feeding or intravenous fluids, nothing by mouth, and/or pharma-

cotherapy for GER may be useful. If this therapy leads to a dramatic improvement in symptoms, a direct relationship between feeding and respiratory symptoms can be inferred. Unfortunately, the converse is not always true, because severe pulmonary inflammation may cause prolonged symptoms even when ongoing aspiration is prevented.

General Strategy

Given the different presentations of respiratory disease related to impaired swallowing and the variety of diagnostic tests available, choosing an approach for an individual patient may be difficult. Literature on the subject often combines groups of patients with several respiratory manifestations of impaired swallowing, such as apnea, recurrent pneumonia, and chronic respiratory symptoms. In choosing a strategy for an individual patient, the clinician must decide what specific questions need to be answered to (a) demonstrate the suspected disorder of swallowing and (b) demonstrate a relationship between the disorder and the resultant respiratory symptoms. In patients with history and physical examination findings that are suggestive of respiratory disease related to impaired swallowing, the former may be sufficient. In many patients, more than one test will be necessary. Suggested approaches to patients with various presentations is suggested in Table 12–3. The approach to patients with respiratory symptoms due to impaired swallowing requires an interdisciplinary approach, with close cooperation between the pediatrician, pulmonologist, swallowing therapist, and gastroenterologist.

Therapy

Apnea

Treatment of apnea due to impaired swallowing is based on treating the underlying

TABLE 12–3. Approach to evaluation of impaired swallowing in children with respiratory symptoms.

Patients	Approach
All patients	History and physical examination
	Observation and chest examination during and after feeding
	Chest roentgenogram
Patients with respiratory symptoms during and/or immediately following feeding	Modified barium swallow
	Trial of NG tube feeding
Patients with respiratory symptoms and frequent spitting or emesis	Esophagram and upper GI series and/or radionuclide milk scan
	Trial of antireflux medication and/or esophageal pH probe study with respiratory recording and/or esophagoscopy with bronchoscopy and BAL for LLM
Patients with respiratory symptoms during sleep	Esophagram
	Esophageal pH probe study with polysomnography
Patients with respiratory symptoms without other manifestations of impaired swallowing; if findings equivocal or lung disease severe or progressive	Evaluationt to exclude other causes of chronic lung disease
	Esophagram
	BAL for LLM, if bronchoscopy being performed in diagnostic evaluation
	Modified barium swallow and/or esophageal pH probe study with respiratory recording and/or radionuclide milk scan

pathology: DA, GER, or GER/AGC. Some patients with GER respond well to medical therapy; those who do not often improve with fundoplication (St. Cyr et al., 1989). We recommend home cardiorespiratory monitoring as an adjunct to therapy for GER because the adequacy of antireflux therapy for this indication cannot be readily assessed and because there is often doubt as to the relationship between GER and ALTE in individual patients. Monitors with a memory are most useful, because respiratory and heart rate pattern during episodes of apnea can be reviewed (Carroll, Marcus, & Loughlin, in press). We often continue monitoring after medical therapy for GER is discontinued to ensure that any recurrence of apnea is promptly recognized. It should be noted that no studies have documented a decrease in mortality in infants who are monitored for ALTE.

Acute Pulmonary Aspiration

Infants or children who are witnessed to aspirate or possibly aspirate food or stomach contents should be evaluated promptly by physical examination, chest roentgenography, and arterial blood gas analysis or pulse oximetry. In the absence of hypoxemia or signs of airway obstruction by food, patients may be observed expectantly. Nothing should be given by mouth. Symptoms may not occur immediately, but usually develop within 12 hours after aspiration. Patients who develop respiratory distress and/or hypoxemia should be cared for in a pediatric intensive care unit where treatment of respiratory failure and hypotension can be initiated as needed. Vigilant assessment for bacterial superinfection, and early use of antibiotics when infection occurs, is important; antibiotic prophylaxis probably does not improve outcome (Hickling & Howard, 1988). Administration of corticosteroids is probably of no benefit. Prevention of recurrence is another goal of therapy; this includes administration of antacids and recognition and treatment of predisposing factors.

Chronic Pulmonary Aspiration

The major goal of therapy for respiratory symptoms related to chronic pulmonary aspiration is to prevent recurrent aspiration, thereby decreasing ongoing pulmonary inflammation. Treatment decisions must take into account both the severity of the pulmonary process and the demonstrated severity of the swallowing disorder. We have found it necessary to treat patients with impaired swallowing and pulmonary dysfunction more aggressively than patients with an apparently similar disorder of swallowing but without pulmonary dysfunction. It is important to recognize that the lung is not completely developed at birth, that lung growth continues into early childhood, and that insults to the developing lung may impair pulmonary function into adulthood. Thus, aggressive prevention of pulmonary insult has the potential to avert permanent pulmonary damage and its sequelae.

In patients with lower respiratory disease related to DA, a trial of nasogastric tube feedings often results in a decrease in symptoms. This suggests that a feeding strategy that bypasses the upper airway is appropriate therapy. Long-term nasogastric tube feeding should be avoided because of the risk of accidental dislodging of the tube with subsequent aspiration. Surgical or percutaneous endoscopic gastrostomy tube placement has been useful in some cases. However, we have often seen recurrence or worsening of symptoms in patients with significant lung disease due to DA after such placement. This presumably results from GER with aspiration. It must be recognized that, in children with severe impairment of upper airway protective mechanisms, even rare episodes of GER may result in significant AGC. Therefore, any child undergoing gastrostomy tube placement for DA resulting in respiratory symptoms should be considered at risk, and strong consideration should be given to medical or surgical antireflux therapy.

Adjuncts to treating the underlying cause of lung disease depend on the specific clinical manifestations and their severity. In patients with atelectasis or infiltrates, chest physiotherapy may be useful. A head-down position should be avoided in patients with GER. Chest physiotherapy should be given when the patient has an empty stomach to avoid promoting GER (Vandeplas, Diericx, Blecker, Langiers, & Deneyer, 1991). Inhaled beta agonist therapy is useful in children with persistent wheezing; theophylline, which may exacerbate GER, should be avoided. Corticosteroids may be beneficial in decreasing pulmonary inflammation in children with wheezing or in those with severe inflammatory parenchymal disease such as bronchiolitis obliterans.

The most critical factor in treatment is close patient followup. Growth, development, and pulmonary symptoms must be monitored closely. Therapeutic plans may need modification either because pulmonary symptoms persist or because the swallowing impairment improves over time. Finally, families of children with pulmonary diseases due to or complicated by impaired swallowing experience significant psychosocial stress and need ongoing support by the professional team.

Outcome

Numerous studies have suggested that respiratory disease due to impaired swallowing improves with treatment. However, studies emphasizing long-term follow-up are not available. The severity of lung disease at the time of initial diagnosis, the presence of neurological or other medical problems, and the ability to effectively treat the underlying disorder undoubtedly influence outcome. Studies of intermediate and long-term outcome are needed to assess current therapy and to counsel families of children with this spectrum of disorders.

References

Alexander, I. G. S. (1968). The ultrastructure of the pulmonary alveolar vessels in Mendelson's (acid pulmonary aspiration) syndrome. British *Journal of Anesthesia, 40,* 408–414.

Ariagno, R. L., Guilleminault, C., Coroblan, R., Owen-Boeddiker, M., & Baldwin, R. (1983). "Near-miss" for sudden infant death syndrome infants: A clinical problem. *Pediatrics, 71,* 726–730.

Bamfor, O., Taciak, V., & Gewold, I. H. (1992). The relationship between rhythmic swallowing and breathing during suckle feeding in term neonates. *Pediatric Research, 31,* 726–730.

Bartlett, D., Jr. (1985). Ventilatory and protective mechanisms of the infant larynx. *American Review of Respiratory Disease, 131* (Suppl.) S49–S50.

Bendig, D. W., Seilheimer, D. K., Wagner, M. L., Ferry, G. D., & Harrison, G. M. (1982). Complications of gastroesophageal reflux in patients with cystic fibrosis. *Journal of Pediatrics, 100,* 536–540.

Berquist, W. E., Rachelefsky, G. S., Kadden, M., Siegel, S. C., et al. (1981). Gastroesophageal reflux-associated recurrent pneumonia and chronic asthma in children. *Pediatrics, 68,* 29–35.

Berquist, W. E., Rachelefsky, G. S., Kadden, M., Siegel, S. C., Katz, R. M., Mickey, M. R., & Ament, M. E. (1981). Effect of theophylline on gastroesophageal reflux in normal adults. *Journal of Allergy and Clinical Immunology, 67,* 407–411.

Berquist, W. E., Rachelefsky, G. S., Rowshan, N., Siegel, S., Katz, R., & Welch, M. (1984). Quantitative gastroesophageal reflux and

pulmonary function in asthmatic children and normal adults receiving placebo, theophylline, and metaproterenol sulfate therapy. *Journal of Allergy and Clinical Immunology, 73,* 253–258.

Boggs, D. F., & Bartlett, D., Jr. (1982). Chemical specificity of a laryngeal apneic reflex in puppies. *Journal of Applied Physiology, 53,* 455–462.

Bond, V. K., Stoetling, R. K., & Gupta, C. D. (1979). Pulmonary aspiration syndrome after inhalation of gastric fluid containing antacids. *Anesthesiology, 51,* 452–453.

Bosma, J. F. (1985). Postnatal ontogeny of the pharynx, larynx, and mouth. *American Review of Respiratory Disease, 131,* S10–S15.

Byrne, W. J., Campbell, M., & Ashcraft, E. (1983). A diagnostic approach to vomiting in severely retarded patients. *American Journal of Diseases of Children, 137,* 259–262.

Carroll, J. L., Marcus, C. L., & Loughlin, G. M. (in press). Disordered control of breathing in infants and children. *Pediatrics in Review.*

Carpenter, D. O. (1989). Central nervous system mechanisms in deglutition and emesis. In S. G. Schultz, J. D. Wood, & B. B. Rauner (Eds.), *Handbook of physiology: The gastrointestinal system* (pp. 685–714). Bethesda, MD: American Physiological Society.

Chrispin, A. R., Friedland, G. W., & Waterston, D. J. (1966). Aspiration pneumonia and dysphagia after technically successful repair of oesophageal atresia. *Thorax, 21,* 104–110.

Christie, D. L., O'Grady, L. R., & Mack, D. V. (1978). Incompetent lower esophageal sphincter and gastroesophageal reflux in recurrent acute pulmonary disease of infancy and childhood. *Journal of Pediatrics, 93,* 23–27.

Danus, O., Casar, C., Larrain, A., & Pope, C. E., II. (1976). Esophageal reflux — An unrecognized cause of recurrent obstructive bronchitis in children. *The Journal of Pediatrics, 89,* 220–224.

Davis R. S., Larsen, G. L., & Grunstein, M. M. (1983). Respiratory response to intraesophageal acid infusion in asthmatic children during sleep. *Journal of Allergy and Clinical Immunology, 72,* 393–398.

Diamant, N. E. (1985). Development of esophageal function. *American Review of Respiratory Disease, 131,* S29–S32.

Downing, S. E., & Lee, J. C. (1975). Laryngeal

chemosensitivity: A possible mechanism for sudden infant death syndrome. *Pediatrics, 55,* 640–649.

Editorial. (1980). Cimetidine and the acid-aspiration syndrome. *Lancet, 1,* 465–466.

Euler, A. R., Byrne, W. J., Ament, M. E., Fonkalsrud, E. W., Strobel, C. T., Siegel, S. C., Katz, R. M., & Rachelefsky, G. S. (1979). Recurrent pulmonary disease in children: A complication of gastroesophageal reflux. *Pediatrics, 63,* 47–51.

Fick, R. B. (1985). Cell-mediated antibacterial defenses of the distal airways. *American Review of Respiratory Disease, 131,* S43–S48.

Fisher M., Roggli, V., Merten D., Mulvihill D., & Spock, A. (1992). Coexisting endogenous lipoid pneumonia, cholesterol granulomas, and pulmonary alveolar proteinosis in a pediatric population. *Pediatric Pathology, 12,* 365–383.

Gibbs, C. F., Schwartz, D. J., Wynne, J. W., Hood, C. I., & Kuck, E. J. (1979). Antacid pulmonary aspiration in the dog. *Anesthesiology, 51,* 380–385.

Guide to diagnosis and management of cystic fibrosis. (1979). p. 14. Rockville, MD: Cystic Fibrosis Foundation.

Gustafsson, P. M., Kjellman, N.-I. M., & Tibbling, L. (1986). Oesophageal function and symptoms in moderate and severe asthma. *Acta Paediatric Scandinavia, 75,* 729–736.

Hardy, K. A., Schidlow, D. V., & Zaeri, N. (1988). Obliterative bronchiolitis in children. *Chest, 93,* 460–466.

Herbst, J. J., Book, L. S., & Bray, P. F. (1978). Gastroesophageal reflux in the "near miss" sudden infant death syndrome. *The Journal of Pediatrics, 92,* 73–35.

Herbst, J. J., Minton, S. D., & Book, L. S. (1979). Gastroesophageal reflux causing respiratory distress and apnea in newborn infants. *The Journal of Pediatrics, 95,* 763–768.

Hickling, K. G., & Howard, R. (1988). A retrospective survey of treatment and mortality in aspiration pneumonia. *Intensive Care Medicine, 14,* 617–622.

Hoyaux, C. L., Forget, P., Lambrechts, L., & Geubelle, F. (1985). Chronic bronchopulmonary disease and gastroesophageal reflux in children. *Pediatric Pulmonology, 1,* 149–153.

Hrabovsky E. E., & Mullet, M. D. (1986). Gastroesophageal reflux and the premature infant. *Journal of Pediatric Surgery, 7,* 583–587.

Huxley, E. J., Viroslav, J., Gray, W. R., & Pierce, A. K. (1978). Pharyngeal aspiration in normal adults and patients with depressed consciousness. *American Journal of Medicine, 65,* 564–568.

Jeffrey, H. E., Rahilly, P., & Read, D. J. C. (1983). Multiple causes of asphyxia in infants at high risk for sudden infant death. *Archives of Disease in Childhood, 58,* 92–100.

Johnson, P., Salisbury, D. M., & Storey, A. T. (1975). Apnea induced by stimulation of sensory receptors in the larynx. In J. F. Bosma & J. Showacre (Eds.), *Development of upper respiratory anatomy and function* (pp. 160–178). Washington, DC: Government Printng Office.

Kahn, A., Montauk, L., & Blue, D. (1987). Diagnostic categories in infants referred for an acute event suggesting near-miss SIDS. *European Journal of Pediatrics, 146,* 458–460.

Kovar, I., Selstam, U., Catterton, W. Z., Stahlman, M. T., and Sundell, H. W. (1979). Laryngeal chemoreflex in newborn lambs: Respiratory and swallowing response to salts, acids and sugars. *Pediatric Research, 13,* 1144–1149.

Leape, L. L., Holder, T. M., Franklin, J. D., Amoury, R. A., & Ashcraft, K. W. (1977). Respiratory arrest in infants secondary to gastroesophageal reflux. *Pediatrics, 60,* 924–928.

Leith, D. E. (1985). The development of cough. *American Review of Respiratory Disease, 131,* S39–S42.

MacFayden, U. M., Hendry, G. M. A., & Simpson, H. (1983). Gastro-oesophageal reflux in near-miss sudden infant death syndrome or suspected recurrent aspiration. *Archives of Diseases of Children, 58,* 87–91.

Mansfield, L. E., Hameister, H. H., Spaulding, H. S., Smith, N. J., & Glab, N. (1981). The role of the vagus nerve in airway narrowing caused by intra-esophageal hydrochloric acid provocation and esophageal distention. *Annals of Allergy, 47,* 431–434.

Mansfield, L. E., & Stein, M. R. (1978). Gastroesophageal reflux and asthma: A possible reflex mechanism. *Annals of Allergy, 41,* 224–226.

Mathew, O. P., Clark, M. L., & Pronske, M. H. (1985). Apnea, bradycardia, and cyanosis during oral feeding in term neonates. *The Journal of Pediatrics, 106,* 857.

Matseche, J. W., Go, V. L. W., & Di Magno, E. P.

(1977). Meconium ileus equivalent complicating cystic fibrosis in postneonatal children and young adults. *Gastroenterology, 72,* 732–736.

Mays, E. E., Dubois, J. J., & Hamilton, G. B. (1976). Pulmonary fibrosis associated with tracheobronchial aspiration. *Chest, 69,* 512–515.

McVeagh, P., Howman-Giles, R., & Kemp, A. (1987). Pulmonary aspiration studied by radionuclide milk scanning and barium swallow roentgenography. *American Journal of Diseases of Children, 141,* 917–921.

Mendelson, C. L. (1946). The aspiration of stomach contents into the lungs during obstetric anesthesia. *American Journal of Obstetrics and Gynecology, 52,* 191–205.

Menon, A. P., Schefft, G. L., & Thach, B. T. (1984). Frequency and significance of swallowing during prolonged apnea in infants. *American Review of Respiratory Disease, 130,* 969–973.

Menon, A. P., Schefft, G. L., & Thach, B. T. (1985). Apnea associated with regurgitation in infants. *The Journal of Pediatrics, 106,* 625–629.

Moran, T. J. (1951). Experimental food-aspiration pneumonia. *Archives of Pathology, 52,* 350–354.

Moran, T. J. (1955). Experimental aspiration pneumonia. IV. Inflammatory and reparative changes produced by intratracheal injections of autologous gastric juice and hydrochloric acid. *Archives of Pathology, 60,* 122–129.

National Institutes of Health Consensus Development Conference Statement. (1987). Infantile apnea and home apnea monitoring (Vol. 6, pp. 3–12) (NIH pub. No. 872905). Washington, DC: U.S. Department of Health and Human Services.

Newman, L. J., Russe, J., & Glassman, M. S. (1989). Patterns of gastroesophageal reflux in infants presenting with apparent life-threatening events. *Journal of Pediatric Gastroenterology and Nutrition, 8,* 157–160.

Nussbaum, E., Maggi, J. C., Mathis, R., & Galant, S. P. (1987). Association of lipid-laden alveolar macrophages and gastroesophageal reflux in children. *Journal of Pediatrics, 110,* 190–194.

Ogura, J. H., Kawasaki, M., & Takenouchi, S. (1964). Neurophysiologic observations on the adaptive mechanisms in deglutition.

Annals of Otology, Rhinology and Laryngology, 73, 1062–1082.

Pearson, J. E. G., & Wilson, R. S. E. (1971). Diffuse pulmonary fibrosis and hiatus hernia. *Thorax, 26,* 300–305.

Plaxico, D. T., & Loughlin, G. M. (1981). Nasopharyngeal reflux and neonatal apnea. *American Journal of Diseases of Children, 135,* 793–794.

Putman, P. E., Ricker, D. H., & Orenstein, S. R. (1992). Gastroesophageal reflux. In R. C. Beckerman, R. T. Crouillette, & C. E. Hunt (Eds.), *Respiratory control disorders in infants and children* (pp. 322–341). Baltimore, MD: Williams & Wilkins.

Ramenofsky, M. L., & Leape, L. L. (1981). Continuous upper esophageal pH monitoring in infants and children with gastroesophageal reflux, pneumonia, and apneic spells. *Journal of Pediatric Surgery, 16,* 374–378.

Schwartz, D. J., Wynne, J. W., Gibbs, C. P., et al. (1980). The pulmonary consequences of aspiration of gastric contents at pH values greater than 2.5. *American Review of Respiratory Disease, 121,* 119–126.

Scott, R. B., O'Loughlin, E. V., & Gall, D. G. (1984). Gastroesophageal reflux in patients with cystic fibrosis. *Journal of Pediatrics, 106,* 223–227.

See, C. C., Newman, L. J., Berezin, S., Glassman, M. J., Medow, M. S., Dozor, A. J., & Schwarz, S. M. (1989). Gastroesophageal reflux-induced hypoxemia in infants with apparent life-threatening events. *American Journal of Diseases of Children, 143,* 951–954.

Shermeta D. W., Whitington P. F., Seto D. S., & Haller, J. A. (1977). Lower esophageal sphincter dysfunction in esophageal atresia: Nocturnal regurgitation and aspiration pneumonia. *Journal of Pediatric Surgery, 12,* 871–876.

Simonsson, B. G., Jacobs, F. M., & Nadel, J. A. (1967). The role of autonomic nervous system and the cough reflex in the increased responsiveness of airways in patients with obstructive airway disease. *Journal of Clinical Investigation, 46,* 1812–1818.

Smith, J., Wolkove, N., Colacone, A., & Kreisman, H. (1989). Coordination of eating, drinking, and breathing in adults. *Chest, 96,* 578–582.

Spaulding, H. S., Mansfield, L. E., Stein, M. R., Sellner, J. C., & Gremillion, D. E. (1982).

Further investigation of the association between gastroesophageal reflux and bronchoconstriction. *Journal of Allergy and Clinical Immunology, 69,* 516–521.

Spitzer, A. R., Boyle, J. T., Tuchman, D. N., & Fox, W. W. (1984). Awake apnea associated with gastroesophageal reflux: A specific clinical syndrome. *Journal of Pediatrics, 104,* 200–205.

St. Cyr, J. A., Ferrara, T. B., Thompson, T., Johnson, D. & Foker, J. E. (1989). Treatment of pulmonary manifestations of gastroesophageal reflux in children two years of age or less. *The American Journal of Surgery, 157,* 400–404.

Thach, B. T., & Menon, A. (1985). Pulmonary protective mechanisms in human infants. *American Review of Respiratory Disease, 131* (Suppl.), S55–S58.

Trowitzsch, E., Meyer, G., Schluter, B., Buschatz, D., & Andler, W. (1992). "A life threatening event" in infants. Results of polysomnography and examination of a group of 122 infants. *Monatsschr-Kinderheilkd, 140,* 233–236.

Tuchman, D. N., Boyle, J. T., Pack, A. I., et al. (1984). Comparison of airway responses following tracheal or esophageal acidification in the cat. *Gastroenterology, 78,* 872–881.

Tucker, J. A. (1985). Perspective of the development of the air and food passages. *American Review of Respiratory Disease, 131*(Suppl.), S7–S9.

Vandeplas, Y., & Sacre-Smits, L. (1987). Continuous 24-hour esophageal pH monitoring in 285 asymptomatic infants 0–15 months old. *Journal of Pediatric Gastroenterology and Nutrition, 6,* 220–224.

Vandeplas, T., Diericx, A., Blecker, U., Lanciers, S., & Deneyer, M. (1991). Esophageal pH monitoring data during chest physiotherapy. *Journal of Pediatric Gastroenterology and Nutrition, 13,* 23–26.

Wanner, A. (1985). Mucociliary and mucus secretory function. *American Review of Respiratory Disease, 131,* S36–S38.

Whitington, P. F., Shermeta, D. W., Seto, D. S., Jones, L., & Hendrix, T. R. (1977). Role of lower esophageal sphincter incompetence in recurrent pneumonia after repair of esophageal atresia. *Journal of Pediatrics, 91,* 550–554.

Widdicombe, J. G. (1954). Respiratory reflexes from the trachea and bronchi of the cat. *Journal of Physiology, 123,* 55–70.

Wilson, S. L., Thach, B. T., Brouillette, R. T., & Abu-Osba, Y. K. (1981). Coordination of breathing and swallowing in human infants. *Journal of Applied Physiology, 50,* 851–858.

Wynne, J. W., Reynolds, J. C., Hood, I., et al. Steroid therapy for pneumonitis induced in rabbits by aspiration of foodstuff. *Anesthesiology, 51,* 11.

Zimmerman, I., Ulmer, W. T., & Weller, W. (1979). The role of upper airways and sensoric recepetors on reflex bronchoconstriction. *Respiratory Experimental Medicine* (Berlin), 1974, pp. 253–265.

Gastroesophageal Reflux

CHAPTER 13

David N. Tuchman, M.D.

Gastroesophageal reflux (GER) occurs when dysfunction of the distal esophagus and proximal stomach allow retrograde movement of gastric contents into the distal esophagus (Herbst 1981). This definition is descriptive and reflects the fact that specific mechanisms accounting for the development of reflux remain unclear. GER has been reviewed in detail by others including Herbst (1981), Berquist (1982), Johnson and Jolley (1981), Jewett and Siegel (1984), Sondheimer (1988), and Boyle (1989).

GER and its complications should be considered during evaluation, management, and treatment of the pediatric patient with impaired swallowing. Accordingly, this chapter reviews mechanisms which account for gastroesophageal competence and the pathophysiology, clinical presentation, diagnosis, and management of reflux in the pediatric population with emphasis on those patients with impaired swallowing.

Gastroesophageal Competence: Physiology

The existence of a pressure gradient between the intra-abdominal cavity (posi-

tive) and the intra-thoracic cavity (negative) tends to promote reflux. In fact, any condition that increases intra-abdominal pressure, such as the Valsalva maneuver, coughing, or use of an abdominal binder, increases this gradient. However, in normal individuals these maneuvers do not result in reflux. Gastroesophageal competence, which prevents reflux from occurring, is maintained by multiple factors including the lower esophageal sphincter (LES), the diaphragm, the phreno-esophageal ligaments, the acute angle of entry of the esophagus into the stomach (the angle of HIS), the intra-abdominal portion of the esophagus "exposed" to positive pressure, and the loose areolar tissue of the esophageal lumen which tends to act as a pinch-cock mechanism. Anatomy of the gastroesophageal region is shown in Figure 13–1. At present, the LES and the diaphragm are considered the most important mechanisms for maintaining gastroesophageal competence (Fisher, Malmud, Roberts, & Lobis, 1977).

The Lower Esophageal Sphincter

Physiology of the LES has been reviewed in Chapter 1 and in standard gastroenter-

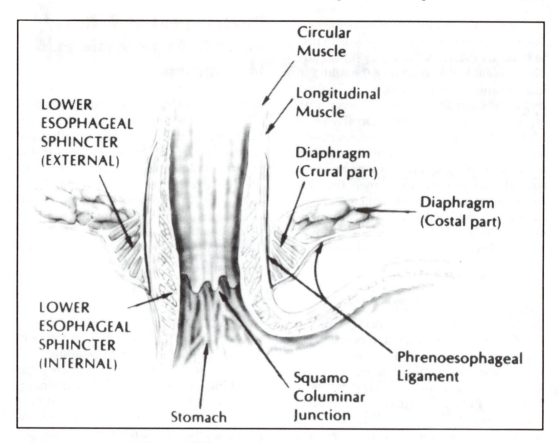

FIGURE 13–1. Anatomy of the gastroesophageal junction. (From Heine, K. J., & Mittal, R. K. [1991]. Crural diaphragm and lower esophageal sphincter as antireflux barriers. *Viewpoints on Digestive Diseases, 23,* 1–6, p. 2, with permission.)

ology texts. Briefly, the LES is identified as a physiologic region of high pressure located at the distal end of the esophagus, generating a "squeeze" pressure of 15 to 30 mm Hg (compared to an intra-gastric pressure of 0). LES pressure, which is maintained by a combination of myogenic and neurogenic factors (Goyal & Rattan, 1978), is subject to hormonal, neurologic, and pharmacologic influences (Goyal & Rattan, 1978) (Table 1–2).

The Diaphragm

During coughing and other conditions that increase intra-abdominal pressure, the pressure gradient between the stomach and thorax may exceed pressures generated by

the LES. In addition, during forceful inspiration, the pressure difference between the esophagus and stomach may reach levels of 70 to 80 mm Hg or greater (i.e., increased negative intra-thoracic pressure) (Heine & Mittal, 1991). Since these maneuvers typically do not result in reflux, factors other than pressures generated by the LES have been sought to account for gastroesophageal competence. It has been hypothesized that, during conditions associated with increased intra-abdominal pressure resulting from contraction of muscles of the abdominal wall, the right crus of the diaphragm plays an important role in preventing reflux (Heine & Mittal, 1991; Mittal & Fisher, 1990). In animal studies, it has been demonstrated that in response to abdominal compression the right crus of the diaphragm contracts and contributes the necessary force at the distal esophagus to prevent reflux (Mittal & Fisher, 1990) (Figure 13–2). Hence, it is currently thought that gastroesophageal competence is maintained by two mechanisms working synergistically: the LES and the diaphragm (Heine & Mittal, 1991). The pressure gradient generated by smooth muscle structures (stomach and esophagus) are counteracted by a smooth muscle structure, namely the LES. Pressures generated by skeletal muscles of the thoracic and abdominal wall are counteracted by the skeletal muscles of the diaphragm (i.e., the right crus of the diaphragm).

Development of GER: Possible Pathophysiologic Mechanisms

Although the LES is an important contributor to gastroesophageal competence, infants and children with GER usually have normal resting LES pressures (Moroz, Espinoza, Cumming, & Diamant, 1976). Very low LES pressure (less than 5 mm Hg) is usually found only in patients with severe esophagitis. Currently, spontaneous relaxation of the LES (also termed inappropriate or transient relaxation) is considered the

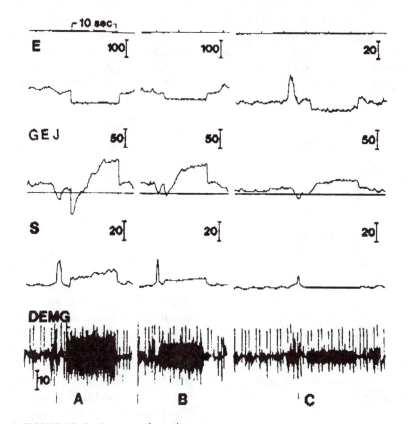

FIGURE 13–2. Gastroesophageal junction pressure increases in response to intra-abdominal pressure. The intra-abdominal pressure is increased by straight leg raises (SLR). Two SLRs are shown in the picture. Each SLR is associated with an increase in gastroesophageal junction pressure that is much greater than the increase in intragastric pressure. Also note an increase in crural diaphragm electromyographic activity during each SLR. (From Mittal, R. K., & McCallum, R. W. [1988]. Characteristics and frequency of transient relaxations of the lower esophageal sphincter in patients with reflux esophagitis. *Gastroenterology, 95,* 593–599, p. 594, with permission.)

major mechanism for the development of reflux in normal adult subjects (Dent et al., 1980), patients with reflux esophagitis (Mittal & McCallum, 1988), and possibly children (Werlin, Dodds, Hogan, & Arndorfer, 1980).

Spontaneous relaxation of the sphincter, which may be demonstrated during esophageal manometry, is characterized by a decrease in sphincter pressure to gastric baseline (zero pressure) unassociated with a swallow (i.e., relaxation is not associated with esophageal peristalsis). This is in contrast to normal function of the sphincter which relaxes in response to swallowing. Duration of sphincter relaxation during spontaneous episodes exceeds that which occurs in response to swallowing. During spontaneous LES relaxation, there is a "common cavity" phenomenon, and gastric contents may move freely into the distal esophagus. Factors leading to the development

of spontaneous sphincter relaxation remain unknown. Interestingly, the crural diaphragm not only relaxes during deglutition, but also during spontaneous relaxation of the LES (Mittal, Rochester, & McCallum, 1989).

Another mechanism for development of gastroesophageal reflux involves transient increases in intra-abdominal pressure that exceed pressures generated at the gastroesophageal junction. In children, episodes of increased intra-abdominal pressure may occur during crying, coughing, sneezing, or defecating. Finally, severe esophagitis may be associated with very low LES pressures (less than 5 mm Hg) so that spontaneous reflux occurrs across an incompetent sphincter (Figure 13–3).

It has been suggested that patients with chronic pulmonary disease, including asthma, may have abnormalities of diaphragmatic function. Dysfunction of the diaphragm

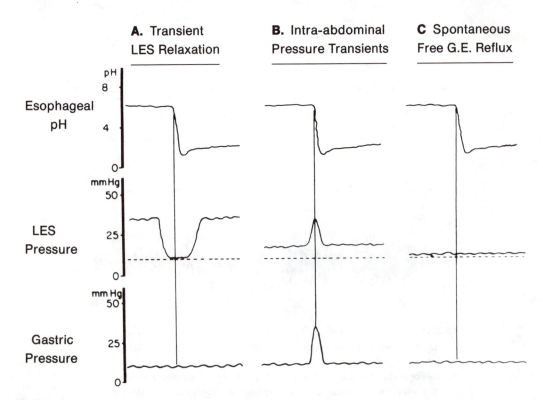

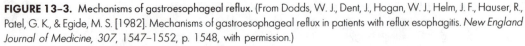

FIGURE 13–3. Mechanisms of gastroesophageal reflux. (From Dodds, W. J., Dent, J., Hogan, W. J., Helm, J. F., Hauser, R., Patel, G. K., & Egide, M. S. [1982]. Mechanisms of gastroesophageal reflux in patients with reflux esophagitis. *New England Journal of Medicine, 307,* 1547–1552, p. 1548, with permission.)

may interfere with anti-reflux mechanisms and account for the high prevalence of GER seen in patients with chronic pulmonary disease (see below and Chapter 12).

Esophageal Function, Saliva, and Deglutition

Material that enters the esophagus following a pharyngeal swallow is mainly cleared by primary peristalsis of the esophageal

body. Helm et al. (1984) investigated other esophageal clearance mechanisms by simultaneously performing esophageal manometry and nuclear scintigraphy while measuring intra-esophageal pH with a probe. This technique allows correlation of motor events with movement of intraluminal substances. These investigators demonstrated that an esophageal bolus is cleared with one swallow. However, multiple swallows may be required to alter intraluminal pH (Figures 13–4 and 13–5). Repeated swallows are needed to deliver a sufficient amount of saliva into the esophageal lumen which buffers small volumes of acid. Swallowed saliva also plays an important role in the clearance of refluxed material by maintain-

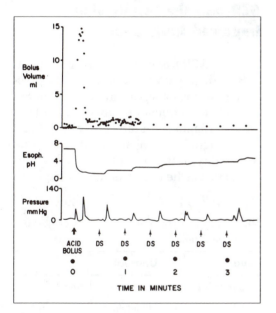

FIGURE 13–4. Relations among esophageal acid clearance, motor activity, and emptying of fluid volume. The top graph shows clearance of a radio-labeled acid bolus from the esophagus using radionuclide imaging. The middle tracing demonstrates sequential increase in esophageal pH measured by a pH probe. Concurrent manometry measures esophageal motor activity. Only peristaltic pressure complexes from the distal esophagus are shown. DS denotes dry swallows. Despite clearance of the injected bolus volume to less than 1 ml by the secondary peristaltic sequence, esophageal pH did not begin to rise until the first dry swallow 30 seconds after bolus injection. (From Helm, J. F., Dodds, W. J., Pelc, L. R., Palmer, D. W., Hogan, W. J., & Teeter, B. C. [1984]. Effect of esophageal emptying and saliva on clearance of acid from the esophagus. *New England Journal of Medicine, 310*, 284–288, p. 286, with permission).

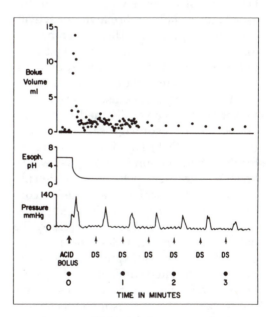

FIGURE 13–5. Effect of oral aspiration of saliva on esophageal acid clearance and emptying of fluid volume. During this swallow, to minimize entry of saliva into the esophagus, saliva was aspirated from the mouth. Despite nearly complete emptying of the bolus volume by the initial secondary peristaltic sequence, saliva aspiration effectively abolished esophageal acid clearance. Only peristaltic pressure complexes from the distal esophagus are shown. DS denotes dry swallows. Despite nearly complete emptying of the bolus volume by the initial secondary peristaltic sequence, saliva aspiration effectively abolished esophageal acid clearance. (From Helm et al. [1984], p. 286, with permission.)

ing intraluminal esophageal pH in the neutral range (Sonnenberg et al., 1982; Helm et al., 1984; Helm, Dodds, & Hogan, 1987). The beneficial effects of saliva extend beyond its buffering action. Saliva contains epidermal growth factor, a polypeptide hormone, which may be important in ameliorating the effects of acid-induced mucosal injury (Dutta, Meirowitz, Vengurlekar, & Resau, 1990; Dutta, Orth, Dukehart, & Vaith, 1986).

Infants and children with impaired swallowing, particularly those with cerebral palsy, may have oral phase abnormalities that compromise the delivery of saliva into the esophagus. As a result, these patients may have impaired clearance of swallowed and refluxed material secondary to (1) inadequate delivery of saliva into the esophagus and (2) abnormal motor activity of the esophageal body. These and other factors may predispose this group of patients to the development of reflux esophagitis.

Acidification of the esophageal mucosa has been shown to cause an increase in salivary flow via a vagally mediated reflux known as the esophago-salivary reflex. (Dutta et al., 1992.) The clinical correlation for this phenomenon is known as "waterbrash," described by patients as sudden filling of the mouth with saliva. A similar condition may occur in cognitively impaired children with cerebral palsy and reflux. The patient or parents may describe an unexplained increase in salivation or oral secretions not associated with clinical deterioration of swallowing function. In this setting, the presence of reflux esophagitis should be suspected, even if clinical regurgitation and emesis are lacking.

Clinical Manifestations of GER

Common and uncommon clinical presentations of GER are shown in Table 13–1. For the clinician, reflux may be characterized as nonpathologic or pathologic. Nonpathologic reflux occurs in infants with episodes of regurgitation and vomiting that

are not clinically significant and do not lead to complications. This type of reflux, by definition, generally resolves by 18 to 24 months of age or sooner (Carre, 1959; Herbst, 1981). Pathologic GER, or gastroesophageal reflux disease (GERD), may be defined as reflux which is associated with significant clinical complications such as protein-energy malnutrition (failure to thrive), reflux esophagitis, chronic pulmonary disease, and apnea. Unfortunately, the patient with impaired swallowing is at risk for developing pathologic reflux.

GER and the Swallowing Impaired Individual

Because GER frequently occurs in individuals with impaired swallowing, its presence may have a significant impact on the clinical evaluation and management of the patient. Diagnosis of reflux may be difficult in the cognitively impaired individual due to inability of the patient to report symptoms such as heartburn and dysphagia. In

TABLE 13–1. Clinical manifestations of gastroesophageal reflux.

Usual	Unusual
Regurgitation	Sandifer syndrome
Vomiting	Rumination
Failure to thrive	Finger clubbing and protein-losing enteropathy
Aspiration	
Reactive airway disease	Neuropsychiatric symptoms
	Apnea
Esophagitis	Acute life-threatening event
Heartburn	Reflux and aspiration mimicking bronchopulmonary dysplasia
Anemia	
Hemetemesis	
Melena	
Stricture	

Sources: Adapted from Herbst, J. J. (1981). Gastroesophageal reflux. *Journal of Pediatrics, 98,* 859–870, p. 860, with permission.

this group of patients, the clinician should be aware that signs and symptoms of reflux may develop even when regurgitation and vomiting are minimal. Clinical presentation of reflux (particularly reflux esophagitis) may include a change in feeding behavior or feeding ability characterized as refusal to feed and/or gagging and retching during feeding. In some patients, it may be difficult for the clinician to distinguish between decompensation of an impaired swallow and development of symptomatic reflux. Other clinical clues suggesting the development of GER in cognitively impaired patients include significant, unexplained loss of weight, increase in oral secretions not associated with deterioration of swallowing function, and unexplained irritability or a significant change in behavior.

Reflux may contribute to the development of protein-energy malnutrition with resultant compromise of muscle strength and function. This may lead to decompensation of swallowing by adversely affecting head and neck control, postural control, and possibly the function of the muscles of deglutition.

Clinical experience suggests that the pediatric patient with impaired swallowing is unable to protect the airway against a reflux event. The specific pathophysiologic mechanisms accounting for this phenomenon remain undefined. It is unclear whether swallowing-impaired patients exhibit abnormalities of upper esophageal sphincter (UES) function such as altered tone or pressure, impaired responsiveness to stimuli such as acid, or incoordination with other phases of swallowing. Specifically, the effect of acid reflux on upper esophageal sphincter (UES) function remains controversial. In unimpaired adults, early studies suggested that acid perfusion of the esophageal mucosa resulted in a reflexive increase in UES pressure (Gerhardt et al., 1978). However, more recent studies, using improved methodology, have not confirmed these findings (Kahrilas et al., 1987; Vakil, Kahrilas, Dodds, & Vanagunas, 1989). Sondheimer (1983) found no difference in resting UES pressure when comparing infants with GER to a control group. Furthermore, UES response to esophageal acidification was variable; in some infants, the UES did not respond to an acid stimulus.

GER and Protein-Energy Malnutrition (PEM)

Patients with pathologic reflux may develop PEM as a result of decreased energy intake secondary to: (1) refusal to feed because of pain and discomfort resulting from reflux esophagitis and (2) loss of nutrients secondary to regurgitation and vomiting. Most pediatric patients with reflux-related PEM become marasmic; that is, they have "balanced starvation" associated with normal visceral protein stores (i.e., normal serum albumin). Rarely, patients with reflux esophagitis and malnutrition may develop kwashiorkor (malnutrition associated with hypoalbuminemia) secondary to loss of protein (i.e., protein-losing enteropathy) from an inflamed esophageal mucosa. Finger clubbing may also be seen in this syndrome (Herbst, Johnson, & Oliveros, 1976).

The patient with an impaired swallow and GER may be unable to meet fluid and energy requirements. Efforts to increase energy and fluid intake by the oral route may "overwhelm" swallowing ability and lead to decompensation of swallowing function.

Reflux Esophagitis

The term "reflux esophagitis" refers to histologic alteration of the esophageal mucosa secondary to acid injury. Criteria for chronic changes of reflux esophagitis include an increase in the thickness of the proliferative or basal cell layer of the epithelium, increased size of the rete pegs, and thinning of the epithelial layer (Ismail-Beigi, Horton, & Pope, 1970). In infants and children, the mucosal response to acid reflux may involve infiltration of the esophageal mucosa with eosinophils (Winter et al., 1982). Chronic reflux esophagitis may lead to the development of gastric metaplasia of the squamous epithelium of the esophagus, a condition known as Barrett's esophagus. This is thought to be a pre-malignant state in adults (Hamilton & Smith, 1987). Barrett's esophagus has been described in children with chronic GER (Dahms & Rothstein, 1984). Hoeffel, Nihovi-Fekete, and Schmitt (1989) reported two children with adenocarcinoma of the lower esophagus which developed in a Barrett's esophagus.

The prevalence rate of reflux esophagitis in patients referred to pediatric gastroenterology centers ranges from 61% to 83% (Shub et al., 1985; Hyams, Ricci, & Leichtner, 1988). Infants and children with reflux esophagitis may present with refusal to feed, unexplained irritability, unusual posturing (torticollis or Sandifer's syndrome), and unexplained iron deficiency anemia in association with occult blood loss in the stool. Esophagitis may also lead to esophageal spasm, or simultaneous contractions of the esophageal body. In older children and adolescents, the more classic complaints or retrosternal discomfort or heartburn occur. On some occasions, older children and adolescents complain of dysphagia localized to the region of the supra-sternal notch or report that food "goes down slowly." Interestingly, some children with histologic findings of reflux esophagitis may be asymptomatic.

Multiple factors may lead to acid-induced inflammation of the esophageal mucosa (Dodds et al., 1981). The nature of the refluxate may influence the degree of mucosal injury. Pepsin, a proteolytic enzyme in gastric juice, when combined with gastric contents of pH less than 3 is particularly injurious. A second factor that may preserve mucosal integrity is the ability of the esophagus, via normal peristaltic mechanisms, to clear refluxed materials. The importance of esophageal motor function in clearing the esophageal lumen was demonstrated by Kahrilas, Dodds, and Hogan (1988). Using simultaneous manometry and radiography,

these workers demonstrated that simultaneous, nonpropagating esophageal contractions which follow a swallow do not effectively deliver a bolus through the lumen of the esophageal body (see Figures 13–6 and 13–7). Esophageal clearance mechanisms, such as altered esophageal peristalsis, may be abnormal in the swallowing impaired patient and lead to prolonged contact of acid with the esophageal epithelium. In addition, acid injury to the esophagus may lead to esophageal dysmotility and further compromise the ability of the esophagus to clear refluxed material.

GER and Central Nervous System Dysfunction

The reported incidence of GER in neurologically impaired children ranges from 15% to 75% (Byrne, Euler, & Ashcraft, 1982; Sondheimer & Morris, 1979). Predisposing factors for development of GER in this patient population include (1) injury of vagal nerve nuclei in the central nervous system leading to alteration of LES function (Vane, Shiffler, & Grosfield, 1982), (2) impaired oral and pharyngeal phases of swallowing associated with poor esophageal clearance mechanisms, (3) increased intra-abdominal pressure secondary to scoliosis or spasticity of abdominal musculature (Kassen, Groen, & Fraenkel, 1965), and (4) effect of body position such as prolonged time in the supine position (Guttman, 1972). Reflux may respond poorly to medical therapy in patients with central nervous system impairment such as cerebral palsy and mental retardation, and as a result, these patients frequently become candidates for anti-reflux surgery (Wilkinson, Dudgeon, & Sondheimer, 1981). However, with the introduction of potent acid inhibitors such as omeprazole and the development of new pro-kinetic agents such as cisapride (see below), medical therapy may become more effective and obviate the need for surgery.

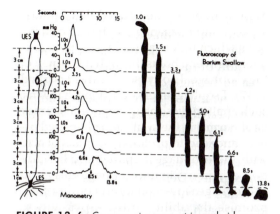

FIGURE 13-6. Concurrent manometric and video recording of a 5-ml barium swallow. The tracings from the video images on the right show the distribution of the barium column at the times indicated above the individual tracings and by arrows on the manometric record. In this example, a single peristaltic sequence completely cleared the barium bolus from the esophagus, resulting in 100% volume clearance. Pharyngeal injection of barium into the esophagus occurs at the 1.0-s mark. The entry of barium causes distention and a slightly increased intraluminal pressure, as indicated by the *downward-pointing arrows* marked "1 s." Shortly thereafter, esophageal peristalsis is initiated. During esophageal peristalsis, luminal closure and hence the tail of the barium bolus passed each recording site concurrent with the onset of the manometric pressure wave. Hence, at 1.5 s, the peristaltic contraction had just reached the proximal recording site and barium had been stripped from the esophagus proximal to that point. Similarly, at 4.2 s, the peristaltic contraction was beginning at the third recording site and, correspondingly, the tail of the barium bolus was located at the third recording site. Finally, after completion of the peristaltic contraction (time 13.8 s), all of the barium had been cleared into the stomach. (From Kahrilas, P. J., Dodds, W. J., and Hogan, W. J. [1988]. Effect of peristaltic dysfunction on esophageal volume clearance. *Gastroenterology, 94*, 73–80, p. 75, with permission.)

GER and Chronic Pulmonary Disease

Gastroesophageal reflux may complicate the clinical course of patients with chronic pulmonary disease including broncho-pulmonary dysplasia (BPD) (Herbst et al., 1979; Sindel, Maisels, & Ballantine, 1989), chronic aspiration pneumonia and reactive airway disease (Mansfield & Stein, 1978;

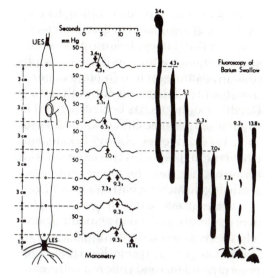

FIGURE 13-7. The tracings from the video recording on the right depict the distribution of the barium bolus at the times indicated by arrows on the manometric record. This is an example of a failed peristaltic contraction resulting in impaired barium clearance. The stripping wave progressed to beyond the aortic arch with the peristaltic sequence terminating with a simultaneous contraction in the distal esophagus. On videofluoroscopy, the simultaneous contraction was seen as a tertiary contraction that trapped small collections of barium in the distal esophageal body, while forcing the remainder either distally into the stomach or retrograde up the esophagus (9.3-s image). (From Kahrilas et al. [1988], p. 75, with permission.)

Shapiro & Christie, 1983; Wilson, Charette, Thomson, & Silverman, 1985), apnea (Downing & Lee, 1975; Menon, Scheffft, & Thach, 1985; Spitzer, Boyle, Tuchman, & Fox, 1984; Walsh, Farrell, Keenan, Lucas, & Kramer, 1981), apparent life-threatening events (Sindel, Maisels, & Ballantine, 1989), and cystic fibrosis (Giuffre, Rubin, & Mitchell, 1987). The association between GER and chronic pulmonary disease has been reviewed in detail by Boyle et al. (1985) and Pack (1990). (See Chapter 12 for a detailed discussion of reflux-associated pulmonary disease.)

There are a number of mechanisms which may explain the relationship between reflux and chronic lung disease. Alteration of diaphragmatic function in individuals with asthma may impair gastro-esophageal competence and lead to increased GER. Use of broncholytic agents such as theophylline may decrease LES pressure, although it is unclear whether this effect is clinically significant (Hubert, Gaudric, Guerre, Lockhart, & Marsac, 1988). In addition, patients with asthma may have an increase in the pressure differential between the abdominal and thoracic cavities (increased negative intra-thoracic pressure), a situation which may promote reflux.

Alternatively, reflux of gastric contents may adversely affect pulmonary function. It has been demonstrated in animal and human studies that acidification of the esophageal mucosa may result in a vagally mediated reflex leading to bronchospasm. Entry of small volumes of acid into the large airways (microaspiration) may stimulate irritant receptors and cause wheezing (Tuchman et al., 1984). In addition, apnea may result if regions of the laryngeal mucosa come into contact with acid or other fluids. This effect is mediated by the superior laryngeal nerve.

Enteral Tube Feeding and the Development of Gastroesophageal Reflux

Placement of a gastrostomy tube, either surgically or by endoscopy, becomes an important option for management in infants and children with impaired swallowing who are unable to meet energy and fluid requirements by the oral route. However, it has been reported that 12 to 50% of patients may develop significant GER following placement of either a surgical or endoscopic gastrostomy tube (Berezin, Schwartz, Halata, & Newman, 1986; Gauderer, 1991; Grunow, al-Hafidh, & Tunnell, 1989; Mollitt, Galladay, & Seibert, 1985), a potentially dangerous situation particularly in the patient unable to protect the airway. Reflux tends to develop within 6 to 12 months following tube placement. The mechanism

leading to the development of this complication remains unknown. It has been hypothesized that following tube placement, fixation of the anterior gastric wall may change the angle of HIS, decrease LES pressure, and impair gastroesophageal competence (Canal, Vane, Goto, Gardner, & Grosfeld, 1987; Jolley et al., 1986).

GER may also occur following tube placement because of alteration of the feeding regimen. Delivery of increased enteral volumes by tube may exceed the ability of the stomach to empty, particularly in individuals with GER complicated by delayed gastric emptying (Hillemeier, Lange, McCallum, Seashore, & Grybowski, 1981) or in patients with malnutrition. Patients unaccustomed to receiving large volumes of enteral feeding may have decreased gastric compliance and be unable to tolerate larger gastric volumes.

Unfortunately, there are no well-documented methods enabling the clinician to predict "at-risk" patients. Post-gastrostomy tube reflux may occur in the absence of clinical emesis and in those patients with negative pH monitoring prior to tube placement (Berezin et al., 1986; Grunow et al., 1989). In patients with central nervous system dysfunction, Wesley, Coran, Sarahan, Klein, and White (1981) suggest investigation for GER prior to placement of a feeding gastrostomy. However, these investigators relied primarily on the barium esophagram to diagnose reflux, a test known to have low sensitivity and specificity (Arasu et al., 1980).

In spite of the high incidence of reflux following gastrostomy tube placement, Wheatley and co-workers (Wheatley, Wesley, Thach, & Coran, 1991) do not recommend that a protective surgical anti-reflux procedure be performed at the time of gastrostomy tube placement. In the majority of their patients, an anti-reflux procedure would have proven unnecessary. In addition, these workers and others have shown that there is no significant difference in early morbidity or mortality in patients undergoing gastrostomy alone versus those having a gastrostomy with simultaneous, or a subsequent, anti-reflux procedure (Langer et al., 1988).

Response to a trial of nasogastric tube feeding in the preoperative period has been advocated by some as a useful prognostic sign for predicting postgastrostomy tube reflux (Gauderer, 1991). It is possible that nasogastric tube feeding may also have therapeutic implications favorably affecting gastric compliance and nutritional status, and thereby lessening the risk of postgastrostomy tube reflux (Boyle, 1989).

Currently, the author uses the following approach in the swallowing-impaired patient who is a candidate for a gastrostomy tube: If the patient has clinical reflux at presentation (regurgitation and/or vomiting) and is unresponsive to a 4 to 6 week course of medical therapy, then an anti-reflux operation is considered at the time of gastrostomy tube placement. In patients without clinical reflux, a 2 to 4 week trial of nasogastric tube feeds is given to determine tolerance for enteral feeding. This also serves to improve the patient's nutritional status. The choice of enteral formula and feeding schedule are determined following consultation with a pediatric dietician. If nasogastric tube feeding is successful, a percutaneous endoscopic gastrostomy tube is placed. If reflux develops post-tube placement, anti-reflux medical therapy is started. In the event that symptoms persist despite adequate medical therapy, an anti-reflux operation is recommended if clinically indicated based on the patient's underlying disorder, prognosis, and wishes of the family.

Diagnosis of Gastroesophageal Reflux

In the pediatric patient, reflux is a clinical diagnosis, although other causes of vomiting must be excluded based on medical history, physical examination, and specific laboratory tests. A complete discussion of the differential diagnosis of the vomiting infant and child is beyond the scope of this chapter. For a more detailed review, the reader is referred to standard pediatric texts. The various diagnostic tests used in the evaluation of the patient with suspected reflux are outlined in Table 13–2.

Treatment of GER

Infants with nonpathologic GER should be treated with conservative measures as outlined below. Based on clinical experience, pediatric patients with impaired swallowing generally have pathologic reflux and do not respond solely to conservative therapy.

Conservative Therapy

Conservative, or nonpharmacologic, nonsurgical, therapy for GER includes modifying body position in the postprandial period and modifying the consistency and volume of feeds. The prone position has been shown to decrease reflux compared to the seated (Orenstein & Whitington, 1983), supine, and lateral positions (Vandenplas & Sacre-Smits, 1985). It is unclear whether upright angled prone is advantageous to flat prone (Orenstein, 1990). Use of the prone position for treatment of reflux is somewhat controversial. The American Academy of Pediatrics recently released a statement suggesting that, during sleep, infants should be placed supine or on their sides to lessen the risk of the sudden infant death syndrome (SIDS) (American Academy of Pediatrics, Task Force on Infant Positioning and SIDS, 1992). However, the Academy also stated that "For ... infants with symptoms of gastroesophageal reflux ... prone may well be the position of choice" (p. 1125).

The efficacy of thickening formula with rice or other types of cereal as treatment for GER has recently been studied by pH monitoring (Bailey, Andres, Daneki, & Pinciro-Carrero, 1987) and scintigraphy (Orenstein, Magill, & Brooks, 1987). Although

TABLE 13-1. Diagnostic tests for gastroesophageal reflux.

Test	Indications	Advantages	Limitations
Radiographic studies (upper gastrointestinal series)	Exclude an anatomic etiology for persistent vomiting, dysphagia	Best test to evaluate anatomy of GI tract May provide information regarding esophageal motility	High false positive and negative rate for reflux Radiation exposure
Intra-esophageal pH monitoring	Temporally relate a reflux edpisode to symptoms and/or a pulmonary event (apnea, wheezing) Quantify amount of acid reflux Relate episodes of reflux, body position, sleep state	Most sensitive test for detecting episodes of acid reflux	"Invasive" In practice, it may be difficult to correlate symptomatic events and a reflux episode in a study limited to 24 hours
Upper endoscopy	Confirm diagnosis of reflux esophagitis Evaluate for lesions that may present with dysphagia	Best test for evaluating mucosa of upper GI tract Obtain histologic diagnosis May be therapeutic (dilate strictures and rings)	Invasive Requires intravenous sedation and/or general anesthesia Small risk of bleeding and perforation
Scintigraphic studies	Evaluate gastric emptying Assess aspiration Quantify extent and severity of GER	Can measure gastric emptying of liquids and solids	Radiation exposure (equivalent to one chest film) Insensitive to small amount of aspiration
Esophageal manometry	Diagnose an esophageal motor disorder Locate LES Confirm relaxation of UES and LES	Evaluate esophageal motor function	Invasive Requires sedation which may alter results in infants and children

thickened formula does not appear to favorably affect pH values, the amount of clinical emesis decreases and infants demonstrate increased weight gain (Orenstein et al., 1987). Use of thickened formula increases the caloric density of the feeding, increases sleep time, and decreases crying time, conditions that may reduce energy expenditure by the infant.

Interestingly, nasogastric tube feeding has been used as treatment for GER (Ferry, Selby, & Pietro, 1983). In infants with reflux, a 7 to 10 day course of nasogastric tube feeding may improve the nutritional status and resolve symptoms of vomiting.

Pharmacologic Therapy

Pharmacologic therapy in the infant with GER is indicated if (a) there is poor symptomatic response following a course (2–4 weeks) of conservative management and/or (b) significant complications of reflux disease are noted at presentation or during the clinical course of the disease. In the older child with GER, medical therapy is used in combination with conservative measures at presentation.

The two drugs most commonly used to treat reflux disease in pediatric patients are bethanechol (Urecholine®) and metoclopramide (Reglan®). These drugs are classified as pro-kinetic agents affecting the motility of the gastrointestinal tract. In spite of their widespread use, there are no well-controlled, double-blind, long-term clinical studies demonstrating therapeutic efficacy for either of these medications. Other pro-kinetic agents, not yet clinically available as treatment for GER in children, include domperidone and cisapride. The reader is referred to Spino (1991) for a more detailed discussion of pharmacologic treatment of motility disorders.

Bethanechol

Bethanechol (Urecholine®) is a cholinergic agonist that stimulates the parasympathetic nervous system and acts primarily on postganglionic parasympathetic receptors. This drug has been shown to affect esophageal function by (1) increasing LES pressure (Orenstein, Lofton, & Orenstein, 1986) and (2) improving esophageal clearance. Bethanechol is thought to act by direct stimulation of the sphincter muscle. Improved esophageal clearance time may occur as a result of changes in esophageal peristaltic amplitude, duration, and velocity; increased frequency of swallowing; or increased sali-

vation. Although the pharmacologic effect of bethanechol on esophageal function has been well-documented, there are conflicting studies regarding its effect on specific reflux intervals as measured by pH monitoring (Orenstein, et al., 1986; Strickland & Chang, 1983). Bethanechol has been shown to be effective in infants with reflux and poor weight gain (Euler, 1980), although double-blind, placebo-controlled trials are lacking in the pediatric age group.

At present, bethanechol is not available in liquid form, so it may be necessary for the pharmacist to prepare bethanechol in suspension. Unfortunately, data regarding the bioavailability of the drug in this form are not available. The dose of bethanechol is 600 micrograms (or 0.6 milligrams/kg/day) given orally in three divided doses approximately 15–30 minutes prior to meals. For older children, the dose is 5 milligrams/dose given three times per day.

The use of bethanechol is generally contraindicated in patients with chronic pulmonary disease because of the possibility that this cholinergic agonist may precipitate bronchospasm. The author has used bethanechol in patients with pulmonary disease (following consultation with pulmonary colleagues) without noting adverse effects on lung function or clinical deterioration. The presence of a seizure disorder is another relative contraindication to the use of bethanechol. Bethanechol also is contraindicated in the presence of peptic ulcer disease and hyperthyroidism. Side effects, which are generally uncommon, include nausea, increased salivation, flushing, and hypotension.

Metoclopramide

Metoclopramide (Reglan®) is a dopamine antagonist which has been shown to (a) increase the amplitude of peristaltic contractions in the esophagus, gastric antrum, and small intestine, (b) elevate the resting tone of the LES, and (c) stimulate gastric emptying. Although metoclopramide blocks some actions of dopamine on tissues of the intestine, its pro-kinetic effect on the gastrointestinal tract occurs mainly by sensitizing gut muscle to cholinergic influences (Schulze-Delrieu, 1981).

In spite of its frequent use as an anti-reflux drug, there is little scientific evidence confirming the clinical effectiveness of metoclopramide as an anti-reflux drug. In fact, metoclopramide may actually worsen reflux measurements as determined by pH monitoring of the distal esophagus (Hyams, Leichtner, Zamett, & Walters, 1986; Machida, Forbes, Gall, & Scott, 1988). Tolia, Calhoun, Kuhns, and Kauffman (1989) found that metoclopramide decreased clinical reflux and improved rate of weight gain in infants less than 1 year of age. Additional studies are needed to further evaluate the therapeutic efficacy of this drug.

The dose of metoclopramide is 0.3 to 0.5 mg/kg/day divided three times a day given 15–30 minutes prior to feeding. Side effects of metoclopramide include drowsiness, irritability, headache, insomnia, dizziness, agitation, and nausea. Dystonic reactions including trismus, torticollis, and oculo-gyric crises are uncommon but tend to occur more often in children and in patients with impaired renal function. Extrapyramidal symptoms respond to discontinuation of the drug, a process which may take 24 hours. Rapid termination can be accomplished by the use of diphenhydramine (Benadryl®) at a dose of 1–2 mg/kg per dose given slowly intravenously. Metoclopramide is contraindicated in patients with pheochromocytoma because of possible stimulation of catecholamine secretion. The drug is also contraindicated in patients with gastrointestinal bleeding, obstruction, or perforation.

H₂-Receptor Antagonists

The H₂-receptor antagonists are used in patients with reflux-related complications that occur secondary to the effects of acid such as reflux esophagitis, reflux-related pulmonary disease, and apnea. The author generally uses an H₂-receptor antagonist in conjunction with either bethanechol or metoclopramide. Commercially available H₂-receptor antagonists include cimetidine (Tagamet®), ranitidine (Zantac®), famotidine (Pepcid®), and nizatidine (Axid®). These drugs block gastric histamine H₂-receptors and inhibit basal, stimulated, and nocturnal acid secretion. As a result, a non-acid refluxate should decrease mucosal injury and allow healing of the esophageal mucosa. In adults, subjective improvement of reflux symptoms occurs in approximately 85 to 90% of patients while histologic resolution of esophagitis occurs in only about 65% (DeMeo & Sontag, 1992).

Acid suppressing agents are also used in patients with reflux-related pulmonary disease because gastric acid, when aspirated, may result in (a) a chemical pneumonitis leading to a bacterial pneumonia, (b) episodes of bronchospasm in patients with reactive airway disease, and, (c) in infants, result in apnea secondary to acid stimulation of chemoreceptors located on the surface of the larynx.

In general, the H₂ blockers have a low incidence of toxicity. Shaw-Stiffel (1991) has reviewed the pharmacology, clinical use, and adverse effects of these agents.

Other Pharmacologic Agents

Omeprazole

Omeprazole is a potent inhibitor of gastric acid secretion and acts by blocking secretion of hydrogen ions by the proton pump (H+/K+ ATPase) located at the luminal surface of the parietal cell.

Omeprazole is more effective than the H₂ blockers in the treatment of reflux esophagitis, probably due to its greater inhibitory effects on acid secretion. Subjective improvement of reflux symptoms occur in 95% of patients and histologic improvement is noted in 90%. At present, omeprazole is indicated for use in adult patients with moderate to severe reflux esophagitis unresponsive to the use of H₂ receptor antagonists. It is recommended that therapy be discontinued after 8 weeks due to animal data showing an increased incidence of carcinoid tumor following long-term therapy. This is felt to occur as a result of potent acid inhibition leading to an increase in the secretion of the (trophic) hormone gastrin. The author has used omperazole in older children and adolescents with good results.

Antacids

With the advent of H_2 antagonists, the use of antacids in pediatric reflux disease has lessened. At present, antacids are used in the older patient to provide symptomatic relief of heartburn and in the patient who is not a candidate for treatment with an H_2 blocker. The dose of antacid is 30 milliliters/1.73 m^2/dose given 1 and 3 hours postprandial and one dose before bedtime. An alternate dosage is as follows: for infants 2–5 ml/dose and children 5–12 ml/dose to a maximum dose of 80 ml/day.

Domperidone

Domperidone is a benzimidazole derivative with the properties of a peripheral dopamine antagonist. This drug has been shown to promote gastric emptying and improve antroduodenal coordination in adult humans. In general, clinical experience using domperidone in pediatric patients with GER is limited (Grill, Hillemeier, Semararo, McCallum, & Grybowski, 1985).

Surgical Therapy for Gastroesophageal Reflux

The indications for surgical treatment of pediatric gastroesophageal reflux disease include (a) the presence of pathologic reflux unresponsive to medical therapy (severe failure to thrive), (b) an esophageal peptic stricture, and (c) significant pulmonary disease secondary to reflux such as apnea or chronic aspiration pneumonia.

Several surgical procedures are available for treatment of reflux, although the Nissen fundoplication appears to be favored by most surgeons in the United States. In this procedure, the gastric fundus is wrapped around the distal esophagus. Other anti-reflux operations include the Belsey and Hill procedures which provide lesser degrees of wrap and gastropexy. The fundoplication has been shown to be an effective anti-reflux barrier (Leape & Ramenofsky, 1980; Tunell, Smith, & Carson, 1983) and is thought to retain its effectiveness during growth and development. The mechanism of action for the fundoplication is not clear, although an increase in LES (Euler, Fonkalsrud, & Ament, 1977) and an increase in the length of the high-pressure zone occurs following operation. One theory is that the wrap "pulls" a greater length of the distal esophagus into the abdominal cavity allowing it to be exposed to positive intra-abdominal pressure, thereby providing an effective "valve." Another possibility is that following the wrap the fundus loses the ability to adaptively relax resulting in an increase in the rate of gastric emptying.

In neurologically impaired children, anti-reflux surgery has been demonstrated to successfully control symptoms and result in a significant increase in weight gain (Rice, Seashore, & Touloukian, 1991). However, surgery offers only partial relief to patients with respiratory symptoms such as recurrent bronchospasm (Perrin-Fayolle, 1989). Specific complications of anti-reflux surgery include para-esophageal herniation, small bowel obstruction, poor wrap alignment, inadvertent vagotomy, the "gas-bloat" syndrome, and the dumping syndrome (Meyer, Deckelbaum, Lax, & Schiller, 1981; Zaloga & Chernow, 1983).

Another troublesome complication in the post-operative period is retching and gagging during gastrostomy feeding (Jolley, Tunnell, Leonard, Hoelzer, & Smith, 1987). The mechanism for this complication remains unclear, although gastric dysmotility may play a role. The patient may appear very uncomfortable during retching, and parents find this complication particularly difficult to manage. Treatment is directed toward modifying the enteral feeding regimen either by changing the feeding rate (bolus to continuous) and/or increasing the percentage of calories contributed by fat and thereby slow gastric emptying. Post-wrap retching is usually transient and resolves spontaneously after a number of weeks to months.

In the swallowing-impaired child, it has been the author's experience that, following anti-reflux surgery, there may be a significant change in feeding behavior characterized by a decrease, or cessation, of oral feeding. A case of oral dysfunction following fundoplication has recently been reported (Borowitz & Borowitz, 1992). Feeding difficulties usually occur in patients undergoing fundoplication and a newly placed gastrostomy tube. The mechanism for this phenomenon is unknown, although it is interesting to speculate that this may be a learned response; that is, delivery of nutrition by tube may be more pleasant and less uncomfortable than attempts at oral feeding. Others have suggested that the (sudden) delivery of adequate nutrition may decrease appetite and the desire for food (G. Putnam, personal communication). The differential diagnosis for feeding difficulties following anti-reflux surgery includes a wrap that is too tight, the dumping syndrome, and post-operative depression.

References

Ament, M. E., & Vargas, J. (1991). Fiberoptic upper intestinal endoscopy. In W. A. Walker, P. R. Durie, J. R. Hamilton, J. A. Walker-Smith, & J. B. Watkins (Eds.), *Pediatric gastrointestinal disease* (pp. 1247–1256). Philadelphia: B. C. Decker.

American Academy of Pediatrics, Task Force on Infant Positioning and SIDS. (1992). Positioning and SIDS. *Pediatrics, 89*, 1120–1126.

Arasu, T. S., Wyllie, R., Fitzgerald, J. F., Franken, E. A., Siddiqui, A. R., Lehman, G. A., Eigen H., & Grossfeld, J. L. (1980). Gastroesophageal reflux in infants and children — Comparative accuracy of diagnostic methods. *Journal of Pediatrics, 96*, 798.

Bailey, D. J., Andres, J. M., Danek, G. D., & Pineiro-Carrero, V. M. (1987). Lack of efficacy of thickened feeding as treatment for gastroesophageal reflux. *Journal of Pediatrics, 111*, 187–189.

Berezin, S., Schwarz, S. M., Halata, M. S., & Newman, L. J. (1986). Gastroesophageal reflux secondary to gastrostomy tube placement. *American Journal of Diseases of Childhood, 140*, 699.

Berquist, W. E. (1982). Gastroesophageal reflux in children. A clinical review. *Pediatric Annals, 11*, 135–142.

Borowitz, S. M., & Borowitz, K. C. (1992). Oral dysfunction following Nissen fundoplication. *Dysphagia, 7*, 234–237.

Boyle, J. T. (1989). Gastroesophageal reflux in the pediatric patient. *Gastroenterology Clinics in North America, 18*(2), 315–337.

Boyle, J. T., Tuchman, D. N., Altschuler, S. M. Nixon, T. E., Pack, A. I., & Cohen, S. (1985). Mechanisms for the association of gastroesophageal reflux and bronchospasm. *American Review of Respiratory Diseases, 131*, S16–S20.

Byrne, W. J., Euler, A. R., & Ashcraft, E. (1982). Gastroesophageal reflux in the severely retarded who vomit. Criteria for and results of surgical intervention in twenty-two patients. *Surgery, 91*, 95–98.

Canal, D. F., Vane, D. W., Goto, D. W., Gardner, G. P., & Grosfeld, J. L. (1987). Changes in lower esophageal sphincter pressure (LES) after Stamm gastrostomy. *Journal of Surgical Research, 42*, 570.

Carre, I. J. (1959). The natural history of the partial thoracic stomach ("hiatal hernia") in children. *Archives of Diseases in Childhood, 34*, 344.

Dahms, B., & Rothstein, F. C. (1984). Barrett's esophagus in children. A consequence of chronic gastroesophageal reflux. *Gastroenterology, 86*, 318–323.

DeMeo, M. R., & Sontag, S. J. (1992). Controversies in the management of gastroesophageal reflux disease. *Gastrointestinal Journal Club, 1*, 3–13.

Dent, J., Dodds, W. J., Friedman, R. M., Sekiguchi, T., Hogan, W. J., Arndorfer, R. C., & Petrie, D. J. (1980). Mechanism of gastroesophageal reflux in recumbent asymptomatic subjects. *Journal of Clinical Investigation, 65*, 256–267.

Dodds, W. J., Dent, J., Hogan, W. J., Helm, J. F., Hauser, R., Patel, G. K., & Egide, M. S. (1982). Mechanisms of gastroesophageal reflux in patients with reflux esophagitis. *New England Journal of Medicine, 307*, 1547–1552.

Dodds, W. J., Hogan, W. J., Helm, J. F., & Dent, J. (1981). Pathogenesis of reflux esophagitis. *Gastroenterology, 81*, 376–394.

Downing, S. E., & Lee, J. C. (1975). Laryngeal chemosensitivity: A possible mechanism for sudden infant death. *Pediatrics, 55*, 640–649.

Dutta, S. K., Matossian, H. B., Meirowitz, R. F., & Vaeth, Jr. (1992). Modulation of salivary secretion by acid infusion in the distal esophagus in humans. *Gastroenterology, 103*, 1833–1841.

Dutta, S. K., Meirowitz, R. F., Vengurlekar, S., & Resau, J. (1990). Localization and characterization of epidermal growth factor receptors in human esophageal epithelium. *Gastroenterology, 98*, A38.

Dutta, S. K., Orth, D., Dukehart, M., & Vaith, J. (1986). Evidence for the presence of epidermal growth factor in human parotid saliva. *Clinical Research, 34*, 349.

Euler, A. R. (1980). Use of bethanechol for the treatment of gastroesophageal reflux. *Journal of Pediatrics, 96*, 321–324.

Euler, A. R., Fonkalsrud, E. W., & Ament, M. E. (1977). Effect of Nissen fundoplication on the lower esophageal sphincter pressure of children with gastroesophageal reflux. *Gastroenterology, 72*, 260–262.

Ferry, G. D., Selby, M., & Pietro, T. J. (1983). Clinical response to short-term naso-gastric feeding in infants with gastroesophageal reflux and growth failure. *Journal of Pediatric Gastroenterology and Nutrition, 2*, 57–61.

Fisher, R. S., Malmud, L. S., Roberts, G. S., & Lobis, I. F. (1977). The lower esophageal sphincter as a barrier to gastroesophageal reflux. *Gastroenterology, 72*, 19–22.

Gauderer, M. W. L. (1991). Percutaneous endoscopic gastrostomy: A 10 year experience with 220 children. *Journal of Pediatric Surgery, 26*, 288–292.

Gerhardt, D. C., Shuck, T. J., Bordeaux, R. A., & Winship, D. H. (1978). Human upper esophageal sphincter — Response to volume, osmotic, and acid stimuli. *Gastroenterology, 75*, 268.

Giuffre, R., Rubin, S., & Mitchell, I. (1987). Antireflux surgery in infants with BPD. *American Journal of Diseases of Children, 141*, 648.

Goyal, R. K., & Rattan, S. (1978). Neurohormonal, hormonal, and drug receptors for the lower esophageal sphincter. *Gastroenterology, 74*, 598–619.

Grill, B. B., Hillemeier, A. C., Semeraro, L. A., McCallum, R. W., & Gryboski, J. D. (1985). Effects of domperidone therapy on symptoms and upper gastrointestinal motility in infants with gastroesophageal reflux. *Journal of Pediatrics, 106*(2), 311–316.

Grunow, J. E., al-Hafidh, A. S., & Tunell, W. P. (1989). Gastroesophageal reflux following percutaneous endoscopic gastrostomy in children. *Journal of Pediatric Surgery, 24*, 42–44.

Guttman, F. M. (1972). On the incidence of hiatal hernia in infants. *Pediatrics, 50*, 325–342.

Hamilton, S. R., & Smith, R. L. (1987). The relationship between columnar epithelial dysplasia and invasive adenocarcinoma arising in Barrett's esophagus. *American Journal of Clinical Pathology, 87*, 301–312.

Heine, K. J., & Mittal, R. K. (1991). Crural diaphragm and lower esophageal sphincter as antireflux barriers. *Viewpoints on Digestive Diseases, 23*(1), 1–6.

Helm, J. F., Dodds, W. J., & Hogan, W. J. (1987). Salivary response to esophageal acid in normal subjects and patients with reflux esophagitis. *Gastroenterology, 93*, 1393–1397.

Helm, J. F., Dodds, W. J., Pelc, L. R., Palmer, D. W., Hogan, W. J., & Teeter, B. C. (1984). Effect of esophageal emptying and saliva on clearance of acid from the esophagus. *New England Journal of Medicine, 310*, 284–288.

Herbst, J. J. (1981). Gastroesophageal reflux. *Journal of Pediatrics, 98*, 859–870.

Herbst, J. J., Johnson, D. G., & Oliveros, M. A. (1976). Gastroesophageal reflux with protein-losing enteropathy and finger clubbing. *American Journal of Diseases of Childhood, 130*, 1256.

Herbst, J. J., Minton, S. D., & Book, L. S. (1979). Gastroesophageal reflux causing respiratory distress and apnea in newborn infants. *Journal of Pediatrics, 95*, 763–768.

Hillemeier, A. C., Lange, R., McCallum, R., Seashore, J., & Grybowski, J. D. (1981). Delayed gastric emptying in infants with gastroesophageal reflux. *Journal of Pediatrics, 98*, 190–193.

Hoeffel, J. D., Nihovi-Fekete, C., & Schmitt, M. (1989). Esophageal adenocarcinoma after gastroesophageal reflux in children. *Journal of Pediatrics, 84*, 259–261.

Hubert, D., Gaudric, M., Guerre, X. X., Jr., Lockhart, A., & Marsac, J. (1988). Effect of the-ophylline on gastroesophageal reflux in patients with asthma. *Journal of Allergy and Clinical Immunology, 81*, 1168–1174.

Hyams, J. S., Leichtner, A. M., Zamett, L. D., & Walters, J. K. (1986). Effect of metoclopramide on prolonged intraesophageal pH testing in infants with gastroesophageal reflux. *Journal of Pediatric Gastroenterology and Nutrition, 5*(5), 716–720.

Hyams, J. S., Ricci, A., & Leichtner, A. M. (1988). Clinical and laboratory correlates of esophagitis in young children. *Journal of Pediatric Gastroenterology and Nutrition, 7*, 52–56.

Ismail-Beigi, F., Horton, P. F., & Pope, C. E., II. (1970). Histological consequences of gastroesophageal reflux in man. *Gastroenterology, 58*(2), 163–174.

Jolley, S. G., Tunnell, W. P., Hoelzer, D. J., Thomas, S., & Smith, E. I. (1986). Lower esophageal pressure changes with tube gastrostomy: A causative factor in gastroesophageal reflux in children? *Journal of Pediatric Surgery, 21*, 624–627.

Jolley, S. G., Tunell, W. P., Leonard, J. C., Hoelzer, D. J., & Smith, E. I. (1987). Gastric emptying in children with gastroesophageal reflux. II. The relationship to retching symptoms following antireflux surgery. *Journal of Pediatric Surgery, 22*(10), 927–930.

Kahrilas, P. J., Dodds, W. J., Dent, J., Haeberle, B., Hogan, W. J., & Arndorfer, R. C. (1987). The effect of sleep, spontaneous gastroesophageal reflux and a meal on UES pressure in humans. *Gastroenterology, 92*, 466–471.

Kahrilas, P. J., Dodds, W. J., & Hogan, W. J. (1988). Effect of peristaltic dysfunction on esophageal volume clearance. *Gastroenterology, 94*, 73–80.

Kassen, N. Y., Groen, J. J., & Fraenkel, M. (1965). Spinal deformities and oesophageal hiatus hernia. *Lancet, 1*, 887–889.

Langer, J. C., Wesson, D. E., Ein, S. H., Filler, R. M., Shandling, B., Superina, R. A., & Papa, M. (1988). Feeding gastrostomy in neurologically impaired children: Is an anti-reflux procedure necessary? *Journal of Pediatric Gastroenterology and Nutrition, 7*, 837–841.

Leape, L. L., & Ramenofsky, M. L. (1980). Surgical treatment of gastroesophageal reflux in children. *American Journal of Diseases of Childhood, 134*, 935–938.

Machida, H. M., Forbes, D. A., Gall, D. G., &

Scott, R. B. (1988). Metoclopramide in gastroesophageal reflux of infancy. *Journal of Pediatrics, 112*, 483–487.

Mansfield, L. E. (1989). Gastroesophageal reflux and diseases of the respiratory tract: A review. *Journal of Asthma, 26*, 271–278.

Mansfield, L. E., & Stein, M. R. (1978). Gastroesophageal reflux and asthma: A possible reflex mechanism. *Annals of Allergy, 41*, 224–226.

Menon, A. P., Schefft, G. L., & Thach, B. T. (1985). Apnea associated with regurgitation in infants. *Journal of Pediatrics, 106*, 625–629.

Meyer, S., Deckelbaum, R. J., Lax, E., & Schiller, M. (1981). Infant dumping syndrome after gastroesophageal reflux surgery. *Journal of Pediatrics, 99*(2), 235–237.

Mittal, R. K., & Fisher, M. J. (1990). Electrical and mechanical inhibition of the crural diaphragm during transient relaxation of the lower esophageal sphincter. *Gastroenterology, 99*, 1265–1268.

Mittal, R. K., & McCallum, R. W. (1988). Characteristics and frequency of transient relaxations of the lower esophageal sphincter in patients with reflux esophagitis. *Gastroenterology, 95*, 593–599.

Mittal, R. K., Rochester, D. F., & McCallum, R. N. (1989). Sphincteric action of the diaphragm during a relaxed lower esophageal sphincter. *American Journal of Physiology, 256*, G139–G144.

Mollitt, D. L., Golladay, E. S., & Seibert, J. J. (1985). Symptomatic gastroesophageal reflux following gastrostomy in neurologically impaired patients. *Pediatrics, 75*, 1124–1126.

Moroz, S. P., Espinoza, X. X., Jr., Cumming, W. A., & Diamant, N. E. (1976). Lower esophageal sphincter function in children with and without gastroesophageal reflux. *Gastroenterology, 71*, 236–241.

Orenstein, S. R. (1990). Prone positioning in infant gastroesophageal reflux: Is elevation of the head worth the trouble? *Journal of Pediatrics, 117*(2), 184–187.

Orenstein, S. R., Lofton, S. W., & Orenstein, D. (1986). Gastroesophageal reflux: A prospective, blind, controlled study. *Journal of Pediatric Gastroenterology and Nutrition, 5*, 549–555.

Orenstein, S. R., Magill, H. L., & Brooks, P. (1987). Thickening of infant feedings for therapy of gastroesophageal reflux. *Journal of Pediatrics, 110*, 181–186.

Orenstein, S. R., & Whitington, P. F. (1983). Positioning for prevention of infant gastro-esophageal reflux. *Journal of Pediatrics, 103,* 534–537.

Pack, A. I. (1990). Acid: A nocturnal broncho-constrictor? *American Review of Respiratory Diseases, 141,* 1391–1392.

Perrin-Fayolle, M., Gormand, F., Braillon, G., Lombard-Platet, R., Vignal, J., Azzar, D., Forichon, J., & Adeleine, P. (1989). Long-term results of surgical treatment for gas-troesophageal reflux in asthmatic patients. *Chest, 96*(1), 40–45.

Rice, H., Seashore, J. H., & Touloukian, R. J. (1991). Evaluation of Nissen fundoplication in neurologically impaired children. *Journal of Pediatric Surgery, 26*(6), 697–701.

Schulze-Delrien, J. (1981). Metoclopramide. *New England Journal of Medicine, 305,* 28–33.

See, C. C., Newman, L. J., Berezin, S., Glassman, M. S., Medow, M. S., Dozor, A. J., & Schwarz, S. M. (1989). Gastroesophageal reflux-in-duced hypoxemia in infants with apparent life-threatening event(s). *American Journal of Diseases of Children, 143,* 951–954.

Shapiro, G. G., & Christie, D. L. (1983). Gastro-esophageal reflux and asthma. *Clinical Review of Allergy, 1*(1), 39–56.

Shaw-Stiffel, T. A. (1991). Treatment of acid-peptic disease. In W. A. Walker, P. R. Durie, J. R. Hamilton, J. A. Walker-Smith, & J. B. Watkins (Eds.), *Pediatric gastroenterology* (pp. 1702–1715). Philadelphia: B. C. Decker.

Shub, M. D., Ulshen, M. H., Hargrove, C. B., Siegal, G. P., Groben P. A., & Askin, F. B. (1985). Esophagitis: A frequent consequence of gastroesophageal reflux in infancy. *Journal of Pediatrics, 107,* 881–884.

Sindel, B. O., Maisels, M. J., & Ballantine, T. V. N. (1989). Gastroesophageal reflux to the primal esophagus in infants with broncho-pulmonary dysplasia. *American Journal of Diseases of Childhood, 143,* 1103–1106.

Sondheimer, J. M. (1983). Upper esophageal sphincter and pharyngoesophageal motor function in infants with and without gas-troesophageal reflux. *Gastroenterology, 85,* 301–305.

Sondheimer, J. M. (1988). Gastroesophageal reflux: Update on pathogenesis and diag-nosis. *Pediatric Clinics of North America, 35,* 103–115.

Sondheimer, J. M., & Morris, B. A. (1979). Gas-troesophageal reflux among severely retard-ed children. *Journal of Pediatrics, 94,* 710.

Sonnenberg, A., Steinkamp, U., Weise, A., Berges, W., Wienback, M., Rohner, H. G., & Peter, P. (1982). Salivary secretion in reflux esoph-agitis. *Gastroenterology, 98,* 889–895.

Spino, M. (1991). Pharmalogic treatment of gastrointestinal motility. In W. M. Walker, P. R. Durie, J. R. Hamilton, J. A. Walker-Smith, & J. B. Watkins (Eds.), *Pediatric gas-troenterology* (pp. 1735–1746). Philadelphia: B. C. Decker.

Spitzer, A. R., Boyle, J. T., Tuchman, D. N., & Fox, W. W. (1984). Awake apnea associat-ed with gastroesophageal reflux: A specific clinical syndrome. *Journal of Pediatrics, 104* (2), 200–204.

Strickland, D. A., & Chang, J. H. T. (1983). Re-sults of treatment of gastroesophageal re-flux with bethanechol. *Journal of Pediatrics, 103,* 311–315.

Tolia, V., Calhoun, Jr., Kuhns, L., & Kauffman, R. E. (1989). Randomized, prospective double-blind trial of metoclopramide and placebo for gastroesophageal reflux in infants. *Jour-nal of Pediatrics, 115,* 141–145.

Tuchman, D. N., Boyle, J. T., Pack, A. I., Schwartz, J., Spitzer, A. R., & Cohen, S. (1984). Com-parison of airway responses following tra-cheal or esophageal acidification in the cat. *Gastroenterology, 87,* 872–881.

Tunell, W. P., Smith, E. I., & Carson, J. A. (1983). Gastroesophageal reflux in childhood. *An-nals of Surgery, 197*(5), 560–565.

Vakil, N. B., Kahrilas, P. J., Dodds, W. J., & Vanagu-nas, A. (1989). Absence of an upper esopha-geal sphincter response to acid reflux. *Ameri-can Journal of Gastroenterology, 84,* 606–610.

Vandenplas, Y., & Sacre-Smits, L. (1985). Sev-enteen hour continuous pH monitoring in the newborn: Evaluation of the influence of position in asymptomatic and sympto-matic babies. *Journal of Pediatric Gastroenter-ology and Nutrition, 4,* 356–361.

Vane, D. W., Shiffler, M., & Grosfield, J. L. (1982). Reduced lower esophageal sphinc-ter pressure after acute and chronic brain in-jury. *Journal of Pediatric Surgery, 17,* 960–969.

Walsh, J. K., Farrell, M. K., Keenan, W. J., Lucas, M., & Kramer, M. (1981). Gastroesophage-al reflux in infants: Relation to apnea. *Jour-nal of Pediatrics, 99*(2), 197–201.

Werlin, S., Dodds, W., Hogan, W., & Arndorfer, R. (1980). Mechanisms of gastroesophage-al reflux in children. *Journal of Pediatrics, 97,* 244–248.

Wesley, J. R., Coran, A. G., Sarahan, T. M., Klein, M. D., & White, S. J. (1981). The need for evaluation of gastroesophageal reflux in brain-damaged children referred for feeding gastrostomy. *Journal of Pediatric Surgery, 16*, 866.

Wheatley, M. J., Wesley, J. R., Tkach, D. M., & Coran, A. G. (1991). Long-term follow-up of brain-damaged children requiring feeding gastrotomy: Should an antireflux procedure always be performed? *Journal of Pediatric Surgery, 26*, 301.

Wilkinson, J. D., Dudgeon, D. L., & Sondheimer, J. M. (1981). A comparison of medical and surgical treatment of gastroesophageal reflux in severely mentally retarded children. *Journal of Pediatrics, 99*, 202–205.

Wilson, N. M., Charette, L., Thomson, A. H., Silverman, M. (1985). Gastro-oesophageal reflux and childhood asthma: The acid test. *Thorax, 40*, 592–597.

Winter, H. S., Madara, J. L., Stafford, R. J., Grand, R. J., Quinlan, J., & Goldman, H. (1982). Intraepithelial eosinophils: A new diagnostic criterion for reflux esophagitis. *Gastroenterology, 83*, 818–823.

Zaloga, G. P., & Chernow, B. (1983). Postprandial hypoglycemia after Nissen fundoplication for reflux esophagitis. *Gastroenterology, 84*, 840–842.

The Multidisciplinary Approach to Management of Swallowing Disorders in the Pediatric Patient

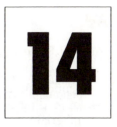

CHAPTER

Rhonda S. Walter, M.D.

Dysphagia, or impaired swallowing, can compromise nutrition, gastrointestinal function, or respiration and lead to serious illness. In an attempt to improve medical care for children with dysphagia, many institutions have already established or are moving toward establishing pediatric feeding and swallowing teams. Such teams invariably encompass professionals from many disciplines already in a given clinical setting.

The multidisciplinary approach to children with disordered swallowing advocates that early recognition is essential and close monitoring is necessary, given the dynamic developmental baseline in the pediatric patient. Clinical information can be gathered that may help predict aspiration, reflux, and failure to thrive. In addition, treatment parameters can be defined, such as those necessary for effective safe introduction (or re-introduction) of oral feeds in tube dependent children.

Pediatric patients with feeding and swallowing disorders are a widely diverse group with multiple etiologies, often dissimilar underlying medical conditions, and the need for individualized recommenda-

tions for identification, care, and management. It is true that "the pediatric swallowing team must expand to encompass the complexity of the child's dysphagia and associated disabilities" (Christensen, 1989), with all members familiar with normal and abnormal development.

No one subspecialty in the field of medical training, physician or support personnel, currently exists that is solely dedicated to disorders of swallowing (Ravich et al., 1985). Given this lack of "formalized" centralization of knowledge, the patient with dysphagia may "suffer from the fundamental and arbitrary division of the swallowing mechanism" among consultant caretakers. The team approach to diagnosis, treatment, and education about swallowing difficulties is often tailored to the clinical setting within which it exists. For example, some institutions have adopted a "swallowing center" approach (Christensen, 1989; Ravich et al., 1985), while others have concentrated on more inpatient referrals in acute or rehabilitation settings (Bach et al., 1989; Emmick-Herring & Wood, 1990; Hynak-Hankinson et al., 1984; Jones & Altschuler, 1987). Several, most notably in the pediatric population, have utilized home- and family based treatment intervention strategies in children at high risk for feeding and swallowing disorders (Chamberlain, Henry, Roberts, Sapsford, & Courtney, 1991; Crane, 1987; Lierman, Wolff, Hazelton, Pesquera, & Wilson, 1987). The common theme among these approaches is a sharing of information germane to the patient's inability to manage feeding and swallowing tasks.

One of the most detailed descriptions of the organization and philosophy behind the swallowing center concept can be found in *The Multidisciplinary Approach to Dysphagia* published by the Johns Hopkins Swallowing Center (Donner & Jones, 1985). A series of articles, contributed by various disciplines, detail the physiology of the swallowing mechanisms through review of clinical experience and radiologic presentation. The point is made throughout the series that symptoms of swallowing abnormalities often were nonspecific, with both patient and physician initially unable to determine which medical specialist should be primarily consulted (Ravich et al., 1985). Thus, a multidisciplinary approach to the adult with dysphagia was adopted, and a swallowing center formed.

In this model, patients are referred by their physicians to a coordinator, prior medical records are accumulated, and a primary physician (gastroenterologist, neurologist, or otolaryngologist) is selected. After evaluation by the primary physician, an imaging study (e.g., cineradiograph) is generally ordered and reviewed, and pertinent subsequent consultations arranged. Weekly case conferences then are held in which the principal care providers review the pertinent data for each patient. Further workup and case disposition is determined, and therapeutic options are discussed and relayed to the patient. As articulated by Ravich et al. (1985), "the swallowing center approach, by assuring face to face communication between clinicians from different subspecialties, is an attempt to improve communication among subspecialists and draw upon their combined expertise" (p. 257). Research opportunities exist as a data base is accumulated. As noted above, many medical institutions have moved toward adoption of such multidisciplinary or "swallowing center" approaches, adapting the process to their particular patient population and clinical personnel.

Team Members and Their Roles

The establishment of a swallowing program in the adult population has been well described (Groher, 1984; Logemann, 1986). Pediatric feeding and swallowing team members must minimally include those with clinical pediatric expertise, as well as "back-up" from pediatric surgical and radiologic subspecialties. Table 14–1 lists the professionals ideally involved in pediatric dysphagia assessment and management. Often, not all members of the team need to consult on a given patient. Core team members, as described, consist of a developmental (or similarly trained) pediatrician, gastroenterologist, occupational therapist, and/or speech-language pathologist (optimally both), nutritionist, and nursing personnel. These members serve to evaluate both inpatient and outpatient populations.

Consultation from a behavioral psychologist and support from social services are often found to be essential. Should videofluoroscopy or other diagnostic tests be deemed necessary, the radiologist becomes integral to delineating the potential anatomic underpinning of the child's dysphagia. Finally, referral to surgery for potential supplemental gastrostomy tube placement, otolaryngology for evaluation of airway competency and/or oral apparatus abnormalities, and dentistry are often utilized. It almost goes without saying that family members and school personnel involved in care-taking roles are the most

TABLE 14–1. Pediatric dysphagia team members and their roles.

Team Member	Roles
Developmental Pediatrician	Coordinates the multidisciplinary diagnosis and treatment of dysphagia in the disabled. Also can be served by physiatrist, pediatric neurologist, or general pediatrician with academic strengths in area of feeding/swallowing problems.
Gastroenterologist	Contributes to the diagnosis and treatment of disordered swallowing and its medical sequelae.
Occupational Therapist	Aids in determining which phases of swallowing are disordered, the safety and feasibility of oral feeds, and the role of positioning.
Speech-Language Pathologist	Contributes to the oro-motor evaluation coupled with direction of concomitant communication deficits, along with treatment recommendations.
Nutritionist	Evaluates nutritional status and requirements, suggests adequate nutrition guidelines.
Nurse	Medical support and educational training to families of patients with complex medical needs.
Radiologist	Delineates radiographically anatomic and functional abnormalities.

Consulting Dysphagia Team Members		
Social Worker	General Surgeon	Family
Behavioral Psychologist	Dentist	School personnel
ENT Surgeon/Otolaryngologist	Pulmonologist	

pivotal components in providing history and implementing management strategies in the child with a feeding disorder.

Indications for Referral

Referrals to a pediatric feeding and swallowing disorders' team may include children with failure to thrive, inadequate nutrient intake for growth, aspiration, gastroesophageal reflux, decompensation on a metabolic or genetic basis, enteral feeding, and gastrostomy tube management (see prior chapters). Other issues may include chronic eating problems related to oral motor dysfunction, intolerance to upgrading food texture, and disruptive mealtime behavior in the presence or absence of one of the above. The referral process can be facilitated by the use of a standardized intake referral form, a condensation of which is included as Table 14–2. The clinical information can be elicited at the initial telephone call by a clinic coordinator or secretary (outpatient basis) or designated team member contact person (inpatient basis). The availability of previous medical records for review prior to patient evaluation is essential to facilitate problem identification, allot personnel, and guide further medical workup.

Assessing Effectiveness of the Multidisciplinary Approach

Clinical efficacy as well as cost efficiency must be considered when utilizing the multidisciplinary team approach to pediatric dysphagia. Intuitively, it makes sense to

TABLE 14–2. Pediatric Feeding and Swallowing Referral Form.

Patient Profile

(Name, DOB, Hospital ID No.) _____

Referred by: _____

Reason Referred: _____

Prior Medical Diagnosis: ☐ MR   ☐ CP   ☐ Seizures   ☐ Behavioral problems
☐ Orthopedic problems   ☐ Failure to Thrive   ☐ Other: _____

Prior Radiologic Studies/Diagnostic Procedures:

☐ Barium Swallow   ☐ Videoesophagram   ☐ Upper GI   ☐ Endoscopy   ☐ pH Probe
☐ Other: _____

Current Medications: _____

Current Height: _____   Current Weight: _____

Usually fed by mouth:

☐ Solids   ☐ Liquids   ☐ Purees   ☐ NPO

Tube Supplementation and date begun:

☐ NG _____   ☐ GI _____   ☐ Button _____   ☐ J-tube _____

History of:	Yes	No
☐ Emesis/regurgitation	☐	☐
☐ Choking/coughing with feeding		
☐ Solids	☐	☐
☐ Liquids	☐	☐
☐ Prior aspiration/other type pneumonias	☐	☐
☐ Prior weight loss or FTT	☐	☐
☐ Food refusal	☐	☐

gather expertise about a given patient into a clinical forum for sharing information and recommendations. However, little literature exists critically evaluating the team process, especially as it applies to pediatric feeding and swallowing disorders. Most reports have described the team model or utilized case studies to illustrate efficacy of multidisciplinary efforts.

Hynak-Hankinson et al. (1984), working with dysphagic geriatric VA population,

documented the need for identification of dysphagic patients in an inpatient setting where such patients often are not isolated in specific units. They argued that a dysphagia team "has the opportunity to influence wide-spread quality changes in the ways that health care providers meet the basic needs of people with disparate health problems" (p. 35). Although this theme echoes throughout the dysphagia literature, it should be recognized as subjective, biased by those already involved in a multidisciplinary approach. Perhaps one of the greatest services an inpatient dysphagia team can provide is in influencing nursing competence, skill, and interest in feeding persons with dysphagia (Emmick-Herring & Wood, 1990; Penington & Krutsch, 1990). This concept of increasing staff expertise is then often translated to mean increased quality of patient care; however, this is very difficult to quantify objectively either in inpatient or outpatient settings.

Bach et al. (1989) supported the impression that patient care is improved by more comprehensive (team-based) assessment for determining the risks of aspiration and the resultant management strategies aimed at decreasing these risks. In *Dysphagia Teams: A Specific Approach to a Nonspecific Problem,* Jones and Altschuler (1987) similarly reported that this approach to care can be utilized by others in a cost-effective manner to alleviate malnutrition and aspiration. A recent prospective study on the effects of multidisciplinary management program on neurologically impaired patients with dysphagia, utilizing a time series design, supported the notion that institution of a multidisciplinary team to manage dysphagia resulted in improvement in patients' weight and caloric intake (Martens, Cameron, & Simonsen, 1990). Interestingly, no effect was found on the incidence of aspiration pneumonia because none occurred in their relatively small sample. As these authors pointed out, the majority of the dysphagia literature has not utilized controlled studies on the efficacy of instituting dysphagia treatment teams. Critical review is further hampered by the disparate nature of diagnostic categories in treatment groups discussed, as well as the small sample size. Finally, as mentioned previously, the pediatric population differs from the adult population in dysphagia etiologies and developmental considerations. Clearly, although team approach has many anecdotal champions, as the field grows, more work needs to be done in the utilization of this approach as a health care model for pediatric feeding and swallowing disorders.

Role of Dysphagia Team in Education

Although no current figures are available estimating the number of children with transient and long-term feeding difficulties, it is clear that the vast majority of patients are cared for in the home, in the context of their families and/or utilize some community resources. Even that portion of the pediatric population with feeding and swallowing disorders that requires in-hospital dysphagia management eventually transitions to families, schools, or chronic care facilities that may not have professionals with dysphagia expertise available. Thus, it is imperative that the pediatric dysphagia team assume the role of educators to those involved in caring for children with dysfunctioning swallow.

Public Law (PL) 99-457 and its predecessor PL99-142 mandate placement of increasing numbers of handicapped children in the public school system, as well as movement of some children with disabilities into less specialized (i.e., more mainstreamed) school settings. This has increased the requests for dysphagia training in the schools. Teachers, school nurses, and therapists need to know not only what route of feeding is "safe" for a given child with swallowing problems, but also how to carry through with therapeutic goals that are proposed by feeding and swallowing teams. In addition, school and community caretakers must have specified access to the various medical specialists involved to report changes in the patients' clinical condition (contingent, of course, on parental consent). Written reports or updates from the school to the clinician can facilitate exchange of information. It is also effective to invite school- or institution-based caretakers to follow-up therapy sessions for practical, hands-on guidance in techniques and explanations. Workshops for school personnel and community professionals involved in the care of children with swallowing disorders are an ideal forum for pediatric dysphagia teams to disseminate information. Teaching materials can include interactive videotapes, directed bibliographies, and summary handouts. Most invaluable are "question and answer" sessions given at schools or facilities where both general and specific issues can be discussed. More formalized dysphagia symposia exist that are generally tailored for those professionals who have clinical interests in pediatric feeding and swallowing disorders.

Although updating professionals is important, the crux of education about feeding problems in children is the training of parents and families. Few areas of development are as emotionally charged as feeding, with parents investing considerable time and effort in nourishment-related activities. Ideally, separate parent conferences can follow dysphagia team evaluations. The goal is to apprise parents of diagnostic impressions, further medical work-up, treatment recommendations, and follow-up goals. Often parents can absorb the information given to them, but find practical application of feeding techniques or nutritive support at home fraught with obstacles. It is here that outpatient nursing and social work is crucial. Access to these team members allows parents to update the team as well as troubleshoot minor problems. Telephone calls and suggestions should be recorded as part of the medical record and reviewed by the team as a whole for comments and/or further recommendations. Parents should receive written instructions whenever possible, and follow-up visits should be scheduled with regular frequency. Finally, parent support groups for children with similar dysphagia problems (e.g., tube dependency, behavior-based feeding problems, the medically fragile child) should be fostered by the outpatient efforts of the multidisciplinary feeding and swallowing team.

Summary

The clinical approach to feeding and swallowing disorders in children relies heavily on input from multiple disciplines. Systematic accumulation of relevant data and sharing of diagnostic impressions and treatment recommendations is facilitated by the team approach. School personnel and parental comfort and expertise in caring for dysphagic children can be aided by consistent continued input from the multidisciplinary team and education regarding both individualized patients and the larger field of swallowing disorders in the pediatric population.

References

Bach, D. B., Pouget, S., Belle, K., Kilfoil, M., Alfieri, M., McEvoy, J., & Jackson, G. (1989, Fall). An integrated team approach to the management of patients with oropharyngeal dysphagia. *Journal of Allied Health*, 450–468.

Chamberlin, J. L., Henry, M. M., Roberts, J. D., Sapsford, A. L., & Courtney, S. E. (1991). An infant and toddler feeding program. *The American Journal of Occupational Therapy*, 45, 907–911.

Christensen, J. R. (1989). Developmental approach to pediatric neurogenic dysphagia. *Dysphagia*, 3, 131–134.

Crane, S. (1987). Feeding the handicapped child — Overview of intervention strategies. *Nutrition and Health*, 5, 109–118.

Donner, M. W., & Jones, B. (1985). The multidisciplinary approach to dysphagia. *Gastrointestinal Radiology*, 10, 193–261.

Emmick-Herring, B., & Wood, P. (1990). A team approach to neurologically based swallowing disorders. *Rehabilitation Nursing*, 15, 126–132.

Groher, M. (Ed.) (1984). *Dysphagia: Diagnosis and management* (p. 1–258). Boston: Butterworths.

Hynak-Hankinson, M. T., Agin, M., Gardner, C., Jones, P. L., Lichtenstein, S., Peiffer, S., & Rao, P. (1984). Dysphagia evaluation and treatment: The team approach, Part I and Part II. *Nutritional Support Services*, 4(5/6), 33–41 and 32–33.

Jones, P. L., & Altschuler, S. L. (1987). Dysphagia teams: A specific approach to a nonspecific problem. *Dysphagia, 1,* 200–205.

Lierman, C., Wolff, R., Hazelton, J., Pesquera, K., & Wilson, E. (1987). Multidisciplinary treatment of feeding disorders in the home. *Pediatric Nursing, 13,* 266–270.

Logemann, J. A. (1986). *Manual for the videofluorographic study of swallowing.* San Diego, CA: College-Hill Press.

Martens, L., Cameron, T., & Simonsen, M. (1990). Effects of multidisciplinary management program on neurologically impaired patients with dysphagia. *Dysphagia, 5,* 147–151.

Mody, M., & Nagai, J. (1990). Multidisciplinary approach to the development of competency standards and appropriate allocation for patients with dysphagia. *The American Journal of Occupational Therapy, 44,* 369–372.

Penington, G. R., & Krutsch, J. A. (1990). Swallowing disorders: Assessment and rehabilitation. *British Journal of Hospital Medicine, 44,* 17–22.

Ravich, W. J., Donner, M. W., Kashima, H., Bucholz, D. W., Marsh, B. R., Hendrix, T. R., Kramer, S. S., Jones, D., Bozma, J. F., Siebens, A. A., & Linden, P. (1985). The swallowing center: Concepts and procedures. *Gastrointestinal Radiology, 10,* 255–261.

Index